V. Schulz   R. Hänsel   V. E. Tyler

Rational Phytotherapy

A Physicians' Guide to Herbal Medicine

Springer

Berlin
Heidelberg
New York
Barcelona
Budapest
Hong Kong
London
Milan
Paris
Santa Clara
Singapore
Tokyo

Volker Schulz   Rudolf Hänsel   Varro E. Tyler

Rational Phytotherapy

A Physicians' Guide to Herbal Medicine

Third edition, fully revised and expanded

With 81 figures and 42 tables

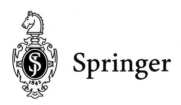

Springer

Prof. Dr. med. Volker Schulz
Oranienburger Chaussee 25
13465 Berlin
Germany

Prof. Dr. rer. nat. Rudolf Hänsel
formerly Institut für Pharmakognosie und
Phytochemie der Freien Universität Berlin
Private address:
Westpreußenstraße 71
81927 München
Germany

Prof. em. Varro E. Tyler, Ph. D., Sc. D.
Purdue University
Present address:
P. O. Box 2566
West Lafayette, Indiana 47906
USA

Translator:
Terry C. Telger
6112 Waco Way
Fort Worth, TX 76133, USA

ISBN 3-540-62648-4 Springer-Verlag Berlin Heidelberg New York

Library of Congress Cataloging-in-Publication Data
Schulz, Volker, Prof. Dr. med. [Rationale Phytotherapie. English] Rational phytotherapy : a physician's guide to herbal medicine / Volker Schulz, Rudolf Hänsel, Varro E. Tyler. – 3rd ed., fully rev. and expanded. p. cm. Includes bibliographical references and index.
    ISBN 3-540-62648-4. – ISBN 0-387-62648-4 (U.S.)
1. Herbs–Therapeutic use. I. Rudolf, Hänsel, 1920– . II. Tyler, Varro E. III. Title. RM666.H33S3813 1997 615.321–dc21

© Springer-Verlag Berlin Heidelberg 1998
Printed in Germany

The use of general descriptive names, registered names, trademarks, etc. in this publication does not imply, even in the absence of a specific statement, that such names are exempt from the relevant protective laws and regulations and therefore free for general use.

Product liability: The publishers cannot guarantee the accuracy of any information about dosage and application contained in this book. In every individual case the user must check such information by consulting the relevant literature.

Typesetting: Appl, Wemding
SPIN: 10570007   14/3133 - 5 4 3 2 1 0 – Printed on acid-free paper

Preface to the English Edition

Rational Phytotherapy adds a truly significant dimension to the practice of science-based herbal medicine. Detailed examination of the original German edition led to the conclusion that the book simply had to be translated into English to make the valuable information it contained available to a broader audience. That desire has now been realized, and the results of scientific studies and clinical trials of therapeutically useful botanical drugs are now placed before interested readers in the universal language of science.

Even the most cursory acquaintance with phytotherapy, herbal treatment, botanical medicine – whatever you choose to call it – causes one to recognize that throughout most of the world, and especially in the United States and the United Kingdom, the practice is at best an imperfect art. In Germany, the use of plant drugs is a science. There are many reasons for this. Tradition can certainly not be discounted. However, the principal reason is, without question, the enlightened system of laws and regulations governing the sale and use of such products in that country.

Basically, the regulations in Germany permit phytomedicines to be sold either as self-selected or prescription drugs provided there is absolute proof of their safety and reasonable certainty of their efficacy. The words "reasonable certainty" are extremely important here. They require that some scientific and clinical evidence be provided prior to approval, but the requirements are not the same as would be necessary for a new chemical entity. Because patent protection it not ordinarily available for these ancient drugs, pharmaceutical companies are generally unwilling to invest the hundreds of millions of dollars required to prove them effective by the same standards applied to totally new, synthetic drugs. They are, however, willing to invest more modest amounts in the scientific and clinical testing needed to establish reasonable certainty of efficacy.

That has been and continues to be done in Germany. Data regarding safety and efficacy submitted to a special scientific body designated Commission E of the German Federal Health Agency (now the Federal Institute for Drugs and Medical Devices) have resulted in judgments validating the utility of several hundred different phytomedicines. The brief summaries of these Commission E findings, as well as its conclusions on about 100 different botanicals that were not approved, were

originally published in German in the *Bundesanzeiger*, the counterpart
of the U.S. *Federal Register*, but they have now been published in English translation by the American Botanical Council in Austin, Texas.
The Commission E monographs are based, in part, on proprietary information so, unfortunately, they are not referenced. If one wants to review
the detailed information which they summarize – or to examine additional studies conducted since their publication – one must seek elsewhere. Presentation and comprehensive analysis of such data, resulting
from pharmacological studies in animals and, especially, from clinical
trials in humans, is the new dimension provided by this book.

Much of the knowledge contained in *Rational Phytotherapy* has never
before been made available in the English language. Summaries of the
numerous clinical trials on some of the popular phytomedicines will as-
tonish many readers who were not only unaware of the results but in
many cases were unaware that such studies had even been conducted.
There is, of course, a reason for this lack of awareness. Studies on the
botanical, chemical, and pharmacological aspects of plant drugs are often published in English, even in journals originating in non-English
speaking nations. Those that do appear in other languages are rapidly
made available in summary form through such publications as *Chemical
Abstracts*. German medial literature, on the other hand, is much less
available to English-only readers. Yet it is in just this literature where
many of the clinical studies on phytomedicines are published. In the
United States, even those who can read German have considerable difficulty in locating the journals, many of which are often unavailable in
major medical libraries. Relatively few of the pertinent articles are currently indexed on MEDLINE. Personally, I have always found it much
easier to request photocopies of such medical studies from colleagues
in Germany rather than to attempt to acquire them here in the United
States.

Of the hundreds of medicinal plants used therapeutically in Europe
today, a relatively small number account for a very large percentage of
the total sales. Interestingly, those enjoying the greatest popularity are
those which, by and large, have been most thoroughly investigated.
These are the ones that are discussed in detail in this book. The tables
in the Appendix provide details on the popularity of both individual
and combination phytomedicines in Germany.

Members of the conventional medical community who are skeptical
about the utility of phytomedicines often base their skepticism on the
lack of human clinical trials for such products or, more precisely, on
their lack of knowledge of those trials that have been conducted. Now,
by turning to the pages of this book, they can learn just exactly how
many therapeutic trials have been conducted with capsules or tablets
of, for example, garlic powder, the total number of patients involved,
the dosage used, whether the studies were controlled, double-blinded,
and the results compared with those obtained from using placebos. In
short, all of the necessary clinical data, with references, are provided

here in addition to sound scientific information on the botany, chemistry, and pharmacology of the herb itself.

All of the numerous books on herbs written previously lack one or more of these essential components. English-language volumes have usually been deficient in clinical information on the herbs considered. The few which do present some clinical details neglect other necessary aspects of botanicals. In the truest sense of the world, *Rational Phytotherapy* may be called the world's first qualitatively complete, science-based herbal in the English language.

It is my belief that the information presented in this volume will have a considerable impact on the therapeutic use of botanicals in the English-speaking world. Physicians, pharmacists, lawmakers, regulators, scientists, and interested lay persons will no longer be able to disregard the scientific and clinical evidence supporting herbal utility simply by claiming ignorance of data available previously only in a foreign language. The evidence recorded on these pages strongly supports the safety and efficacy of a substantial number of herbs and should facilitate their increased use as desirable conventional drugs for the prevention and treatment of a variety of conditions, syndromes, and illnesses.

For far too long, the use of botanicals in English-speaking countries has depended largely on folklore, hearsay, and even gossip. Now, for the first time, the broad spectrum of scientific and clinical evidence supporting the use of many such products has been collected, summarized, presented and referenced in a concise, intelligible form. Publication of *Rational Phytotherapy* will, without question, become a significant landmark, a milestone of achievement, in the development of phytomedical science and its application to human health.

Varro E. Tyler
West Lafayette, Indiana, U. S. A.

Preface to the Third Edition

In 1995, phytomedicines accounted for approximately 7% of all prescription medications covered by public health insurance in Germany, with total sales of about 2 billion DM. Two-thirds of the prescriptions were for single-herb products, i.e., products whose active ingredients derive from only one medicinal plant. Just 5 herbs account for approximately 60% of these prescriptions, and 28 herbs account for more than 90%. But when Commission E of the former German Health Agency reviewed the efficacy of 363 different medicinal plants from 1982 to 1994, it gave a positive rating to about 250 of them. A comparison of these figures shows that the historical diversity of herbal remedies in Germany is no longer reflected in the present-day practice of prescribing medications. Of course, many family doctors advise their patients on self-medication, and this could easily double the figures on sales and use of the leading plant drugs. Nevertheless, the total number of medicinal plants that are important in medical practice is still only a fraction of those that are listed and described in historical textbooks of herbal medicine.

Despite its special treatment in the 1976 German Drug Law, phytotherapy is not an "alternative medicine" but a scientifically tested and proven treatment modality that is at the very root of modern pharmacotherapy. It is true with herbal medicines as with other drugs that as a remedy becomes more widely used, better information is needed regarding its safety and efficacy. Thus, a basic goal of this third edition of *Rational Phytotherapy* is to take a focused, systematic look at the most important groups of indications in phytotherapy and at herbal products that have been proven safe and effective by scientific standards. Little or no attention is given to preparations that are rarely used or whose safety and efficacy have not been well documented. The evaluation of combination products that contain several medicinal herbs is a particularly difficult task. Most of these products are derived from traditional herbal practices, and very few have been subjected to comparative clinical studies to evaluate the additive or synergistic effects of their individual components. Nevertheless, 49 of the 100 most commonly prescribed herbal medications in 1995 were combination products. Theoretical considerations aside, we believed it important to recognize the authority of medical experience; therefore we included combination herbal products under the Drug Products heading that concludes each of the indication-oriented chapters, considering only those products that are among the 100 most commonly prescribed herbal drugs (see Appendix, Table A3).

The findings of Commission E of the former German Health Agency were very helpful in evaluating the products. References to Commission E findings later in the text are based on the monographs published by the Commission in the Bundesanzeiger (a publication comparable to the Federal Register in the U.S.).

We are deeply indebted to Mrs. Gabriele Voigt, who managed all aspects of technical organization from the initial text entry to the page proofs. We are also grateful to our wives for patiently helping with our work as "assistant instructors."

Berlin and Munich
July 1996

Table of Contents

List of Figures

All figures were taken from „Hänsel/Hölzl, Lehrbuch der Pharmazeutischen Biologie", 1996, Springer-Verlag Heidelberg, unless indicated otherwise.

1 Medicinal Plants, Phytomedicines, and Phytotherapy

1.1
Common Roots of Pharmacotherapy

From a historical perspective, the production of medicines and the pharmacologic treatment of diseases began with the use of herbs. Methods of folk healing practiced by the peoples of the Mediterranean region and the Orient found expression in the first European herbal, De Materia Medica, written by the Greek physician Pedanios Dioscorides in the first century AD. During the Renaissance, this classical text was revised to bring it more in line with humanistic doctrines. The plants named by Dioscorides were identified and illustrated with woodcuts, and some locally grown medicinal herbs were added. Herbals were still based on classical humoral pathology, which taught that health and disease were determined by the four bodily humors – blood, phlegm, black bile, and yellow bile. The humors, in turn, were associated with the elemental principles of antiquity: air, water, earth, and fire. The elements could be mixed in varying ratios and proportions to produce the qualities of cold, moist, dry, or warm – properties that also were associated with various proportions of the four bodily humors. Thus, if a particular disease was classified as moist, warm, or dry, it was treated by administering an herb having the opposite property (Jüttner, 1983). Plant medicines were categorized by stating their property and grading their potency on a four-point scale as "imperceptible," "perceptible," "powerful," or "very powerful." Opium, for example, was classified as grade 4/cold. A line of association that linked sedation with "cooling" allowed the empirically known sedative and narcotic actions of opium to be fitted into the humoral system. Pepper was classified as grade 4/dry and warming. The goal of all treatment, according to Hippocrates, was to balance the humors by removing that which is excessive and augmenting that which is deficient" (H. Haas, 1956). Humoral pathology obviously developed into one of the basic principles of conventional medicine.

The monographs that appeared in herbals typically consisted of an illustration of the healing plant, the name of the plant and its synonyms, its action (potency grade and property), and the indications for its use. Indications were not stated in the modern sense of disease entities but as symptoms. For example, cough, catarrh, and hoarseness were each considered separate illnesses. The monograph concluded with a detailed account of the various preparations that could be made from the herb. By and large, the authors of herbals were not laypersons but doctors trained in conventional medical schools. The herbals were written not just for doctors but also for the "common man," in some cases for the express purpose of serving as a guide "when the doctor is too expensive or too far away" (quoted in Jüttner, 1983).

1.2
Making Medicines Safer by Isolating and Modifying Plant Constituents

In his famous "Account of the Foxglove" published in 1785, William Withering described how he was called to the home of an itinerant salesman in Yorkshire. "I found him vomiting incessantly, his vision was blurred, and his pulse rate was about 40 beats per minute. On questioning, I learned that his wife had boiled a handful of foxglove leaves in a half pint of water and had given him the brew, which he swallowed in one draught to seek relief from asthmatic complaints. This good woman was well acquainted with the medicine of her region but not with the dose, for her husband barely escaped with his life."

Cardiac glycosides of the digitalis type have a very narrow range of therapeutic dosages. Exceeding the full medicinal dose by just 40% can produce toxic effects. The dosage problem is compounded by the large qualitative and quantitative variations that occur in the crude plant material. Depending on its origin, the crude drug may contain a predominance of gitoxin, which is not very active when taken orally, or it may carry a high concentration of the very active compound digitoxin.

Thus, isolating the active constituents from herbs with a narrow therapeutic range (Fig. 1.1) and administering the pure compounds is not simply an end in itself. This scientific method of medicinal plant research is, rather, the means by which very potent constituents can be processed into safe medicinal products. The goal is not to concentrate the key active component but to obtain a pharmaceutical product that has a consistent, uniform composition. Processing the isolated constituent into pills, tablets, or capsules results in a product that is diluted by pharmaceutical excipients. For example, the concentration of digitoxin in a digitoxin tablet is approximately 10 times lower than in the original digitalis leaf.

With the development of the natural sciences and the scientific method in medicine beginning in the early 19th century, herbal remedies became an object of scientific analysis. The isolation of morphine from opium (1803–1806) marked the first time that chemical and analytic methods were used to extract the active principle from a herb. It then became possible to perform pharmacologic and toxicologic studies on the effects of morphine in animals and humans. Various substances isolated from opium, including morphine, codeine, and papaverine, are still in therapeutic use today. In other cases efforts have been made to improve on the natural substance by enhancing its desired properties and minimizing its adverse side effects. One of the first examples of this approach was the development of acetylsalicylic acid from the salicin in willow bark. In an effort to surpass the natural precursors, scientists would sometimes produce medicines with unexpected effects. Modifying the reserpine molecule led to mebeverine, while modifying the atropine molecule led to ipratropium bromide and the powerful meperidine group of analgesics. The develop-

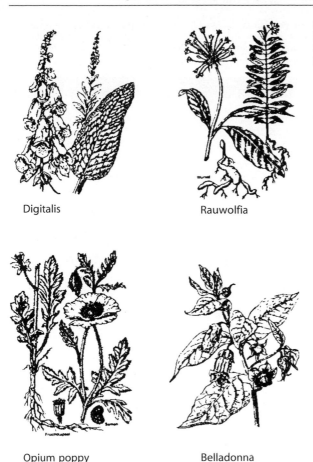

Fig. 1.1.
Potent herbs whose active constituents are isolated for therapeutic use.

Digitalis

Rauwolfia

Opium poppy

Belladonna

ment of cromolyn from khellin is another instance where a plant constituent was modified to obtain a more useful medicine. Medicinal herbs from the New World were another source of important drug substances. The coca shrub yielded cocaine, the prototype for modern local anesthetics, while the bark of Cinchona species yielded quinine, a drug still important in the treatment of malaria. A recent example of an active compound successfully isolated from plants is artemisin, an antimalarial agent derived from a species of Chinese wormwood. Resistance to this compound develops much more slowly than to synthetic antimalarial drugs. Taxol, which is derived from yew bark, has demonstrated cytostatic properties in the treatment of malignant tumors.

A significant portion of all currently used medications are derived, either directly or indirectly, from active principles that have been isolated from plants. Some well-known examples are listed in Table 1.1. Most of these substances do not occur in plants individually but in groups of compounds, such as caffeine in the group of methylxanthines, digoxin in the group of cardiac glycosides, and morphine in the group

Table 1.1. Examples of plant constituents that are isolated for medicinal use. Naturally, these constituents do not occur alone in plants but as fractions accompanied by related chemical compounds. The isolated substances, which generally have strong, immediate actions, are not considered phytomedicines in the strict sense.

Plant constituent	Source	Uses
Atropine	Belladonna	Parasympatholytic
Caffeine	Coffee shrub	Analeptic
Cocaine	Coca leaves	Local anesthetic
Colchicine	Autumn crocus	Gout remedy
Digoxin	Digitalis	Cardiac remedy
Emetine	Ipecac	Emetic
Ephedrine	Ephedra herb	Antihypotensive
Ergotamine	Ergot	Migraine remedy
Kawain	Kava	Anxiolytic
Morphine	Opium poppy	Analgesic
Penicillin	Penicillium spp.	Antibiotic
Physostigmine	Calabar bean	Cholinesterase inhibitor
Pilocarpine	Jaborandi leaves	Glaucoma remedy
Quinidine	Cinchona bark	Antiarrhythmic
Quinine	Cinchona bark	Antimalarial
Reserpine	Rauwolfia	Antihypertensive
Salicin	Willow bark	Anti-inflammatory
Scopolamine	Datura spp.	Antispasmodic
Taxol	Pacific yew bark	Cytostatic
Theophylline	Tea shrub	Bronchial dilator

of opium alkaloids. These isolated compounds and groups of compounds generally produce strong, immediate effects and are in the strict sense not classified as phytomedicines (phytomedicinals).

1.3
Extracts as Pharmacologically Active Components of Phytomedicines

Phytomedicines are medicinal products that contain plant materials as their pharmacologically active component. Keller (1996) may be consulted for an up-to-date overview of experiences with herbal drug products in Germany and Europe. For most phytomedicines, the specific ingredients that determine the pharmacologic activity of the product are unknown. The crude drug (dried herb) or a whole extract derived from it is considered to be the active ingredient. Thus, phytomedicines are complex mixtures of compounds that generally do not exert a strong, immediate action, and whose effect would be classified as imperceptible to perceptible in the historical grading system. Due to the large part of patient and consumer expectations (see Sect. 1.5.5), it is essential that phytomedicines in the strict sense have a wide margin of safety. Most liquid dosage forms are produced from fluidextracts, and most solid dosage forms are solid extracts. Relatively few herbal drug products are made with powdered herbs or oil distillates (see Appendix, Table A 3, p. 288).

1.3.1
What are Extracts?

Extracts are concentrated preparations of a liquid, powdered, or viscous consistency that are ordinarily made from dried plant parts (the crude drug) by maceration or percolation. Fluidextracts are liquid preparations that usually contain a 1:1 ratio of fluidextract to dried herb (w/w or v/w). Ethanol, water, or mixtures of ethanol and water are used exclusively in the production of fluidextracts. Solid or powdered extracts are preparations made by evaporation of the solvent used in the production process (raw extract). Further details on pharmaceutical preparation and extraction techniques for herbal medications are shown in Fig. 1.2.

In some cases it is necessary to remove unwanted components from the raw extract and increase the concentration of the therapeutically active ingredients. Standardized ginkgo powdered extract (50:1) is an example of this process. The 50:1 ratio means that, on average, 50 parts of crude drug must be processed to yield 1 part extract. Potentially allergenic ginkgolic acids are eliminated from the extract along with pharmacologically inert substances.

Volatile oils are also concentrates of active plant constituents. They are generally obtained by direct distillation from the crude drug material or, less commonly, by lipophilic extraction. The ratio of herb to concentrate (known technically as the HER, or herb-to-extract ratio) for volatile oils is usually in the range of 50:1 to 100:1 (w/v), corresponding to a volatile oil content of 1–2 % in typical herbs that contain such oils.

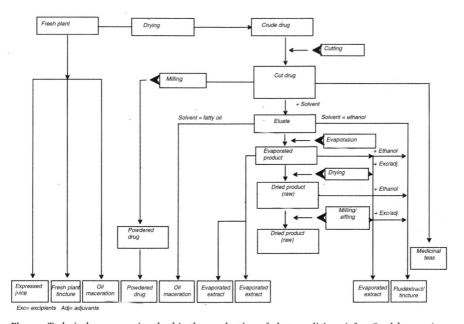

Fig. 1.2. Technical processes involved in the production of phytomedicines (after Gaedcke, 1991)

1.3.2
Standardization of Extracts

Two key factors determine the internal composition of an extract: the quality of the herbal raw material and the production process.

1.3.2.1
Quality of the Herbal Material

Herbs are natural products. Nature does not supply its products with a consistent, standardized composition. We know from daily experience that there are different vintages of wines and different qualities of black teas, there are high-acid and low-acid coffees, and there are sweet and bitter types of fennel. Similarly, the constituents of medicinal herbs can vary greatly as a result of genetic factors, climate, soil quality, and other external factors. The material derived from cultivated medicinal plants shows smaller variations than material gathered from the wild. Another advantage of cultivation is that the increase in relevant constituents can be monitored during plant growth, making it possible to determine the optimum time for harvesting. Quality irregularities caused by variable growth conditions can be controlled in part by culling out materials that do not meet strict quality standards. This ensures that further processing is limited to plant materials that are sufficiently standardized in their relevant constituents. Thus, standardization of the extract begins with the selection and mixing of the herbal raw materials.

1.3.2.2
Production Methods

The nature of the solvent and of the extraction and drying processes critically affects the internal composition of the finished product. Polar compounds are soluble in water, while lipophilic constituents are soluble in alcohol. An aqueous extract of valerian has a fundamentally different spectrum of ingredients than a solid extract that has been processed with ethanol. Even when identical solvents are used, the extraction technique itself can yield products that have different pharmacologic actions. This principle can be illustrated by a simple example:

A total of 107 volunteers were randomly assigned to 3 groups after a 3-week "run-in" phase. Group A drank 4–6 cups of coffee daily that had been brewed by boiling (pharmaceutically a decoction, filtered or decanted). Group B drank the same amount of coffee that had been brewed by filtering (pharmaceutically a percolate), and Group C drank no coffee. The test period lasted a total of nine weeks. The subjects in Group A showed a significant rise in serum cholesterol averaging 0.48 nmol/L. Their LDL level also rose by 0.39 mmol/L. There was no significant difference between Groups B and C, and there were no significant changes in HDL or apolipoprotein levels in any of the groups. Thus, adverse effects were associated with the consumption of coffee brewed by boiling but not with coffee brewed by filtering (Bak et al., 1989).

The above study illustrates that differences in the preparation process – in this case decoction versus percolation – can significantly alter the action of the preparation in the human body. This particularly applies to commercially produced extracts, which are manufactured by a variety of processes using various solvents. All extracts are not the same!

Commercially available extracts vary greatly in their quality. Like many other products, plant extracts are sold in free markets and "spot markets" that offer surplus goods at a premium price. Strict standards usually are not applied to the phytochemical ingredients of these extracts, so there is no guarantee that processing of the extracts will yield an herbal medicine of consistent and acceptable quality (Hänsel and Trunzler, 1989).

1.3.2.3
Adjustment of Quality

Another approach to achieving consistent pharmaceutical quality is to blend selected batches of the primary extracts together in a way that ensures a most consistent concentration of specific ingredients or groups of compounds. The ingredients selected for this "quality adjustment" process should be those that are important for the actions and efficacy of the product, to the extent that such constituents are known. If therapeutic efficacy is critically influenced by a single group of compounds (e. g., anthranoids in anthranoid laxatives, see Sect. 5.6.4), the quality adjustment can be accomplished with therapeutically inert excipients. With most phytomedicines, however, the contribution of specific components to therapeutic efficacy is either speculative or unknown. In these cases the extracts are adjusted to certain marker compounds to ensure pharmaceutical quality. Often these marker compounds are chemicals that are merely characteristic components of the herb in question. In many cases these substances have not been tested for their actions or therapeutic efficacy in pharmacologic test models or in clinical studies.

Since individual plant species are genetically determined, their chemical composition is also determined to some degree. It is reasonable to assume, then, that correlations exist between the marker compounds of plants and other therapeutically relevant ingredients that occur in whole extracts. The strength of these correlations is unknown for most phytomedicines, however, so the quality adjustment of whole plant extracts based on selected marker constituents remains questionable from a therapeutic standpoint. Technological means are needed to compensate for the biologic variability of herbal medicines.

1.3.2.4
Analytical Quality Control

Besides the controlled cultivation of herbs and the use of standardized production methods, chemical analysis is necessary to ensure the optimum homogeneity of plant extracts. This applies to the raw materials themselves (dried herbs and extracts) as well as the finished products. In contrast to the chemically defined constituents of synthetic drugs, which can be quantitatively measured, a lack of knowledge about the specific chemical constituents of phytomedicines forces us to rely on qualitative and semiquantitative chromatographic methods of separation and analysis.

Figure 1.3 shows a typical profile of the ingredients in a St. John's wort extract that was fractionated by high-performance liquid chromatography (HPLC). Depending on the technology and solvent used, this technique can generate chemical spectra that characterize the multicomponent active principle as uniquely as a fingerprint.

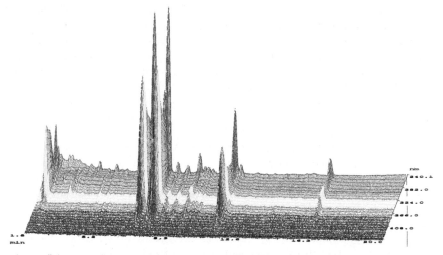

Fig. 1.3. "Fingerprint" spectrum showing the chemical composition of a St. John's wort extract. Each peak represents a chemical compound or group of compounds. The basic spectral pattern is stored electronically to determine the identity of the sample. The spectrum covers a range of wavelengths from 201.0 to 601.0 nm with a resolution of 2.00 nm. Indicated retention times: 1.50 to 19.97 min. Displayed wavelengths: 240.1 to 450.0 nm.

When a "fingerprint chromatogram" covering a broad range of ingredients is stored electronically and its basic pattern is compared with a given test sample to determine a "match factor," this technique can define the identity of active plant constituents with greater accuracy than the conventional practice of measuring selected key constituents. This is particularly true when little is known about the relation of these constituents to actions and efficacies or about the quantitative makeup of the remaining components.

1.4
Phytomedicines

1.4.1
Liquid Dosage Forms

Phytomedicines are drug products made from botanicals (herbs), whole extracts, or concentrates of active plant constituents. They are available in solid and liquid form. The liquid dosage forms include:

- Tinctures, glycerites, and related products
- Syrups
- Medicinal oils
- Medicinal spirits
- Plant juices

1.4.1.1
Tinctures, Glycerites, and Related Products

Tinctures are alcoholic or hydroalcoholic solutions prepared from botanicals. If glycerol is used as a solvent, the preparation is known as a glycerite. Increasingly, extractions are performed with a mixture of glycerol, propylene glycol, and water instead of ethanol and water. Polyethylene glycol 400 has recently been used as a solvent. Glycerol is a physiologic substance, occurring as a component of natural glycerides. Propylene glycol is a form of glycerol in which one of the two terminal hydroxyl groups is absent. Polyethyleneglycol is a synthetic product, the number 400 indicating its average molecular weight. It is a clear, colorless liquid that preferentially extracts lipophilic compounds from the crude drug.

The type of solvent used is indicated by the manufacturer; for example, it may appear on the package insert under the heading "Other Ingredients" or "Excipients." There are two methods of producing fixed combinations in tincture form: by mixing individual tinctures or by mixing the crude drug and then performing the extraction. The difference is illustrated by two similar prescription formulas that are used in the treatment of indigestion:

Prescription 1:

Rx	Comp. cinchona tincture	100 mL
Directions:	Take 30 drops, diluted with water,	
	three times daily shortly before meals.	

The preparation is made by extracting an herbal mixture composed of cinchona bark (12 parts), bitter orange peel (4 parts), gentian root (4 parts), and cinnamon bark (2 parts) with 70 % ethanol (v/v) (100 parts).

Prescription 2:

Rx	Cinchona tincture	60.0
	Bitter orange peel tincture	20.0
	Gentian tincture	20.0
	Cinnamon tincture	10.0
Directions:	Take 30 drops, diluted with water,	
	three times daily shortly before meals.	

The pharmacist makes up this prescription by mixing the ready-made tinctures. The preparation may become cloudy or form precipitates, but generally this will not alter its efficacy. One advantage of liquid dosage forms in general is that they provide an alternative for patients who have difficulty swallowing pills and capsules. One disadvantage is their shorter shelf life, which may be further reduced due to improper storage by the patient (open container, too much heat or moisture).

1.4.1.2
Syrups

Already known to ancient Arabic healers, medicinal syrups entered European medicine during the early Middle Ages. The word *syrup* is derived from the Arabic sirab, scharab or scherbet, meaning a sugary juice beverage. Syrups are viscous preparations for internal use containing at least 50 % sucrose and usually 60–65 %. The sugar content of syrups (about 66 %) is essential for extending their shelf life. Microorganisms cannot proliferate in saturated sugar solutions because highly concentrated solutions deprive the microbes of the water necessary for their development. Preservatives must be added to syrups with a lower sugar content to protect them from bacterial growth.

Syrups are used as flavoring agents, especially in pediatric medicine. Marshmallow syrup, fennel syrup, English plantain syrup, and thyme syrup are all commonly prescribed herbal syrups.

1.4.1.3
Medicinal Oils

Medicinal oils are mostly fatty oils or liquid waxes containing solutions or extracts of drug substances. Medicinal oils are used both internally and externally. Examples of medicinal oils prepared by extraction of plant material are St. John's wort oil and garlic oil maceration. Oils containing dissolved drugs are exemplified by solutions of volatile oils in liquid jojoba wax, which are commonly used as massage oils, especially in aromatherapy.

1.4.1.4
Medicinal Spirits

A spirit or essence is a solution of a volatile substance in alcohol or in water and alcohol. Medicinal spirits are made either by dissolving the volatile oil in alcohol, as in the case of Peppermint Spirit BPC made with peppermint oil, or by distillation.

To produce a medicinal spirit by distillation, the crude drug is pulverized, mixed with alcohol, and allowed to stand until the volatile components have dissolved out of the herbal tissue (oil cells, oil glands, oil reservoirs). Finally these components are recovered by distillation.

There is an inherent risk of dependency in the use of medicinal spirits, which may reactivate an old alcohol-related illness or exacerbate an existing one.

1.4.1.5
Plant Juices

Freshly harvested plant parts are macerated in water and pressed. The shelf life of the expressed juice can be extended by conventional pasteurization or by rapid, ultra-high-temperature treatment (flash method). Plant juices are produced only from medicinal plants that do not contain highly potent chemicals. While expressed juices do contain the water-soluble components of the processed plant, they are free of lipophilic constituents. Little is known about the chemical composition of plant juices or their possible reactions in aqueous media. Plant juices are over-the-counter remedies that are used chiefly for self-medication.

Some common sources of plant juices are birch leaves, nettle, watercress, St. John's wort, garlic, dandelion, lemon balm, European mistletoe, radish, English plantain, and horsetail.

1.4.2
Solid Dosage Forms

Powdered extracts and concentrates must be protected from light, oxygen, and moisture. This is best accomplished by processing them into solid dosage forms such as granules, tablets, coated tablets, and capsules. Preparing medications in a form appropriate for their intended use also permits more accurate dosing. In addition to solid dosage forms, there are other forms such as tinctures of fluidextracts, ampules, and semisolid preparations. This section deals exclusively with solid dosage forms. A drug substance becomes a medication through the process of pharmaceutical formulation, in which excipients are added to the drug substance. Physicians can easily access product information to learn about the excipients that have been used in any given product. Solid dosage forms must be taken with an adequate amount of liquid (100–200 mL) to avoid leaving drug residues that may harm the esophagus. This is a particular concern in the elderly and in patients with preexisting damage to the esophageal mucosa (alcohol).

1.4.2.1
Granules

Granules are aggregates of powdered material held together with binders. Their production involves the use of various excipients such as gelatin solution, methyl cellulose, povidone, simple syrup, lactose, and sucrose. Granules are usually processed into tablets but also may be used as a separate dosage form. Drug substances used in the treatment of gastrointestinal complaints are often produced in granulated form.

1.4.2.2
Uncoated Tablets

Tablets are made by the compression of powdered or granulated material (compressed tablets). Besides the active ingredients, which may amount to only a few milligrams, tablets contain diluents, binders, lubricants, coloring and falvoring agents, and desintegrators to help the compressed tablet dissolve in an aqueous medium.

1.4.2.3
Coated Tablets

Coated tablets are compressed tablets covered with a coating of sugar, dyes, fat, and wax. The function of the coating is to protect the medicinal core. Tablets can also be coated with film-forming agents, usually polymers (e.g., cellulose acetate phthalate), to produce a film-coated tablet (FCT). Several advantages of coated tablets are indicated below:

- Release of the medication can be controlled or delayed (enteric-coated tablets, controlled-release tablets).
- Shelf life is extended, as the coating protects against external influences such as light, moisture, and mechanical stresses.
- They are easier to swallow than uncoated tablets.
- The coating masks any unpleasant taste from the medicinal core.

1.4.2.4
Capsules

Hard gelatin capsules consist of a two-part cylindrical shell whose halves are fitted together after the medication – a powdered or granulated drug substance – has been placed inside. Besides gelatin, the capsule shell contains glycerin or sorbitol as a softening agent, water, aromatics, dyes, and antimicrobial additives. Volatile oils may be encapsulated by adding them first to a powdered excipient; the oils will subsequently be released in the gastrointestinal tract.

Soft gelatin capsules are spherical, oval, oblong, or teardrop-shaped capsules with a gelatin shell enclosing semisolid or liquid contents that must be free of water (e.g., oily garlic extracts or peppermint oil).

The material of the capsule shell can be designed to delay the release of the drug substance until the capsule has entered the stomach or intestine. A chemically modified cellulose, hydroxypropylene methylcellulose phthalate (HPMCP), makes an effective enteric (gastric-acid-resistant) coating. Insoluble while in the acidic milieu of the stomach, this compound dissociates when the pH rises above 7 and becomes soluble under physiologic conditions.

Enteric coatings on capsules and tablets offer several advantages:

- They protect the drug substance from deactivation or decomposition by gastric juices.
- They shield the stomach lining from drug substances that could cause irritation or nausea (salicylates, emetine).
- They prevent dilution of the drug substance before it reaches the bowel (intestinal antispasmodics or antiseptics).

Enteric-coated capsules or tablets that release the drug substance after entering the bowel should never be taken during or after meals, but approximately 1 hour before meals.

Particles larger than 3 mm in diameter do not leave the stomach with the chyme; they are retained in the stomach until the subsequent interdigestive phase. One danger of enteric-coated capsules is that they may remain in the stomach for some time while the pH of the gastric juice rises, leading to premature release of the drug inside the stomach.

1.4.2.5
Lozenges

Lozenges (troches, pastilles) have a tablet-like appearance (round, oblong, etc.) but differ from tablets in that they are not made by compression but are molded or cut from pliable masses of varying composition. Lozenges are designed to release the active ingredient slowly into the oral cavity while sucked or chewed. The base is composed of sucrose (usually more than 90 %), acacia (about 7 %), gelatin, tragacanth, and water (e.g., Echinacea Capsettes).

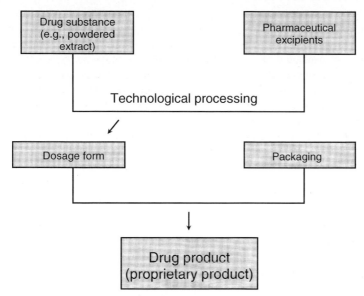

Fig. 1.4. Relationship between drug substance, dosage form, and finished drug product.

1.4.3
Packaging

The package is an essential part of any medication. Packaging turns a pharmaceutical preparation into a product ready for consumer use. It encloses and protects the contents from the environment. The package is labeled to designate its contents and convey other information such as the expiration date and the batch number in case the product must be recovered or recalled. Package inserts provide detailed information on contents, actions, usage, indications, contraindications, and side effects (Fig. 1.4).

In the United States where most botanical products are sold as dietary supplements, not as approved drugs, therapeutic claims cannot be made on the label or in the package insert (technically part of the labelling). A statement can be made regarding the effect of the product followed by a disclaimer indicating the claim has not been approved by the Food and Drug Administration. An additional statement must then appear noting the the product is not intended to diagnose, treat, cure, or prevent any desease.

1.4.4
Herbal Combination Products

The active ingredient of an herbal medication as defined by the German Drug Law is a preparation (e. g., a whole extract) made from one herb. If the product contains no additional herbal ingredients, it is classified as a single-herb product. This type of product is preferred in the practice of rational phytotherapy. For products that contain a fixed combination of several active ingredients, meaning a combination of several whole extracts in the case of herbal remedies, the German Drug Law requires proof that ". . . every pharmacologically active ingredient contributes to the positive evaluation of the remedy." Although a number of herbal combinations are still currently on the market in Germany, proof of efficacy has been furnished only for a small minority of these products.

From a historical perspective, the preference for multi-herb formulations in phytomedicine has several roots. One factor dating from antiquity is the "magic of numbers" principle. Galen (131–201 AD) taught that, while the nature and dosage of a remedy were important, it was also important to prescribe the correct number of medicines to achieve the desired curative effect (Haas, 1956). Another historical idea was the "theriaca" principle, which states that since we do not know what ingredient will work in any given case, it is best to try as many drugs as possible so that a potentially effective ingredient will not be omitted. A theriaca was a mixture of 50–100 different substances; there were 65 ingredients in the theriaca dispensed by Valerius Cordus (1511–1544). A theriaca with 12 ingredients was still listed in the German pharmacopeias of 1882 and 1926 (including 1% opium). Theriaca-like mixtures are still being marketed today under various brand names (Swedish Herbs).

As a reaction against the polypharmacy movement, Paracelsus (1490–1541) categorically rejected the use of remedies composed of many drugs. By recognizing the importance of administering a component that exerts a specific, desired therapeutic action, Paracelsus became the father of modern pharmaceutical research. Four centuries later there are still remedies that contain 10–20 separate components. Considering the thousands of possible combinations that can be made and the endless product variations that result, the pharmacologist Forth (1984) wrote: "This is what accounts for the alienation of experimental pharmacology from phytotherapeutic products. It is not caused by the disdain of science for natural products."

The "more is better" concept has survived to this day and has even found its way into homeopathic medicine, in which combinations of drugs are alien to the theoretical concept of Hahnemann. In addition to complex homeopathic remedies, there are products on the market that combine homeopathic and phytotherapeutic agents. Meanwhile, phytotherapy has been largely removed from the canon of conventional, academically recommended treatment modalities, a development that reached its culmination when phytotherapy was declared an alternative medicine by the German Drug Law of 1976. The establishment of phytotherapy as an alternative medicine is tantamount to segregating the entire class of herbal remedies from orthodox medicine (Bock, 1993). Unfortunately, this stigmatization affects rational phytomedicines in addition to less rational herbal remedies. Rational phytomedicines are herbal medicines whose safety and efficacy conform to current testing standards as fully as conventional drugs. The group of scientifically proven single-extract products (Table 1.2) satisfy approval standards without qualification. Placing these drugs in the category of alternative medicine or complementary medicine hampers the effort to gain acceptance and recognition by mainstream medical science.

The fifth amendment to the German Drug Law of August 9, 1994, laid the groundwork for drawing a distinction between rational and irrational plant medicines. This amendment states that scientifically proven phytomedicines (most likely single-herb

Table 1.2. Examples of phytomedicines that have undergone state-of-the-art pharmacologic testing, and whose efficacy has been established by controlled studies and well-documented reports of physician experience.

Herb or extract	Key constituents	Pharmacologic actions	Uses
Ginkgo biloba leaf extract (50:1)	Bilobalide, ginkgolides, flavonoids	Anti-ischemic, antihypoxidotic, PAF-antagonistic, antihemorrheologic	Symptomatic treatment of cognitive deficits due to organic brain disease. Other uses see p. 126
St. John's wort herb	Hypericins and hyperforin are presumably involved	Antidepressant	Mild and moderate depression, anxiety, and nervous unrest
Chamomile flowers	Chamazulene, bisabolol, lipophilic flavonoids	Anti-inflammatory, antispasmodic	Inflammatory disorders of the gastrointestinal tract with spasticity; other uses see p. 252, 255
Kava rhizome and roots	Methysticin and chemically related pyrones	Local anesthetic, anticonvulsant, central muscle relaxant	States of nervous anxiety, tension, and restlessness
Garlic cloves	Alliin (ca. 1 %), alliinase	Lowers lipid levels, inhibits platelet aggregation, fibrinolytic, antibacterial, antihypertensive	To support dietary measures in patients with high serum lipid levels; prevention of age-related vascular changes
Milk thistle fruits	Silymarin (flavono-lignans), especially silybinin	Antihepatotoxic; at the cellular level, promotes ribosome formation and protein synthesis	Dyspeptic complaints, toxic liver diseases
Horse chestnut extract	Aescin (triterpenoid saponins)	Astringent, antiedemic	Complaints due to lower extremity venous disease
Senna leaves	Sennosides, especially sennoside B	Stimulates bowel motility, antiabsorptive, stimulates secretions	Constipation, or to cleanse the bowel before diagnostic procedures
Hawthorn extract	May consist of glycosyl flavonoids and proanthocyanidins	Positive inotropic, antiarrhythmic, improves hypoxic tolerance, reduces afterload	Mild heart failure (stage II of NYHA)

products) will be evaluated for pharmaceutical quality, efficacy, and safety in a normal approval process and will be given a corresponding approval number that physicians can recognize. A special provision of the Drug Law mandates that old products having the status of de facto approval be phased out of the drug market by the year 2005. The possible continuing approval of largely untested products designated as traditional remains a problem, although these products have been declared non-reimbursable according to the August 1994 guidelines issued by the Federal Commission of Physicians and Health Insurers.

The 100 most commonly prescribed herbal medications in Germany (see Appendix) still include 49 combination products. Twenty-two of these products each contain two active ingredients. Most of these combinations have reproducible efficacy based on known pharmacologic actions and, in some cases, clinical therapeutic studies. Of the remaining 26 combination products, it is noteworthy that 21 contain an odd number of components (3-, 5-, 7- or 9-herb combinations) while only 5 contain an even number (4) – a throwback, perhaps, to the old medical teachings of Galen.

In evaluating multicomponent herbal products, however, it would be unfair to ignore practical therapeutic experience, especially that gained by family doctors and other private physicians in their daily experience with medicinal products. Thus, despite theoretical considerations, our review of drug products at the end of each chapter is not limited to the preferred single-herb remedies but includes combination products that are among the 100 most commonly prescribed herbal medications in Germany (see Appendix).

1.5
Phytotherapy

1.5.1
Pharmacologic Characteristics

1.5.1.1
Therapeutic Range

Phytomedicines are considered to have a broad therapeutic range (see Sect. 1.2 and 1.5.4). It is difficult or nearly impossible to ingest a toxic or lethal dose of an herbal remedy that is administered orally. The difference between an extract and an isolated compound is illustrated by the difference between caffeine-containing beverages and caffeine itself. About 10 g of pure caffeine, taken at one time, is a life-threatening dose for humans (Wirth and Gloxhuber, 1982). This is the equivalent of drinking about 20 liters of strong coffee (82 mg caffeine/150 mL) or 400 bottles of a cola beverage (25 mg caffeine/200 mL) in one sitting. An acutely lethal caffeine dose could not be ingested with these beverages, especially since caffeine is rapidly broken down to harmless metabolites within the body.

When it comes to the prescribing of phytomedicines by physicians, it should be common knowledge among patients and consumers that every herbal remedy approved as a drug can be taken with confidence in its inherent safety (see Sect. 1.5.5).

1.5.1.2
Onset of Action

Most phytomedicines do not produce immediate effects but act only after a latent period of variable duration. While a number of phytomedicines can be shown to produce acute effects in pharmacologic experiments, the desired therapeutic result often appears only after the product has been used for a period of weeks or months. This is illustrated by the following example.

The long-term use of bulk laxatives is very widely prescribed for the treatment of irritable colon (Bär, 1987). An immediate effect is an increase in the quantity of the stool. There may be increased flatulence, bloating, and constipation at the start of therapy due to gases such as hydrogen, methane, and carbon dioxide that are released by the anaerobic breakdown of indigestible carbohydrates. The initial increase in complaints is an undesired immediate effect. It takes 1–3 months to establish a new intestinal flora that is well adapted to the anaerobic fermentation of bulk materials and can induce the fecal volume expansion that leads to the desired effect (see Sect. 5.6.2).

Latent periods for the onset of therapeutic efficacy are not unique to phytotherapy. The phenomenon is well known in mainstream pharmacotherapy and is illustrated by a number of psychotherapeutic drugs, especially the neuroleptics and antidepressants. It is not surprising, therefore, that some psychoactive herbal drugs must be taken for several weeks before there is a demonstrable response (see Chap. 2).

1.5.2
Pharmacologic and Clinical Research

Therapeutically oriented pharmacologic research and up-to-date clinical studies are still the exception in phytotherapy. But increasingly, the phytomedicine industry is showing the practical value of theoretical research and clinical testing in herbal medicine, as the list in Table 1.2 illustrates.

A distinctive feature of phytomedicines compared with synthetic drugs lies in the priority of clinical testing over pharmacologic research. Almost all synthetic drugs are first tested in laboratory animals before they are tried in subjects and patients. Phases I–III of clinical drug testing are designed to show whether pharmacologically documented effects are obtained in human patients to a significant and acceptable degree. By contrast, the actions of phytomedicines have usually been observed empirically in human patients treated with the herbs. It is often difficult to devise an experimental model in which the therapeutically relevant actions of an herb can be demonstrated in an animal model. This can be done with extracts that have acute effects, such as anthranoid laxatives, but it is far more difficult with extracts that have a long latent period, such as valerian extract. There is a need to develop new methods of pharmacologic research that can further elucidate the modes of action of many herbal remedies. Another problem in the pharmacologic testing of plant drugs is the difficulty of obtaining accurate pharmacokinetic data for extracts that have a complex composition. Unless we can prove that the unknown constituents of the extract responsible for effects in laboratory animals actually reach the potential site of action in humans, we cannot know for certain that pharmacologic findings have therapeutic relevance. For example, the flavonoids that occur in many extracts produce a variety of effects in vitro (Cody et al., 1986; Gabor, 1975; Havsteen, 1983), but they are so poorly absorbed in vivo and are broken down so rapidly by microbial and endogenous enzymes that the contribution of flavonoid constituents to the efficacy of plant extracts in humans is very difficult to evaluate.

One interim result is clear. The kind of rational evidence that supports pharmacologic therapy in orthodox medicine has not yet been furnished for all herbal medicines. It is proper to demand, at the very least, evidence that unequivocally documents the therapeutic efficacy of herbal remedies in human patients.

For drugs whose active ingredients are known, including the medicines used in phytotherapy, health authorities evaluate therapeutic efficacy on the basis of scientific findings. In Germany this includes empirical data gained through scientific methods, as illustrated by articles in professional journals or statements from professional societies. Apparently there are marked differences in the validity of criteria that are used to evaluate efficacy. It is not uncommon for the same criteria to be applied to phytomedicines as are applied to drugs with different synthetic components. This implies a greater emphasis on objective parameters. "Subjective assessments by the patient or physician are apt to be imprecise" (Immich, 1988). Meanwhile, however, it has become clear that, in patients with pain as well as in numerous pathologic conditions and treatment situations, carefully elicited subjective assessments (e. g., self-rating by the patient) can be far more useful for evaluating treatment response and monitoring progress than the "hard data" furnished by objective biochemical, radiologic, and other technically sophisticated procedures (Saller and Feiereis, 1993).

The relative value of subjective and objective parameters as study criteria is illustrated by an example from phytotherapy: Eucalyptus oil, menthol, mint oil, and peppermint oil produce a pleasant, fresh cooling sensation when inhaled or applied topically to the nasal mucosa, and many patients with colds are convinced that they can breathe more easily. For many years this effect was widely attributed to a reduction in mucosal swelling. Then Naumann (1967), using instruments that accurately measured the volume and pressure of nasal airflow, showed that the topical application of menthol in oily solution in concentrations up to 7% either had no objective effect or actually caused a slight swelling of the mucosa, resulting in constriction of the airway. Similarly, rhinomanometric measurements after 5 min of vapor inhalation showed no increase in nasal volume. Remarkably, however, a decrease in nasal airflow resistance was measured in subjects who performed standard physical exercise (120 Watts on a bicycle ergometer for 5 min) after inhaling the vapors. It seems paradoxical that the objective improvement shown by bicycle ergometry was not perceived subjectively, whereas the lack of objective improvement was perceived subjectively as a significant increase in nasal airflow (Burrow et al., 1983). These results were found to be reproducible under varying conditions (Fox, 1977; Eccles et al., 1987a, b).

The failure of peppermint and eucalyptus oils to increase objectively nasal volume does not mean that these medications lack therapeutic benefit. In the case of a cold, which is self-limiting, it is better to treat the subjective symptoms without interfering with the body's normal, salutary inflammatory response. While certain types of intranasal surgery will objectively improve nasal airflow, the discomfort will persist if the surgery causes nerve damage that makes the patient unable to perceive the improved inflow of air (Burrow et al., 1983).

1.5.3
Indications for the Use of Phytomedicines

Phytomedicines are, with few exceptions (e. g., see Sect. 5.7.1.6), not appropriate for use in emergency or acute-care situations; consequently they have little or no role in the hospital setting. They are mainly prescribed by family doctors in the office setting or used for self-medication. The frequency with which phytomedicines are used in a given practice depends largely on the type of patients that are seen and the nature of their illnesses. A large percentage of patients treated with herbal medicines have relatively mild and ambiguous symptoms that often defy a clear-cut diagnosis. Herbal remedies are also commonly used in patients with chronic illnesses and complaints.

Chapters 2 through 9 in this book cover specific organ systems that represent key indications for the use of phytomedicines. Their systematic arrangement reflects the relative frequency with which herbal medicines are prescribed in the physician's office. The 100 most commonly prescribed herbal medications in Germany (see Appendix) can be broken down as follows in terms of their frequency of use for specific groups of indications:

- diseases of the respiratory tract (29 products);
- disorders of the central nervous system (19 products);
- urinary tract remedies (11 products);
- cardiovascular disorders (10 products);
- disorders of the digestive tract, liver, and bile (10 products);
- dermatologic remedies and external anti-inflammatory agents (8 products);
- immunostimulants (6 products);
- gynecologic remedies (4 products);
- herbal remedies for internal use in the treatment of rheumatic disorders and inflammatory conditions (3 products).

1.5.4
What Physicians Require from Phytomedicines

The task of the physician is to help the sick. The tools available to physicians in this endeavor are their senses, voices, instruments, medications, and other aids. The emphasis in the choice of the various therapeutic options has changed during the course of the twentieth century. The earliest decades were still marked by epochal advances in medicine and especially in the use of drugs. Small wonder that these advances sparked a fondness for intervention, despite the growing risks, and a declining emphasis on the doctor's word. Many of the new synthetic drugs had such profound and immediate effects that, for a time, it seemed as if there were no longer a need for lengthy explanations by the physician. Spoiled by success, medicine took little interest in such matters as risks and side effects. They were either deemphasized or dealt with in a detached way, e. g., by referring the patient to the package insert accompanying a drug. As a result, physician services in general acquired an impersonal, high-tech image that growing numbers of patients found objectionable, especially during the past 20 years.

This trend has sparked a countermovement in which patients by the millions are turning to alternative fields of medicine. Meanwhile, many physicians, motivated in large part by economic pressures, have changed their thinking with a view toward keeping their remaining patients within the bounds of orthodox medicine and regaining patients who have strayed. One change has been a renewed emphasis on the doctor-patient consultation, especially in the office setting. In approximately

50 % of the patients who see a general practitioner, a definitive diagnosis cannot be established within the physician's office. The primary goal in these cases after the initial interview is to provide treatment that will alleviate the patient's discomfort, physical complaints, or specific symptoms (Mader and Weissgerber, 1993). To be successful despite diagnostic uncertainties, the treatment must take into account the basic attitudes of the patient, such as an aversion to synthetic drugs (see Sect. 1.5.6), as well as the potential risks and benefits of therapeutic agents that are considered acceptable.

Remedies prescribed by family doctors continue to rank highly in this regard. In Germany, general practitioners and internists in private practice write about two-thirds of all prescriptions, issuing most of them to patients over 60 years of age. Indeed, every insured patient over age 60 takes an average of about 3 medications on a long-term basis (Schwabe and Paffrath, 1995). But the treatment of chronic illnesses in older patients seldom requires the use of drugs that produce strong, acute effects with rapid onset. The priority concerns in this population are long-term efficacy and a large therapeutic range to ensure that errors of compliance, for example, will not pose an immediate health risk. The gentler and more gradual actions of most phytomedicines are appealing in this regard.

On the other hand, the emphasis on safety and tolerance does not alter the responsibility of the physician to provide treatment that is adequate, appropriate, and necessary. (Especially in the case of reimbursable prescription drugs, these criteria are mandated by German law.) Phytotherapy is by no means exempt from these requirements (see Sect. 1.5.7). The qualities of adequate and appropriate pertain mainly to efficacy, which must be supported by proper documentation. The traditional use of herbal remedies, mainly in the form of medicinal teas, generally does not furnish proof of therapeutic efficacy that is adequate by present-day standards. Moreover, in making the change from traditional tea preparations to ready-made products, it is common for manufacturers to reduce dosages to a therapeutically inactive range. Thus, therapeutic efficacy remains an unproven claim for most ready-to-use herbal medications, and controlled clinical studies in particular are needed to furnish the necessary proof.

In the absence of sufficient product-specific studies, the physician must give close attention to the pharmaceutical quality of the herbal product (see Sect. 1.3) and to its dosage. As a general rule, the equivalent dosage of an herbal product compared with a traditional single dose taken in a cup of medicinal tea would be in the range of 200–500 mg of crude extract. Large capsules or coated tablets are the only practical means of delivering such a dose. Much of the critical attitude toward combination products stems from this inherent practical limitation on dosing. Despite the immense number of herbal remedies that line the shelves of German pharmacies, there are still only a few phytomedicines that have been satisfactorily documented by scientific and clinical research. Consequently, physicians have but a limited selection of products from which to choose, especially when prescribing within insurer-imposed guidelines. The choice is limited not just in terms of pharmaceutical quality and adequate dosing but also in terms of safety and efficacy.

1.5.5
Hopes and Expectations of the Patients

The Allensbach Institute of Demoscopy recently conducted a public opinion survey to explore attitudes toward natural remedies. They surveyed a total of 2647 people ranging from 16 to 90 years of age. Thirty five percent of the those surveyed rejected natural remedies; the remaining 65% used natural remedies occasionally or regularly. When asked whether natural remedies were effective, only 8% said no; 43% had no opinion, and 49% believed that the effectiveness of natural remedies should be judged differently than that of chemical drugs. Opinions on product safety were even more revealing. Eighty percent of all those surveyed rated the risk of treatment with natural remedies as low, while 84% rated the risks of synthetic drugs as moderate to high. (IfD survey 6039, 1997) (Fig. 1.5).

Thus, the demand of many patients for herbal remedies is rooted partly in the emotional perception that natural products are gentler and less hazardous than chemical products. Even a conference with their physician would be unlikely to shake patients from this preconceived notion. A more reasonable approach is to base the prescription and recommendation of herbal remedies on the way in which patients actually use these products, which presupposes that the products have a wide, safe therapeutic range. Potent phytomedicines like the galenical preparations made from cardiac glycoside-containing plant parts, belladonna, or colchicum species do not meet the safety standards to which herbal medicines must conform. Use of the isolated plant constituents (digitalis glycosides, atropine, colchicine) is definitely preferred in cases where such drugs are indicated (Table 1.1).

At the same time, confidence in a remedy is the best foundation for its successful use, especially in older patients with chronic health problems. It is not sensible, nor

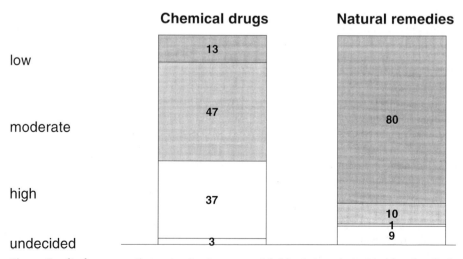

Fig. 1.5. Result of a representing review in 2627 german inhabitants to evaluate the risks of medical supplies. In general for herbal remedies a great margin of safety is assumed (Allensbacher Archiv, 1997).

is it sound medical practice, to give such patients an academic lecture on pros and cons. Once the treatment decision has been made, it is better to bolster patients' confidence by educating them about the selected medication in positive terms. The basic background information about a synthetic drug mainly involves its chemical structure, which is of little interest to most patients. But with an herbal medication, the patient can be shown a picture of the medicinal plant and told its history, providing an excellent context for the treatment interview. Thus, those who recommend phytomedicines should become familiar with the plants from which they are derived. They should also know something about their traditional uses, botanical characteristics, the parts that are used therapeutically, and the preparation of the product.

1.5.6
Benefits and Risks of Phytomedicines Compared with Other Therapies

For medications with a known active ingredient, drug approval laws in Germany require documentation that allows the therapeutic efficacy and safety of the drug to be evaluated for the dosage indicated. The scientific documentation may consist of toxicologic, pharmacologic, and clinical data in the following order of importance: controlled studies, uncontrolled studies, empirical observations, and collections of anecdotal reports. If methods and procedures have progressed since the studies were last performed, this fact must be duly considered in interpreting the results (Feiden, 1995).

These criteria make it clear that tradition and past experience, while crucial to advocates of herbal remedies, play a minor role in the modern-day assessment of therapeutic efficacy. As a result, phytotherapy lags well behind orthodox medicine in a scientific sense, especially when it comes to testing the efficacy of plant remedies by controlled clinical studies. The marked placebo effect and the relatively mild, gradual actions of plant drugs add to the difficulty of subjecting phytomedicine to this level of research. Nevertheless, this type of research is essential if phytomedicines are to gain acceptance in critical professional circles. It should be added that older synthetic drugs sometimes have the same deficiencies, yet they are tolerated by professional orthodoxy to a much higher degree than herbal medicines.

It must be acknowledged, of course, that the therapeutic efficacy of synthetic drugs is generally better than that of phytomedicines. The advantages of herbal remedies include greater trust on the part of the patients, based on their high expectations of safety and tolerance. For many products, however, the lower incidence of side effects is a claim that has yet to be proven by modern statistical standards. For this type of claim, controlled comparative studies matching phytomedicines against standard synthetic products are of relatively little value. There is a strong suggestive effect that may cause patients informed of potential side effects to experience the types of effects that are known to be associated with synthetic drugs.

Empirical observations are of much greater value for inquiries of this kind. In one observational study, for example, it was found that, in a group of 10,815 patients who had been treated with a ginkgo preparation for senile dementia, only 183 (1.69%) spontaneously reported side effects. In another group of 2141 patients treated for the same condition with a synthetic psychotropic drug, a total of 116 (5.42 %) reported side effects (Burkard and Lehrl, 1991).

Even greater differences have been noted in the pharmacotherapy of patients with depression. The tricyclic antidepressants, which have been used for more than 30 years, cause troublesome side effects such as sedation, dry mouth, and accommodation difficulties in 20–50 % of all patients, especially during initial use. While newer synthetic antidepressants have reduced the incidence of side effects to about 20 %, this is still a very high percentage (Linden et al., 1992). An herbal antidepressant based on St. John's wort extract, recently used therapeutically with great success, is associated with about a 10 times lower incidence of objectionable side effects (Woelk et al., 1993).

The latter two examples may be taken as proof that empirical medical knowledge as well as patient expectations regarding the excellent tolerance of herbal remedies can be documented for a single product. There is a need for further studies of this kind.

1.6
Medicinal Teas Today

> *Persons who prefer their daily coffee, cocoa, or tea to caffeine tablets are unknowingly accepting and enjoying the pleasures of gentle-acting phytomedicines.*
>
> Reinhard Ludewig, 1989

1.6.1
Origin of the Word *Tea*. Medicinal and Nonmedicinal Teas

The word tea is of relatively recent origin. In 1601 a captain with the Dutch East India Company took several sacks of tea on board from a Chinese junk in Java and brought them to Holland, also bringing the name of the product, *t'e*, as it was called in the Amoy dialect of southern China. When Chinese tea found its way into other countries via Dutch and then British seaports, it retained the southern Chinese name that is familiar to us. Countries that first imported the herb by the land route through Russia adopted the name *chai*. Tea first reached Russia with a tea caravan in 1638 as *ch'a*, the name by which the herb is called in the Cantonese and Mandarin dialects of Chinese. The meaning of the term tea gradually broadened in the English language, first referring to the dried tea leaf, then to the beverage brewed from it, and soon it was applied to all herbs from which potable infusions can be made. The meaning of the word in any given case is determined by the context or by explanatory modifiers such as black tea, linden blossom tea, or herbal breakfast tea.

A basic distinction is drawn between:

- nonmedicinal teas that are consumed for pleasure, such as black tea and its blends, flavored teas, and tea-like products;
- medicinal teas that are used either as single teas or, more commonly, as tea mixtures (species).

For a product to be called a tea or tea mixture according to German food laws, it must consist of the leaf buds, young leaves and shoots of the tea shrub, *Camellia sinensis,* that have been prepared by methods normally used in the countries of origin (see also Sect. 5.5.1.1). Earl Gray, for example, is a mixture of teas originating from Ceylon, China, and India, to which bergamot oil is added.

Tea-like products are defined by German food laws as nonmedicinal tea substitutes made from the tops, flowers, or fruits of plants. They may bear the name tea only in conjunction with the name of the plant from which they are derived, e. g., apple peel tea, blackberry leaf tea, fennel tea, and rooibos tea. The latter tea, called also red bush tea, is the national drink of South Africa and has long been marketed and consumed in Europe. Rooibos tea consists of the dried leaves and branch tips of Aspalathus linearis, a bushy plant from the legume family distantly related to our Lupi-

Table 1.3.
Indications for the use of medicinal teas.

A. **Psychosomatic disorders**
  A 1 Anxiety and restlessness
  A 2 Nervous sleep disorders
  A 3 Functional cardiac complaints

B. **Colds and congestion**
  B 1 For phlegm congestion (expectorant teas)
  B 2 For dry cough
  B 3 To induce sweating
  B 4 For fever

C. **Gastrointestinal disorders**
  C 1 Digestive problems (flatulence, bloating)
  C 2 Appetite loss
  C 3 Digestive problems associated with biliary tract dyskinesia
  C 4 Mild inflammations of the gastric mucosa
  C 5 Motion sickness

D. **Urinary tract disorders**
  D 1 To promote diuresis
  D 2 To disinfect the urine
  D 3 To prevent stone disease (urolithiasis)

E. **Diarrhetic conditions**
  E 1 Nonspecific, mild, transient forms

F. **Constipation**
  F 1 To promote gentle bowel movements with soft stools, e. g., in patients with anal fissures or hemorrhoids or following anorectal surgery.
  F 2 Chronic constipation, irritable colon.

G. **Local use as mouthwash or gargle**
  G 1 Inflammations of the oropharyngeal mucosa
  G 2 Oral hygiene

H. **Correctives**
  H 1 To improve the odor or flavor of a tea mixture
  H 2 To improve the appearance of a tea mixture

I. **Less common uses**
  I 1 Adjuvant for excessive menstrual bleeding and other menstrual complaints
  I 2 Physical and mental fatigue
  I 3 Adjuvant for rheumatism

nus species. In Germany the following herbs are offered singly or in mixtures as nonmedicinal teas: apple peels, blackberry leaves, rose hips, hibiscus flowers, raspberry leaves, life everlasting, mallow leaves, mallow flowers, peppermint leaves, sunflower blossoms, and calendula flowers. Obviously, it is sometimes difficult to draw a strict dividing line between a tea-like product and a medicinal tea. Even the pharmacodynamic action of a product does not provide a differentiating feature. For example, the effects of a cup of real tea are easier to demonstrate than the effects of a cup of linden blossom tea owing to the caffeine content of the regular tea. Thus, it is not surprising that shrewd businessmen occasionally try to represent a tea as medicinal while circumventing the German Drug Law. The basic determinants of whether a tea is a medicine or a food in any given case are the designated purpose of the product and consumer expectations. The lables of tea-like products are not allowed to mention actions or medicinal uses – a provision that can be formally circumvented by using magazine ads or printed information pamphlets to modify consumer expectations.

1.6.2
Medicinal Teas and Their Actions

Tea infusions can be prepared from single herbs or from herb mixtures. About 1000 single-herb teas and blends have been approved in Germany (Hiller, 1995). Common medicinal tea herbs and their indications are listed in Table 1.3 and 1.4. Exotic single-herb teas like those from the traditional medicine of India, China, or South American countries should not be prescribed if at all possible. The pharmacist may be able to procure exotic herbs, but by law he can dispense the tea only if he can guarantee the pharmaceutical quality of the product. Usually these products have not been properly tested, so they cannot be legally dispensed (see also Sect. 1.6.8).

A typical medicinal tea consists of several herbs; thus, it represents the prototype of a fixed drug combination. It is considered sound pharmaceutical practice to have no more than 4–7 herbs in a blended tea (Wichtl, 1989).

Examples of acceptable tea mixtures can be found in pharmacopeias and in the standard approval criteria established by German health authorities. The compositions and formulations of these tea mixtures are given in the special section of this book dealing with specific indications.

There have been virtually no controlled clinical studies on the efficacy of medicinal teas. One reason for this is that study participants cannot be blinded as they can in a study of solid herbal preparations, so it is extremely difficult to establish a placebo control.

In some cases the efficacy of a medicinal tea is obvious. Anthranoid herbs have a definite laxative action, teas with aromatic bitters stimulate the appetite, and nothing is better for an upset stomach than fasting and peppermint tea. The medicinal value of teas is based largely on empirical evidence. The contribution of the placebo effect to efficacy is probably large. The slogan, "Drink tea, wait and see," can be interpreted as a temporizing measure during the expectant phase of a still-undiagnosed illness that can calm emotions (anxiety) and reduce stress. Similar reasoning applies to patients who live in constant fear of becoming sick: "Health is just undetected disease."

Table 1.4. Herbs used in medicinal teas, and their indications.

Crude herbal drug	Latin name	Indications (keyed to Table 1.3)
Agrimony	Agrimoniae herba	E 1, G 1
Angelica root	Angelicae rad.	C 1, C 2
Aniseseed	Anisi fruct.	B 1, C 1
Avens root	Gei urbani rhizoma	C 1, E 1
Basil	Basilici herb.	C 1
Bearberry leaf	Uvae ursi fol.	D 2
Bilberry	Myrtilli fruct.	E 1, G 1
Birch leaf	Betulae folium	D 1
Bitter orange peel	Aurantii pericarp.	C 1, C 2, H 1
Black currant leaf	Ribis nigri fol.	D 1
Blackberry leaf	Rubi frutic. fol.	E 1
Blessed thistle	Cnici benedicti herb.	A 1, A 2
Blonde psyllium	Plantaginis ovatae sem.	F 2
Broom	Sarothamni scop. herb.	A 3
Buckthorn bark	Frangulae cort.	F 1
Buckthorn berries	Rhamni cathartici fruct.	F 2
Burnet-saxifrage root	Pimpinellae rad.	B 1
Calendula flowers	Calendulae flos	G 1, G 2, H 2
Caraway	Carvi fruct.	C 1, C 2
Cascara bark	Rhamni purshiani cort.	F 1
Chamomile	Matricariae flos	C 1, C 4
Chamomile, Roman	Chamomillae romanae flos	C 1, I 1
Cinchona bark	Cinchonae cort.	C 1, C 2
Cinnamon	Cinnamomi cort.	C 1, C 2, H 1
Cocoa shells	Cacao testis	H 1
Coriander seed	Coriandri fruct.	C 1, C 2
Cornflower	Cyani flos	H 2
Dandelion root and leaf	Taraxaci rad. cum herb.	C 1, C 2
Devil's claw	Harpagophyti rad.	C 1, C 2
Early goldenrod	Solidaginis gig. herb.	D 1, D 3
Elder flowers	Sambuci flos	B 3
Eucalyptus leaf	Eucalypti fol.	B 1
European aspen bark	Populi cort.	I 3
European aspen leaf	Populi fol.	I 3
Fennelseed	Foeniculi fruct.	C 1
Fumitory	Fumariae herb.	C 3
Gentian	Gentianae rad.	C 1, C 2
Ginger	Zingiberis rhizoma	C 1, C 2, C 5
Goldenrod	Virgaureae herb.	D 1, D 3
Hawthorn leaf and flowers	Crataegi fol. cum flore	A 3
Hibiscus flowers	Hibisci flos	H 1, H 2
Hops	Lupuli strob.	A 1, A 2
Horsetail	Equiseti herb.	D 1, D 3
Iceland moss	Cetrariae lichen	B 2, C 2
Immortelle flowers	Stoechados flos	H 2
Juniper berries	Juniperi fruct.	C 1, C 2
Kidney bean pods	Phaseoli pericarpium	D 1, D 3
Knotgrass	Polygoni avicularis herb.	B 1, B 2, G 1
Lady's-mantle	Alchemillae herb.	E 1
Lavender flowers	Lavendulae flos	A 1, A 2, C 1
Lemon balm	Melissae fol.	A 2, C 1, C 2
Lesser centaury	Centaurii herb.	C 1, C 2

Table 1.4. Continued.

Crude herbal drug	Latin name	Indications (keyed to Table 1.3)
Licorice	Liquiritiae rad.	B 2, H 1
Linden flowers	Tiliae flos	B 2, B 3
Linseed	Lini sem.	C 4, F 1
Lovage root	Levistici rad.	D 1, D 3
Mallow flowers	Malvae flos	B 2, H 2
Mallow leaf	Malvae fol.	B 2
Marshmallow leaf	Althaeae fol.	B 2
Marshmallow root	Althaeae rad.	B 2, C 4
Maté	Mate folium	I 2
Meadowsweet flowers	Spiraeae flos	B 3
Milk thistle fruit	Cardui mariae fruct.	C 1, C 2
Mullein flowers	Verbasci flos	B 1, B 2
Nettle leaf	Urticae herba	D 1
Oak bark	Quercus cort.	E 1, G 1
Orange blossoms	Aurantii flos	A 2, H 1
Orange flowers	Aurantii flos	A 1, H 1
Orthosiphon leaf	Orthosiphonis fol.	D 1
Passion flower	Passiflorae herb.	A 1
Peppermint	Menthae pip. fol.	C 1, C 3
Plantain	Plantaginis lanceol. herb.	B 1, G 1
Primula flowers	Primulae flos	B 1
Primula root	Primulae rad.	B 1
Psyllium seed	Psyllii sem.	F 2
Raspberry leaf	Rubi idaei fol.	H 1
Restharrow root	Ononidis rad.	D 1, D 3
Rhubarb	Rhei rad.	F 1
Rose hips	Rosae pseudofructus cum fructibus	H 1
Rosemary	Rosmarini fol.	C 1
Sage	Salviae fol.	C 1, G 1, G 2
Senega snakeroot	Senegae rad.	B 1
Senna leaves	Sennae fol.	F 1
Senna pods	Sennae fruct.	F 1
Shepherd's purse	Bursae pastoris herb.	I 1
Silverweed	Anserinae herb.	E 1, G 1
Sloe berries	Pruni spinosae fruct.	G 1
Sloe blossoms	Pruni spinosae flos	H 2
St. John's wort	Hyperici herb.	A 1
Thyme	Thymi herb.	B 2
Tormentil rhizome	Tormentilliae rhizoma	E 1, G 1
Triticum rhizome	Graminis rhiz.	D 1
Turmeric	Curcumae longae rhiz.	C 1, C 2
Valerian	Valerianae rad.	A 1, A 2
Violet rhizome	Violae rhizoma	B 1, B 2
White deadnettle	Lamii albi herb.	B 1, G 1
White deadnettle flowers	Lamii albi flos	B 1
Wild thyme	Serpylli herb.	B 1
Willow bark	Salicis cort.	B 4
Witch hazel bark	Hamamelidis cort.	E 1
Witch hazel leaf	Hamamelidis fol.	G 1
Wormwood	Absinthii herb.	A 1, A 2, A 3
Yarrow	Millefolii herb.	C 1, C 2

The regimen that surrounds the use of a medicinal tea can positively influence the patient's subjective experience of his or her situation. The process of preparing the infusion and sipping the tea at intervals throughout the day can become a kind of relaxation exercise. A tea infusion differs from a solid dosage form of the same composition in that its sensory effects – smell, taste, and pleasant warming sensation behind the sternum – are fully appreciated. Thus, medicinal teas continue to be an effective, recommended therapy as long as they are made from herbs that are free of toxicologic risk.

1.6.3
Various Forms of Medicinal Teas

Three kinds of tea are distinguished according to their external form:

- blended teas (species),
- tea-bag teas,
- soluble teas.

All three forms are commercially produced and sold as ready-to-use products. Coarse-cut teas and tea-bag teas (filter bags) can also be made and stored in pharmacies. Most of these teas are prepared according to the specifications stated in pharmacopeias or other legal standards. Finally, the pharmacist can compound teas as prescribed by a physician, generally preparing the tea as a mixture of cut herbs.

1.6.3.1
Mixtures of Cut and Dried Herbs
Until a few decades ago, this was the only type of tea that was widely available. An example is the "sedative tea" listed in the German Pharmacopeia, 6th ed. It is prepared from:

- coarsely cut bogbean   4 parts
- coarsely cut peppermint   3 parts
- coarsely cut valerian   3 parts.

One advantage of such products is that the user can check the quality of the mixture by inspecting it for pest infestation, a high content of powdered herb (tea dust), etc.

Tea mixtures composed of various herbs should be shaken vigorously or stirred with a spoon before use. This ensures that small, light components that have settled during storage will not distort the ratio of the ingredients.

1.6.3.2
Tea-bag Teas
Real tea (Camellia sinensis) was the first tea to be packaged in filter bags, and 80 % of it is currently sold in this form (Katalyse Environmental Group, 1981). Tea bags are advantageous in that they simplify dosing and are convenient to use. Their disadvantages relate to the finely chopped condition of the herbal material. This provides a large surface area that is accessible to air, promoting oxidative changes and the evaporation of aromatics and volatile oils. Another disadvantage is that the quality of a powdered

herb is more difficult to assess by simple inspection. For example, chamomile flowers may contain excessive amounts of stem pieces (Schilcher, 1982; Bauer et al. 1989).

1.6.3.3
Soluble Teas

Powdered and instant teas are not teas in the strict sense. They consist of particles of a carrier substance such as lactose or maltodextrin that have been coated with a dry herbal extract. The quality of these products is variable. The filler content ranges from 50% to 92%, so the actual content of herbal extract is only 8–50%. Sucrose is the vehicle used in most instant teas, and the product may contain up to 97% sugar – a fact that should be noted by diabetics.

1.6.4
Standard Approval for Tea Mixtures

Tea mixtures that are prepared in quantity and stored in pharmaceutical laboratories, public pharmacies, and hospital pharmacies are exempt from individual approval according to the German Drug Law, as long as the tea formula is in compliance with official standards. These formulas are constantly modified as new discoveries are made and new knowledge is gained. The physician who prescribes standard teas can be certain that the herbs prescribed do not pose a toxicologic risk.

1.6.5
Teas Compounded as Prescribed by a Physician

Common abbreviations: cort. (cortex, bark); fol. (folium or folia, leaf or leaves); frct. (fructus, fruits); pericarp. (pericarpium, peel); rad. (radix, root); rhiz. (rhizome); sem. (semen or semina, seed); stip. (stipes or stipites, stem); summ. (summitates, branch tips); tub. (tuber or tubera).

Historically, the prescription written by a physician consists of six parts (Bader et al., 1985).

1. The **heading** contains the name and academic degree of the prescriber, the prescriber's address, telephone number and professional title (e. g., general practitioner), and the date on which the prescription is written.

2. The **superscription**, written Rx, is the symbol for the Latin word *recipe* (take) and directs the pharmacist to prepare the medication.

3. The **prescription** (or **inscription**) lists the ingredients and states their individual quantities relatively (in parts) or absolutely (in grams). Usually the total quantity of the prescription is 100 g. The various ingredients of the prescription have different functions and may consist of four distinct parts.

- The **base**, or chief active ingredient, such as a bitter herb in an appetite-stimulating stomach tea.
- The **adjuvant**, or supportive medicine, that acts in the same manner as the base, such as an aromatic bitter in a stomach tea.

- The **corrective**, or substance added to improve odor, flavor, or appearance. For example, calendula flowers, hibiscus flowers, or life everlasting flowers may be added as correctives to carminative teas (Pahlow, 1985).
- The **vehicle** or excipient, such as stabilizing or filling herbs that are added to a tea mixture to give it a suitable form or consistency. Stabilizing herbs keep the tea mixture homogeneous and, with lengthy storage, ensure that the lower third of the package has the same composition as the upper third. For example, hairy leaves can be added to help stabilize plants parts that have a smooth surface. Stabilizing herbs should be pharmacologically and toxicologically inert; an example is raspberry leaves. Coltsfoot leaves were once a popular stabilizing agent but are no longer used today due to their content of pyrrolizidine alkaloids.

4. The **subscription** directs the pharmacist to prepare and dispense the drug in a form suitable for use by the patient. For example, the direction "m.f.spec." stands for "*misce fiat species*," or "mix to yield a tea."

5. The **transcription** gives the necessary directions to the patient. "Take as directed" is satisfactory in most cases. The transcription may indicate when and how many times a day the tea should be consumed (see p.32). If necessary, the physician or pharmacist should also give oral instructions on how the tea is to be prepared (see Sect.1.6.6).

6. The **signature** appears at the bottom of the prescription blank and should be handwritten by the prescribing physician.

Formulas for Tea Mixtures
Tea formulas may be found in textbooks of phytotherapy (e.g., Weiss, 1982), books on medicinal plants (e.g., Braun and Frohne, 1987; Lindemann, 1979; Pahlow, 1979), and handbooks (e.g., Wurm, 1990). The standard approval criteria for medicinal teas (Braun, 1987) provide a reliable information source in Germany, listing tea mixtures that have a prescribed qualitative composition but a variable quantitative composition. The following guidelines are imposed:

- The quantitative composition of the active ingredients can be freely selected within certain ranges;
- free qualitative and quantitative selections can be made from a corresponding list of "other ingredients," as long as the content of these ingredients does not exceed 30% of the tea by weight;
- no single "other ingredient" may exceed 5 percent of the tea mixture by weight.

The standard approval criteria refer to herbs by their common names as listed in Table 1.4. The standard tea mixture designated "cough and bronchial tea I" illustrates how the standard criteria can be used to formulate an individual prescription.

- Active ingredients in percentages by weight: fennel seeds 10.0–25.0, English plantain 25.0–40.0, licorice root 25.0–35.0, thyme 10.0–40.0.
- Other ingredients: marshmallow leaves, rose-hip pulp, Iceland moss, cornflower blossoms, lungwort leaves, mallow leaves, cowslip flowers, pansy.

- *Step 1*

  Choose a composition that is within the ranges specified in the standard monograph, e.g.

  Active ingredients

Fennel seed	10.0 g
English plantain	40.0 g
Licorice root	25.0 g
Thyme	10.0 g

  Other ingredients

Mallow flowers	5.0 g
Wild thyme	5.0 g

- *Step 2*

  If necessary, latinize the common names, using the synonym list in Table 1.4:

Foeniculi fruct.	10.0 g
Plantaginis lanceolatae herb.	40.0 g
Liquiritiae rad.	25.0 g
Thymi herb.	10.0 g
Malvae flos	5.0 g
Serpylli herb.	5.0 g

- *Step 3*

  List the ingredients on the prescription blank in quantitative order (if desired) and state the directions for the patient:

Rx	Date
English plantain	40.0 g
Licorice root	25.0 g
Fennel seed	10.0 g
Thyme	10.0 g
Mallow flowers	5.0 g
Wild thyme	5.0 g
Pectoral tea for Mrs. . . .	
Drink 1 cup in the morning and in the evening.	

Oral instructions from the physician, physician's assistant, or pharmacist

Pour boiling water (150 ml = about 1 large cupful) over 1 tablespoon of tea, cover and steep for about 10 minutes, then pour through a tea strainer. Freshley prepare each cup just before use.

1.6.6
Guidelines for Tea Preparation

There are basically three ways to prepare tea:

- Infusion: Pour boiling water over the amount of herb indicated on the prescription or package (e.g., 1 teaspoon). Cover the vessel, steep for 5–10 minutes, and strain through a sieve.
- Decoction: Cover the designated amount of tea mixture with cold water and bring to a boil. Simmer for 5–10 minutes, then strain.
- Cold maceration: Cover the tea mixture with tap water, let stand for 6–8 hours at room temperature, then strain.

Cold maceration is usually recommended for herbs with a high mucilage content such as marshmallow root, psyllium, linseed, or Iceland moss (cetraria) for fear that heat might reduce the viscosity of the mucilage.

A cold maceration does pose hygienic problems, however. The raw materials for medicinal teas may be heavily contaminated by microorganisms. There are herbs on the market that were harvested and processed under poor hygienic conditions. They harbor large numbers of bacteria such as Escherichia coli, Salmonella spp., Pseudomonas aeruginosa, and Staphylococcus aureus (Hefendehl, 1984). Exposing the herb to boiling water will typically reduce the bacterial count by about 90% (Härtling, 1983; Leimbeck, 1987). In fact, some herbal wholesale firms and suppliers have advised their clients to provide written instructions that consumers always use boiling water when preparing the teas (Wichtl, 1989).

With regard to dosing schedule, the old rule of drinking 1 cup of tea 3 times daily is generally valid (before breakfast, at about 5:00 p.m., and before bedtime), but the following exceptions should be noted.

- Tea used as a laxative or sleep aid should be taken at night.
- Peppermint and chamomile tea for an upset stomach should be taken at the patient's usual meal times or as needed.
- Linden blossom tea and elder flower tea should be consumed hot while the patient is in bed, because much of their diaphoretic effect is based on physical warming. The sensitivity to heat stimuli shows a diurnal pattern; diaphoretic tea has no effect in the morning, but when taken in the afternoon as the body temperature is rising, it promptly induces profuse sweating (Hildebrandt et al., 1954).
- Diuretic tea is taken at breakfast time; 1 liter should be consumed in one sitting if possible.
- Appetite-stimulant teas are taken about 30 min before meals. Note: Liver diseases are often associated with anorexia. Teas for the liver and gallbladder generally contain bitter-tasting herbs, so it may be advisable to take them 30 min before meals as well.

Some authors recommend medicinal teas as an adjunctive therapy in the management of chronic illnesses (Weiss, 1982), with patients drinking 2 or 3 cups daily for a period of 3–4 weeks. Long-term use is not advised due to a lack of experimental studies on the potential long-term toxicity of the herbs used in medicinal teas (see Sect. 1.6.8).

1.6.7
Teas for Infants and Children

A distinction is drawn between teas used for medicinal purposes and teas that are included in the nutritional regimen of infants and children. In practice, there is considerable overlap between the two types; for example, fennel tea can be used medicinally and as a nutritional supplement. A healthy breast-fed or bottle-fed infant normally does not require extra fluids. Potable water may be given as a thirst quencher under hot conditions (summer) or in low-humidity environments (houses with central heating). Fever and diarrhea are exceptional situations. The Nutritional Committee of the German Society of Pediatrics (1988) has published the following recommendation. If tea is given to infants between 10 days and 6 months of age, it should contain no more than 4% carbohydrates, preferably in the form of maltodextrin. Teas for infants over 4 months old who have started teething should not contain carbohydrates. There is no objection to using protein as a vehicle in this age group. Vehicles in the form of hydrolyzed proteins (e.g., from collagen) have a molecular weight less than 5000 D in about 70% of cases, in the range of 5000–10,000 D in 23%, and 10,000–20,000 D in 8%. The glycine content must be less than 25%. If the tea is prepared as directed, using 0.5 g of tea powder per 100 mL of ready-to-drink liquid, there should be a negligible risk of hyperglycinemia (Marfort and Schmidt, 1989). Pediatric teas based on protein hydrolysates should be used only if other foreign proteins are also to be used for infant nutrition, generally after 4 months of age. This is a sound precaution when one considers the high of sensitization to foreign protein during the first months of life.

Instead of instant products, teas can be used in the form of coarsely cut leaves or tea-bag teas. It is always best to use teas from reputable manufacturers whose products are constantly tested for compliance with legally prescribed standards.

Given the past history of popular interest in teas for infants and children, particularly in Germany, remarkably little reliable information is available on the safety and efficacy of these products.

1.6.8
Adverse Effects and Risks

There have been no reports of objectionable side effects for the majority of medicinal teas used in Germany (Table 1.4). Arnica flowers, European mistletoe, and psyllium can trigger allergic reactions. Herbs with a high tannin content such as uva ursi leaves, lady's mantle, and tormentil rhizome can cause stomach discomfort in sensitive individuals, as can herbs with a high content of bitters such as gentian root, dandelion, and wormwood (overacidification of the stomach). The long-term use of anthranoid-containing laxative teas made from buckthorn bark, rhubarb root, senna leaves, or senna pods can lead to electrolyte losses, most notably potassium deficiency. Because the long-term use of laxatives is a form of product abuse, the resulting effects actually constitute a toxic reaction.

Pharmaceutical incompatibilities and pharmacodynamic interactions are important issues due to the common practice of prescribing teas as an adjunct to essential medications. Unfortunately, almost no clinical studies have been done in this area, so we must base our considerations on plausibility. It is conceivable, for example, that tannin-containing teas might delay the absorption of sedatives, hypnotics, antidepressants, and tranquilizers (Ludewig, 1992) and reduce the efficacy of the antidiabetic drug metformin. Tannins would presumably decrease the absorption of products containing iron, calcium, and magnesium.

Proven medicinal teas that have been used in Germany for many years are known to be free of acute toxicity over a large range of doses. Less is known about their possible chronic toxic effects except in the case of herbs that contain pyrrolizidine alkaloids, such as coltsfoot leaves. Pyrrolizidine alkaloids (PA's) are a group of about 200 structurally related compounds that have been found in some 350 plant species including medicinal plants such as Cynoglossum species (hound's tongue), Petasites species (petasite), Tussilago farfara (coltsfoot leaves and flowers), Senecio species (ragwort, liferoot), and Symphytum species (comfrey) (Westendorf, 1992). Toxicity to humans has been particularly well documented for the PA's occurring in Crotolaria species (bush tea). A latent period of weeks or months after exposure is followed by the appearance of nonspecific symptoms such as anorexia, lethargy, and abdominal pain. Further progression is characterized by emaciation, swelling of the abdomen, and liver changes that take the form of acute, subacute, and chronic veno-occlusive lesions. PA's act on the centrilobular hepatocytes of the liver, destroying them in large numbers, and they damage small branches of the hepatic vein, causing endothelial disruption and predisposing to thrombosis.

Coltsfoot leaves contain relatively large amounts of hepatotoxic and hepatocarcinogenic PA's (average concentration 4.3 ppm) and most of these chemicals are released into solution when the tea is prepared (Wiedenfeld et al., 1995). In Austria and other countries, the commercial sale of coltsfoot leaves has been banned since 1994. In Germany, a maximum limit has been imposed that prohibits the consumption of more than 1 µg of pyrrolizidine alkaloids per day (Bundesanzeiger No. III, Vol. 17.6, 1992). Apparently it is assumed that there is a limit for carcinogenic compounds below which the herb can be safely used, but this assumption is controversial. In any case, coltsfoot tea is an expendable commodity that is easily replaced by other mucilaginous herbs such as marshmallow leaves and mallow leaves; hence we would recommend discontinuing any further use of coltsfoot in Germany or elsewhere.

References

Bader H, Gietzen K, Wolf H (eds) (1985) Lehrbuch der Pharmakologie und Toxikologie. 2nd Ed., edition medizin, VCH Verlagsgesellschaft, Weinheim, 87–88.

Bak AAA, Grobbee DE (1989) The effect on serum cholesterol levels of coffee brewed by filtering or boiling. N Engl J Med 321: 142–147.

Bär U (1987) Medikamentöse Therapie des Colon irritabile. In: Hotz J, Rösch W (eds) Funktionelle Störungen des Verdauungstrakts. Springer, Berlin Heidelberg New York, 196–202.

Bauer KH, Frömming KH, Führer C (1989) Pharmazeutische Technologie. 2nd Ed., Thieme Verlag, Stuttgart New York, 450.

Bock KD (ed) (1993) Wissenschaftliche und alternative Medizin. Springer Verlag, Berlin Heidelberg: 43–47.

Braun R (ed) (1987) Standardzulassungen für Fertigarzneimittel. Text und Kommentar. Deutscher Apotheker Verlag, Stuttgart, and Govi-Verlag, Frankfurt am Main.

Braun H, Frohne D (1987) Heilpflanzenlexikon für Ärzte und Apotheker, 5th Ed. Fischer Verlag, Stuttgart.

Burkard G, Lehrl S (1991) Verhältnis von Demenzen vom Multiinfarkt- und vom Alzheimertyp in ärztlichen Praxen. Münch Med Wschr 133 (Suppl 1): 38–43.

Burrow A, Eccles R, Jones AS (1983) The effect of camphor, eucalyptus and menthol vapour on nasal resistance to airflow and nasal sensation. Acta Otolaryngol (Stockholm) 96: 157–161.

Cody V, Middleton R jr., Harborne JB (eds) (1986) Plant flavonoids in biology and medicine. Biochemical, pharmacological and structure-activity relationships. Alan R. Liss Inc. New York.

Eccles R, Lancashire B, Tolley NS (1987b) Experimental studies on nasal sensation of airflow. Acta Otolaryngol (Stockholm) 103: 303–306.

Eccles R, Lancashire B, Tolley NS (1987a) The effects of aromatics on inspiratory and expiratory nasal resistance to airflow. Otolaryngol 12: 11–14.

Ernährungskommission der Deutschen Gesellschaft für Kinderheilkunde (1988) Der Kinderarzt 3: 368.

Feiden K (ed) (Iggo, Supplement 6, 1995) Arzneimittelprüfrichtlinien. Wissenschaftliche Verlagsgesellschaft mbH Stuttgart.

Forth W (1984) Grenzen der rationalen Beurteilung von Arzneistoffen. In: Kleinsorge H, Zöckler CE (eds) Fortschritt in der Medizin – Versuchung oder Herausforderung? TM-Verlag Hameln: 69–80.

Fox N (1977) Effect of camphor, eucalyptol and menthol on the vascular state of the mucous membrane. Arch Otolaryngol 6: 112–122.

Gabor M (1975) Abriß der Pharmakologie von Flavonoiden unter besonderer Berücksichtigung der antiödematösen und antiphlogistischen Effekte. Akademiai Kiado, Budapest.

Gaedcke F (1991) Phytopharmaka. Definition und Erläuterung wichtiger Begriffe zur Beurteilung ihrer Herstellung und Qualität. Dtsch Apoth Z 131: 2551–2555.

Haas H (1956) Spiegel der Arznei. Ursprung, Geschichte und Idee der Heilmittelkunde. Springer, Berlin Göttingen Heidelberg, p 176.

Hänsel R, Trunzler G (1989) Wissenswertes über Phytopharmaka. Taschenbuch Medizin. G. Braun Verlag, Karlsruhe.

Harnack GA (1980) Kinderheilkunde. Springer Verlag, Berlin Heidelberg New York.

Härtling C (1983) Beitrag zur Frage des mikrobiellen Zustandes pflanzlicher Drogen. Fakten und Folgerungen. Pharm Z 132: 643–644.

Havsteen B (1983) Flavonoids, a class of natural products of high pharmacological potency. Biochem Pharmacol 32: 1141–1148.

Hefendehl FW (1984) Anforderungen an die Qualität pflanzlicher Arzneimittel. In: Eberwein B, Helmstaedter G, Reimann J et al. (eds) Pharmazeutische Qualität von Phytopharmaka. Deutscher Apotheker Verlag, Stuttgart, pp 25–34.

Hildebrandt G, Engelbertz P, Hildebrandt-Evers G (1954) Physiologische Grundlagen für eine tageszeitliche Ordnung der Schwitzprozeduren. Z Klin Med 152: 446–468.

Hiller K (1995) Pharmazeutische Bewertung ausgewählter Teedrogen. Dtsch Apoth Z 135: 1425–1440.

IfD survey 6039 (1997) Institut für Demoskopie, Allensbach/Germany, Allensbacher Archiv.

Immich H (1988) Klinische Studien kritisch bewertet. Vortragsreferat von B. M. Ganzer. Pharm Z 46: 22–23.

Jüttner G (1983) Therapeutische Konzepte und soziales Anliegen in der frühen Kräuterheilkunde. In: Imhof AE (ed) Der Mensch und sein Körper. Beck, Munich, pp 118–130.

Keller K (1996) Herbal medicinal products in Germany and Europe: experiences with national and European assessment. Drug Inform J 30: 933–948.

Leimbeck R (1987) Teedrogen: Wie steht es mit der mikrobiologischen Qualität? Dtsch Apoth Z 127: 1221–1224.

Lindemann G (1979) Teerezepte. Verlag Tibor Marczell, Munich.

Linden M, Osterheider M, Schaaf B, Fleckenstein G, Weber Hl (1992) Fluoxetin in der Anwendung durch niedergelassene Nervenärzte. Münch Med Wschr 134: 836–840.

Ludewig R (1992) Tee als Genuß-, Vorbeugungs- und Heilmittel. Ein alltägliches Beispiel für die schulmedizinisch begründete Phytotherapie. Natur- und Ganzheitsmedizin 5: 185–192.

Ludewig R (1989) Schulmedizin und Naturmedizin im Meinungsstreit um Arzneimittel. Plädoyer für einen Modus vivendi. Natur- und Ganzheitsmedizin 2: 40–47.

Mader FH, Weißgerber H (eds) (1993) Allgemeinmedizin und Praxis. Springer Verlag, Berlin Heidelberg.

Merfort I, Schmidt E (1989) Säuglings- und Kindertees. Pharmakologie und Anwendung. In: Schmidt E, Schöch G (Hrsg) Die Ernährung des Säuglings und Kindes. Marseille Verlag, München, S 153–164.

Naumann HH (1967) Die Reaktion der Nasenschleimhaut auf verschiedene Medikamente. In: Döst FH, Leiber B (eds) Menthol and Menthol-Containing External Remedies. Thieme Verlag, Stuttgart.

Pahlow M (1979) Das große Buch der Heilpflanzen. Gräfe und Unzer, Munich.
Pahlow M (1985) Heilpflanzen in der Apotheke. Informationen und Tips aus der Praxis. Dtsch Apoth Z 125: 2663–2664.
Saller R, Feiereis H (eds) (1993) Erweiterte Schulmedizin. Vol. 1: Beiträge zur Phytotherapie. Hans Marseille Verlag, Munich, pp 25–26.
Schilcher H (1982) Gesund durch Kräuter-Tees. Möglichkeiten und Probleme der Arzneikräuter-Tee-zubereitungen. Apotheker-Journal, Heh 7: 36–39.
Schwabe U, Paffrath D (eds) (1995) Arzneiverordnungs-Report `95. Gustav Fischer Verlag, Stuttgart Jena.
Weiss RF (1991) Lehrbuch der Phytotherapie, 7th Ed., Hippokrates, Stuttgart.
Westendorf J (1992) Pyrrolizidine alkaloids – general discussion. In: De Smet PAGM, Keller K, Hänsel R, Chandler RF (eds) Adverse Effects of Herbal Drugs. Vol. 1, Springer Verlag, Berlin Heidelberg New York, pp 193–214.
Wichtl M (ed) (1989) Teedrogen. 2nd Ed. Wissenschaftliche Verlagsgesellschaft, Stuttgart, pp 10, 26.
Wiedenfeld H, Lebada R, Kopp B (1995) Pyrrolizidinalkaloide im Huflattich. Dtsch Apoth Z 135: 1037–1046.
Withering W (1937) An Account of the Foxglove and Some of Its Medicinal Uses, with Practical Remarks on Dropsy and other Diseases. C.G.J. & J.Robinson, London, 1785. Reprinted in Med Class 2: 305–443.
Woelk H, Burkard G, Grünwald J (1994) Benefits and Risks of the Hypericum Extract LI 160: Drug Monitoring Study with 3250 Patients. J Geriatr Psychiatry Neurol 7 (Suppl 1): S 34–38.

2 Central Nervous System

The plant kingdom is replete with compounds and mixtures of compounds that have a stimulating or calmative effect on the central nervous system (CNS). In cases where this action is due to a single high-potency compound that can be chemically isolated, such as morphine, cocaine, or atropine, the plant and its preparations are considered to be outside the realm of phytotherapy (see Sect. 1.2). Herbs that contain caffeine are discussed in Sect. 3.2.1.1. Most other herbs affecting the CNS fall under the broad heading of plant sedatives. However, recent controlled therapeutic studies have identified fairly specific indications for three of the psychotropic plant drugs. Thus, ginkgo biloba extract is considered a nootropic agent that is effective in the symptomatic treatment of cognitive deficits (Hartmann and Schulz, 1991). Extracts from St. John's wort have proven highly effective in the treatment of depression (Harrer, Payk, and Schulz, 1993), and extracts from the kava root (*Piper methysticum* rhizome) have shown efficacy as anxiolytic drugs (Volz and Hänsel, 1994).

Except for ginkgo and kava, the findings on psychotropic plant drugs were compiled by Commission E in 1984 and 1985. Based on information available at that time, the Commission cited similar indications for the majority of these herbs, mentioning the symptom of unrest in nearly all its monographs. Consequently, the indications stated for St. John's wort in Table 2.1 are somewhat outdated. None of the 28 controlled studies conducted since 1984 have confirmed sedative effects useful in treating nervous unrest from alcoholic extracts of St. John's wort, but this therapy

Table 2.1. Indications for herbal remedies with psychotropic actions based on the monographs of Commission E, with the year of publication in the *Bundesanzeiger*.

Herb	Year	Indications
Hops	1984	Mood disorders such as anxiety and restlessness, sleep disturbances
Kava	1990	Nervous anxiety, tension and restlessness
Lavender	1984	Mood disorders such as restlessness, insomnia, functional upper abdominal complaints
Lemon balm	1984	Nervous insomnia, functional gastrointestinal complaints
Passion Flower	1985	Nervous unrest, mild sleeplessness, nervous gastrointestinal complaints
St. John's wort	1984	Psychoautonomic disturbances, depression, anxiety, and/or nervous unrest
Valerian	1985	Restlessness, nervous insomnia

has proven effective for various depressive mood disorders including moderate and severe depression. Commission E published its monographs on ginkgo extracts in the summer of 1994; the therapeutic indications are reviewed below.

2.1
Ginkgo in the Treatment of Cognitive Deficiency

2.1.1
Introduction

The first green growth to appear at the center of Hiroshima in 1946 was the sprout of a ginkgo tree. Like all other flora and fauna in the city, the ginkgo tree originally there was incinerated when the atomic bomb was dropped on August 6, 1945. The new plant showed all the usual traits of its species and grew into a normal, full-size tree.

Extreme hardiness seems to be a characteristic of ginkgo trees, which have lived on earth for approximately 300 million years. They are as resistant to harmful insects and microorganisms as they are to the environmental toxins of modern civilization. They are commonly planted as ornamental trees along the heavily trafficked streets of major cities like Tokyo and New York. Their genetic resistance to mutagenic influences may relate to the ability of some ginkgo constituents to act as free-radical scavengers. This, in turn, may have bearing on the pharmacologic and therapeutic properties of ginkgo extracts.

The ginkgo tree died out in Europe during the Ice Age. The German physician and botanist Engelbert Kaempfer first described the tree in his book Amoenitatum Exoticarum in 1712 following a visit to Japan. The first European ginkgo tree was planted in Utrecht, Holland, in 1730, and by 1800 the gingko had become naturalized throughout Europe. The oldest ginkgo tree in Germany (about 200 years) is believed to stand on the grounds of Wilhelmshöhe Castle near the town of Kassel. Goethe wrote a poem about the bilobed ginkgo leaf in 1815 after walking the grounds of Heidelberg Castle, and he had several ginkgo trees planted near his summerhouse in Weimar.

Ginkgo biloba has no tradition as a medicinal plant in Germany. Therapeutic uses of the ginkgo seed have been described in China and other parts of eastern Asia for 2000 years. Present-day Chinese medicine uses extracts from ginkgo leaves in wound dressings. The vasoactive properties of ginkgo principles may play a role in this application. A major traditional Chinese use of ginkgo is in the treatment of bronchial asthma, presumably owing to its PAF-inhibiting properties (Schmid and Schmoll, 1994).

2.1.2
Botanical Description

Ginkgo biloba (Fig. 2.1) is a dioecious plant, with male and female flowers occurring on different trees. The trees do not blossom until they are 20–30 years old. Young trees are narrow and pear-shaped, later developing a broad crown and eventually

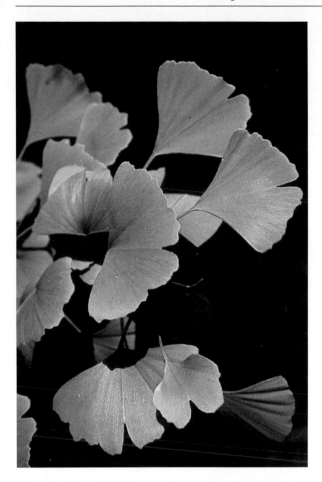

Fig. 2.1.
Branch of *Ginkgo biloba*.

reaching a height of up to 40 m. Ginkgo trees more than 1000 years old and measuring 10–20 m in circumference have been described in China, Korea, and Japan.

The last surviving member of the Ginkgoaceae family, *Ginkgo biloba* is unrelated to any other plant species alive today. The foliage of the ginkgo tree more closely resembles that of certain ferns than that of deciduous trees, its fan-shaped leaves lacking the central rib and cross venation seen in broad-leaf trees.

2.1.3
Crude Drug and Extract

The dried green leaves of the ginkgo tree provide the crude drug from which ginkgo extracts are obtained. Leaves may be gathered from cultivated trees or from the wild. Most of the bulk herb comes from China, Japan, North and South Korea, and from plantations in Europe (southern France) and North America. The content of flavonoid glycosides is highest in fresh ginkgo leaves that are harvested in May shortly after the appearance of new foliage, while the leaves are still a pure green color (Sticher, 1993). The leaves may be gathered by climbing and picking, or they may be stripped from branches that have been cut from the tree. On plantations, leaves are machine-harvested from trees that are pruned to the size and shape of large shrubs. When dried, the leaves lose about three-fourths of their fresh weight. The dried leaves are compacted into large bales to help keep them dry and prevent moisture-related fermentation.

Ginkgo extracts are produced in standard fashion by extracting the milled leaves with polar solvents. These primary extracts, which have about a 4:1 ratio of crude herb to extract, and the dried leaves themselves are no longer marketed in Germany. The monograph published by Commission E in August of 1994 (Bundesanzeiger No. 133) states that the only acceptable extracts are those with an herb-to-extract ratio in the range of 35:1 to 67:1 (average: 50:1) that have been extracted with an acetone-water mixture and then further purified without adding concentrates or isolated constituents. This standardized process eliminates unwanted components, including those that make the product less stable or pose an excessive toxicologic risk – fats, waxes, tannins, proanthocyanidins, biflavonoids, ginkgol, ginkgolic acids, proteins, and mineral components. The extracts suitable for use in drug manufacture are designated in the technical literature as EGb 761 and LI 1370.

2.1.4
Key Constituents, Analysis, Pharmacokinetics

The monograph published by Commission E lists the following characteristics of medicinal ginkgo extracts: 22–27% flavonoid glycosides, determined by high-performance liquid chromatography as quercetin, kaempferol, and isorhamnetin and calculated as acylflavonoids with the molecular weight $M_r = 756.7$ (quercetin glycosides) and $M_r = 740.7$ (kaempferol glycosides); 5–7% terpene lactones, consisting of about 2.8–3.4% ginkgolides A, B, and C and 2.6–3.2% bilobalide; and less than 5 ppm ginkgolic acids. Analytic and production-related variations are included in the ranges indicated.

Other chemicals present in the extracts include hydroxykynurenic acid, shikimic acid, protocatechuic acid, vanillic acid, and p-hydroxybenzoic acid.

For quantitative analysis, the key constituents are separated from the extract by high-performance liquid chromatography. Additionally, gas chromatographic techniques are used for analysis of the ginkgolides and bilobalide. The flavonoid glycosides are hydrolyzed with methanol and hydrochloric acid prior to chromatographic separation. Safe upper limits have been established for the concentration of ginkgolic acids, which are considered toxic and allergenic.

The pharmacokinetics of ginkgo extracts have been studied in experimental animals and in humans. Experiments with the radiolabeled extract EGb 761 in rats showed a 60% absorption rate. Human studies with EGb 761 indicated an absolute bioavailability of 98–100% for ginkgolide A, 79–93% for ginkgolide B, and at least 70% for bilobalide. In studies with the extract LI 1370, the plasma flavonoid levels in healthy subjects showed a dose-dependent rise after the ingestion of 50 mg, 100 mg, and 300 mg and were maximal at 2–3 hours (Nieder, 1991).

2.1.5
Pharmacology and Toxicology

Some 50 original papers have been published on the pharmacologic actions of ginkgo extracts (surveys in: Oberpichler and Krieglstein, 1992; Hänsel et al., 1993; Rupalla et al., 1995). Most of the studies were performed with the extract EGb 761. The 1994 Commission E monograph summarizes the experimentally documented pharmacologic actions of EGb 761 as follows:

- increases tolerance to hypoxia, especially in brain tissue;
- inhibits the development of post-traumatic or toxin-induced brain edema and hastens its resolution;
- reduces retinal edema and retinal lesions;
- inhibits the age-related decline of muscarinic choline receptors and α_2-adrenergic receptors; promotes choline uptake in the hippocampus;
- improves memory and learning capacity and aids in the compensation of disturbed equilibrium, acting particularly at the level of the microcirculation;
- improves the rheologic properties of the blood;
- scavenges toxic oxygen-derived free radicals;
- inhibits platelet activating factor (PAF) and exerts a neuroprotective effect.

As with other phytomedicines, all the constituents of ginkgo extracts are assumed to contribute in their totality to the therapeutic effect. But some pharmacologic actions can be related to specific groups of compounds. For example, the ginkgo flavonoids (mostly rutin derivatives) are the most efficient free-radical scavengers. We know from experimental studies in animals and humans that rutin raises the threshold for the seepage of blood from capillary vessels, an effect generally described as decreased capillary fragility.

The ginkgolides inhibit platelet activating factor (PAF). A bioregulator synthesized in mammalian cell membranes in response to various stimuli, PAF mediates various physiologic responses and, when excessive, can initiate pathophysiologic processes. It induces platelet aggregation in the blood and functions as a key mediator in allergic inflammatory processes. PAF receptors have been detected in various tissues including the brain. PAF-induced platelet aggregation is known to occur in zones of incomplete ischemia, e.g., at the periphery of an infarcted area. The ginkgolides and bilobalide, whose chemical structures are unique in nature, have also demonstrated characteristic neuroprotective properties in various pharmacologic models (Braquet, 1988, 1989; Krieglstein et al., 1995).

The toxicity of therapeutically applied ginkgo extracts is very low. Tests in mice showed an LD_{50} of 7725 mg/kg on oral administration and 1100 mg/kg on intravenous administration. An acute LD_{50} could not be determined in rats. Tests for mutagenic, carcinogenic, and genotoxic effects were negative (Hänsel et al., 1993).

2.1.6
Clinical Efficacy in Patients with Cognitive Deficiency

The symptomatic treatment of cognitive deficits due to organic brain disease is considered the primary indication for ginkgo extracts. There is no single definition for the term cognitive deficits. In medical parlance it has been largely synonymous with cerebral insufficiency, an older term reflecting the etiologic hypothesis that stenotic vascular changes with aging cause a progressive decrease in cerebral blood flow, leading to a decline in mental and physical functioning. The clinical manifestations include impairment of memory and other cognitive functions, affective symptoms such as anxiety and depression, and physical complaints such as tinnitus, vertigo, and headache (Fig. 2.2). The older etiologic concept of cerebrovascular insufficiency has been largely abandoned since it was shown that neuronal degeneration like that occurring in Alzheimer's disease is a more frequent cause of impaired mental functioning in elderly patients (Blaha, 1989; German Federal Health Agency, 1991; Kurz, 1995).

The clinical features of these central nervous system disorders correspond to the syndrome of dementia. Both the broadened classification of mental disorders in the DSM-IV (American Psychiatric Association, 1995) and the 10th revision of the international disease classification of the WHO (ICD 10, German Institute for Medical Documentation and Information, 1994) define dementia as a pattern of disturbance in which several higher mental functions are simultaneously affected. The cardinal symptoms are impairment of memory, abstract thinking, and psychomotor func-

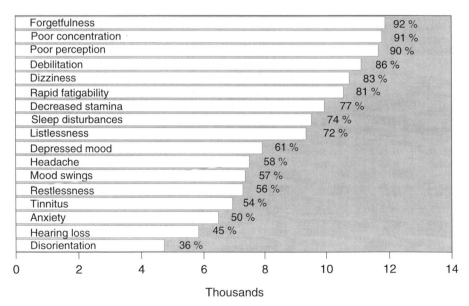

Fig. 2.2. Frequency distribution of typical symptoms in 13,565 patients diagnosed with dementia (multi-infarct dementia, Alzheimer's dementia, mixed type). Results based on a survey of 1357 private physicians (Burkard and Lehrl, 1991).

tions such as speech. Changes in mood, social functioning, and personality may also be present.

Based on its pharmacologic actions and clinical effects, ginkgo extract is closely related to the class of nootropic drugs, i.e., agents that act on the central nervous system and tend to improve cognitive performance. A definite mechanism of action has not yet been established for nootropic drugs. It is generally thought that nootropic drugs act by their ability to stimulate populations of nerve cells that are still functional (stabilization of adapter capacity) or protect them from pathologic influences (neuroprotective effects). Our understanding of the mechanism of action of nootropic drugs is based largely on studies in experimental animals since it is rarely possible to conduct this type of biochemical and pharmacodynamic research in human subjects (Kanowski, 1991; Oberpichler and Krieglstein, 1992; Itil et al., 1996).

The therapeutic efficacy of nootropic drugs can be meaningfully tested only in human subjects, the best subjects being patients with dementia. By the late 1980's, no definite guidelines had yet been established for testing drugs that improve cognitive functions. At the same time, most of the 36 controlled clinical studies on the use of ginkgo special extracts in patients with cognitive deficits (Table 2.2) were conducted in the 1980's (surveys in: Kleijnen and Knipschild, 1992a, b; Hopfenmüller, 1994; Volz and Hänsel, 1994). The criteria used to assess efficacy in these studies were improvements in typical symptoms and complaints (Figs. 2.3 and 2.4) and improved performance in psychometric tests (Fig. 2.5).

In 1991 the German Federal Health Agency established new criteria for testing the efficacy of nootropic drugs (German Federal Health Agency, 1991). Besides the primary goal of improving dementia symptoms or delaying their progression, the new guidelines required that nootropic therapy also improve functioning in daily activities and reduce the patient's care needs. The guidelines limited clinical testing to patients with primary degenerative dementias of the Alzheimer type, vascular dementias, and mixed forms of both; they also required that efficacy be demonstrated on three mutually independent levels of observation (Fig. 2.6).

Measured by the new criteria, few of the studies listed in Table 2.2 would meet minimum requirements from a methodologic standpoint, and none could provide statistical evidence rigorous enough to confirm efficacy. This accounts for the extremely negative attitude of clinical pharmacologists in particular toward the use of ginkgo products. Meanwhile, tens of thousands of practicing physicians have had positive experience with ginkgo therapy over the past 30 years. These physicians have seen marked improvements in their patients' symptoms and complaints, comparable to the highly statistically significant benefits demonstrated by most of the double-blind studies listed in Table 2.2.

Evaluating all these empirical findings and study results against the new, rigorous test criteria ignores the fact that, for patients and their families, the improvement in daily symptoms and complaints is as important as the issue of care needs. Moreover, the requirement that efficacy be proven simultaneously in psychopathologic findings (physician-observed clinical symptoms), psychometric testing (by an independent psychologist), and social functioning (ability to cope with daily activities as assessed by family members and caregivers) poses serious practical difficulties. Valid psychometric testing can be performed only in patients with a Mini-Mental State Examination (MMSE) score of at least 18 (scores in the range of 15–22 are defined as "mild

Table 2.2. The results of 36 controlled clinical studies in dementia patients. The extract EGb 761 was used in 25 of these studies, the extract LI 1370 in 11. A total of 2326 patients were included in the studies. The dose generally ranged from 120 to 160 mg/day, and treatment was generally continued for 8–12 weeks (reviews and original quotes from the studies may be found in Kleijnen and Knipschild, 1992; Volz and Hänsel, 1994; Hopfenmüller, 1994; and Kanowski, 1996).

Year	First Author	Study Design	Cases	mg/d	Weeks	Extract
1975	Moreau	PDB	60	120	12	EGb 761
1976	Augustin	PDB	168	120	24	EGb 761
1977	Israel	POS	48	240	8	EGb 761
1978	Leroy	VDB	60	120	8	EGb 761
1981	Dieli	PDB	40	120	8	EGb 761
1982	Eckmann	PDB	50	120	4	EGb 761
1982	Haan	VOS	60	87,5	2	EGb 761
1982	Krauskopf	VDB	20	120	8	EGb 761
1983	Pidoux	PDB	12	160	12	EGb 761
1985	Geßner	VDB	60	120	12	EGb 761
1986	Hindmarch	PDB	8	120–160 single dose		EGb 761
1986	Arrigo	PDB	80	120	6	EGb 761
1986	Weitbrecht	PDB	40	120	12	EGb 761
1987	Israel	PDB	80	160	12	EGb 761
1987	Wesnes	PDB	54	120	12	EGb 761
1988	Halama	PDB	40	120	12	EGb 761
1989	Hofferberth	PDB	36	120	8	EGb 761
1989	Vorberg	PDB	100	112	12	LI 1370
1990	Eckmann	PDB	58	160	6	LI 1370
1990	Gerhardt	VDB	80	120	6	EGb 761
1990	Schulz	PDB	77	150	12	LI 1370
1990	Rabinovici	PDB	99	150	12	LI 1370
1991	Brüchert	PDB	209	150	12	LI 1370
1991	Schmidt	PDB	99	150	12	LI 1370
1991	Halama	PDB	50	150	12	LI 1370
1991	Hartmann	PDB	45	150	12	LI 1370
1991	Hofferberth	PDB	50	150	6	LI 1370
1991	Maier-Hauff	PDB	50	150	6	LI 1370
1991	Rai	PDB	27	120	24	EGb 761
1992	Gräßel	PDB	72	160	24	EGb 761
1992	Hörr	PDB	40	200	4	EGb 761
1992	Ihl	PDB	20	240	12	EGb 761
1992	Hofferberth	PDB	40	240	12	EGb 761
1992	Michaelis	PDB	52	120	8	EGb 761
1994	Vesper	PDB	86	150	12	LI 1370
1996	Kanowski	PDB	216	240	24	EGb 761

Abbreviations: PBD = placebo-controlled double-blind study; POS = placebo-controlled open study; VDB = double-blind study comparing ginkgo extract with synthetic nootropic drugs; VOS = open study comparing ginkgo extract with synthetic nootropic drugs.

cognitive impairment"). This criterion excludes patients who have moderate to severe cognitive deficits (MMSE < 15), for whom treatment with a nootropic drug is the only therapeutic alternative. Another difficulty is that elderly patients who are accustomed to their family doctor and are limited in their ability to cope with new situations may find it difficult, for the sake of research, to accept repeated psychometric testing by an unfamiliar third party. Assessment on the social level, which is done without the help of the attending physician, is mainly a problem if the family members and other caregivers are close to the patient in age. Most experts agree

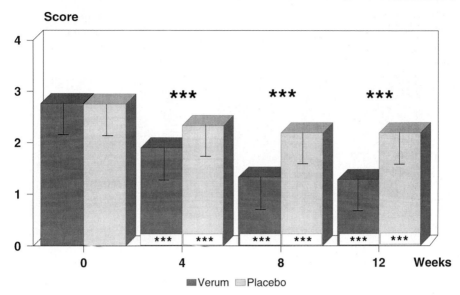

Fig. 2.3. Severity of memory lapses during 12 weeks' therapy with a ginkgo special extract (dark columns) compared with a placebo (light columns). The ginkgo-treated group shows a significantly greater reduction in symptoms (*** = p < 0.001) than the placebo group (Vorberg et al., 1989).

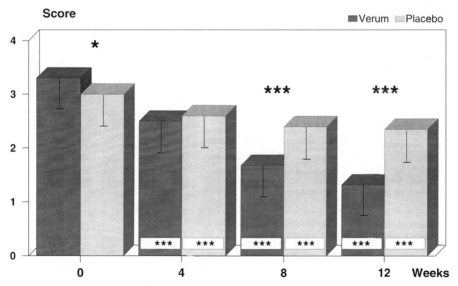

Fig. 2.4. Placebo-controlled double-blind study as in Fig. 2.3, showing the progression of symptom scores for vertigo. Eight to 12 weeks' therapy was needed before the ginkgo-treated patients showed significant improvement (*** = p < 0.001) relative to the placebo (Vorberg et al., 1989).

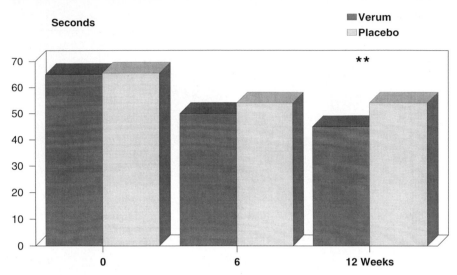

Seconds

■ Verum
□ Placebo

Fig. 2.5. Improvement of mental function in 209 dementia patients as demonstrated by an objective performance test. Dark columns: mean values in patients treated with ginkgo; light columns: mean values in patients treated with a placebo. Improvement in the ginkgo group is relatively marked following 12 weeks' therapy (** = p < 0.01). The age-normal value in this test would have been about 30–40 seconds (Brüchert et al., 1991).

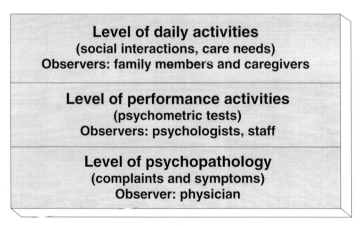

Level of daily activities
(social interactions, care needs)
Observers: family members and caregivers

Level of performance activities
(psychometric tests)
Observers: psychologists, staff

Level of psychopathology
(complaints and symptoms)
Observer: physician

Fig. 2.6. In 1991 the German Health Agency issued new guidelines for the testing of medications for dementia. They require that efficacy be demonstrated concurrently on three mutually independent levels of observation. Treatment periods of at least one year are recommended for evaluations at the daily activities level.

that at least 1 year of observation is needed to assess the impact of therapy on social functioning (German Federal Health Agency, 1991). Placebo-controlled studies of this duration in patients with an average life expectancy of approximately 5 years would raise ethical problems for the physicians conducting the study. Physicians who consider ginkgo to be beneficial would find it unethical to withhold the therapy from elderly patients for such a long period purely for research purposes. Therefore it is no wonder that no long-term studies conforming to the new guidelines have yet been done on ginkgo preparations or other nootropic drugs. It is left to the individual physician to decide whether a lack of rigorous evidence means that ginkgo extracts are without benefit in patients with cognitive deficits.

2.1.7
Indications, Dosages, Risks, and Contraindications

The 1994 Commission E monograph recognizes the following indications for the special extracts defined in Sect. 2.1.3 and 2.1.4 above.

- Symptomatic treatment of deficits due to organic brain disease as part of a comprehensive therapy program in demential syndromes with these principal features: memory impairment, concentration difficulties, depression, vertigo, tinnitus, and headache.
  The primary target group includes demential syndromes in patients with primary degenerative dementia, vascular dementia, and mixed forms of both.
  Note: Before treatment with ginkgo extracts is started, it should be determined whether the patient's symptoms are caused by an underlying disease that would require specific treatment.
- Improvement of pain-free walking distance in patients with Fontaine Stage IIa or IIb peripheral arterial occlusive disease (intermittent claudication) as an adjunct to physical therapy, particularly ambulatory exercise.
- Vertigo or tinnitus of vascular or involutional origin.

The total daily dose is 120–240 mg of crude dry extract is taken in 2 or 3 separate doses. Most of the clinical studies demonstrating efficacy (Table 2.2) employed doses in the range of 120–160 mg/day. A minimal 8-week course of treatment is recommended in patients with dementia (see Fig. 2.3), and the patient should be reevaluated at 3 months to determine whether it is appropriate to continue therapy. The only contraindication to ginkgo is a hypersensitivity to Ginkgo biloba preparations. Side effects are very rare and consist of mild gastric upset, headache, or allergic skin reactions. There are no known interactions with other drugs.

The use of ginkgo extracts for arterial occlusive disease is discussed more fully in Sect. 3.3.2. Several controlled studies have been published on ginkgo in the treatment of vertigo and tinnitus (survey in Hänsel et al., 1993).

2.1.8
Therapeutic Significance

Today there are approximately 1 million elderly persons in Germany who suffer from some form of dementia. The therapeutic mainstays in these patients, besides treatment with nootropic drugs, are physiotherapy, sociotherapy, and cognitive exercises. Critics of nootropic therapy recommend exclusive reliance on nonpharmacologic treatment methods. But there are several arguments against this one-sided approach.

Table 2.3. Frequency of side effects during 3 months' treatment with the ginkgo extract LI 1370 (10,815 patients) and with various synthetic nootropic drugs (2141 patients) (Burkard and Lehrl, 1991).

Patients, side effects	Number (%) with LI 1370	Number (%) with other nootropic drugs
Total number of patients	10,815 (100%)	2141 (100%)
– with no side effects	10,632 (98.31%)	2025 (94.58%)
– with side effects	183 (1.69%)	116 (5.42%)
Nausea	37 (0.34%)	16 (0.75%)
Headache	24 (0.22%)	5 (0.23%)
Stomach problems	15 (0.14%)	15 (0.70%)
Diarrhea	15 (0.14%)	1 (0.05%)
Allergy	10 (0.09%)	2 (0.09%)
Anxiety, restlessness	8 (0.07%)	19 (0.89%)
Sleep disturbances	6 (0.06%)	11 (0.51%)
Other	68 (0.63%)	47 (2.20%)

First, there is considerably less evidence from controlled clinical studies to support the efficacy of nonpharmacologic therapies (Grässel, 1989; Ermini, 1992). Few studies have investigated the additive effects of combining nootropic agents with cognitive exercises (Israel, 1987; Koalick, 1992). Furthermore, nonpharmacologic treatments are time- and personnel-intensive and, at present, are available only to a dwindling minority of patients since moderate to severe cognitive impairments usually are no longer responsive to cognitive training. The broad application of these methods would probably be at least 10 times more costly than pharmacotherapy. Thus, excluding ginkgo from the list of reimbursable drugs would, for the foreseeable future, deny many patients access to treatment for their dementia – a state of therapeutic nihilism that recognized experts have warned us about for some time (Kanowski, 1991; Beske and Kunczik, 1991).

The leading synthetic drugs available for the pharmacotherapy of dementia are piracetam and pyritinol, the ergot alkaloids (ergoloid mesylates), nicergoline, and predominantly vasoactive compounds such as nimodipine. These groups of drugs are considered to have very similar therapeutic efficacies (Kleijnen, 1993; Riederer et al., 1992). The treatment costs in Germany average about $1 to $1.25 per day (Schwabe and Paffrath, 1995) and are relatively constant within this group of indications. The key advantage of ginkgo therapy over the synthetic drugs lies in its significantly lower incidence of side effects, e.g., 1.69% in 10,632 patients treated with ginkgo extract LI 1370 versus 5.42% in 2325 patients treated with synthetic nootropics (Burkard and Lehrl, 1991; Table 2.3).

2.1.9
Drug Products

The *Rote Liste 1995* (Red List – the German equivalent of *Physician's Desk Reference*) contains a total of eight allopathic ginkgo preparations, five of which meet the specifications of the 1994 Commission E monograph (extracts EGb 761 and LI 1370); the three others do not.

References

American Psychiatric Association (ed) (1994) DSM-IV. Diagnostic and Statistical Manual of Mental Disorders. 4th Edition. R.R.Donnelly & Sons Company.

Beske F, Kunczik T (1991) Frühzeitige Therapie kann Milliarden sparen. Der Kassenarzt 42: 36–42.

Blaha L (1989) Differentialdiagnose der zerebralen Insuffizienz in der Praxis. Geriatrie und Rehabilitation 2,1: 23–28.

Braquet P (ed) (1988) Ginkgolides. Chemistry, Biology, Pharmacology and Clinical Perspectives. Vol 1. JR Prous Science, Barcelona.

Braquet P (ed) (1989) Ginkgolides. Chemistry, Biology, Pharmacology and Clinical Perspectives. Vol 11. JR Prous Science, Barcelona.

Brüchert F, Heinrich SE, Ruf-Kohler P (1991) Wirksamkeit von Ll 1370 bei älteren Patienten mit Hirnleistungsschwäche. Münch Med Wschr 133 (Suppl 1): 9–14.

Bundesgesundheitsamt (1991) Empfehlungen zum Wirksamkeitsnachweis von Nootropika im Indikationsbereich "Demenz" (Phase III). Bundesgesundheitsblatt 7: 342–350.

Burkard G, Lehrl S (1991) Verhältnis von Demenzen vom Multiinfarkt- und vom Alzheimertyp in ärztlichen Praxen. Münch Med Wschr 133 (Suppl. 1): 38–43.

Deutsches Institut für medizinische Dokumentation und Information (ed) (1994) ICD-10. Internationale und statistische Klassifikation der Krankheiten und verwandter Gesundheitsprobleme. 10th Revision. Vol. 1. Urban & Schwarzenberg, Munich Vienna Baltimore.

Ermini-Fünfschilling D (1992) Möglichkeiten und Grenzen eines Gedächtnistrainings mit Patienten bei beginnender Demenz. Moderne Geriatrie 12: 459–465.

Gräßel E (1989) Vergleich zweier Personengruppen bezüglich der Auswirkungen des mentalen Trainings ("Gehirn-Jogging") auf die Selbsteinschätzung der Leistungsfähigkeit in Abhängigkeit von der Trainingszeit (Tageszeit der Trainingsdurchführung). Geriatrie & Rehabilitation 2, 1: 44–46.

Hänsel R, Keller K, Rimpler H, Schneider G (eds) (1993) Hagers Handbuch der Pharmazeutischen Praxis, 5th Edition, Drogen E–O. Springer Verlag, Berlin Heidelberg New York, pp 268–292.

Hartmann A, Schulz V (eds) (1991) Ginkgo biloba: Aktuelle Forschungsergebnisse 1990/91 Münch Med Wschr 133:1–64.

Hopfenmüller W (1994) Nachweis der therapeutischen Wirksamkeit eines Ginkgo biloba-Spezialextraktes. Metaanalyse von 11 klinischen Studien bei Patienten mit Hirnleistungsstörungen im Alter. Arzneim Forsch/Drug Res 44: 1005–1013.

Israel L, Dell' Accio E, Martin G, Hugonot R (1987) Extrait de Ginkgo biloba et exercices d'entrainement de la memoire. Evaluation comparative chez personnes agees ambulatoires. Psychologie Medicinale 19: 8, 1431–1439

Itil TM, Eralp E, Tsambis F, Itil Kz, Stein U (1996) Central nervous system effects of Ginkgo biloba, a plant extract. Am J Therap 3:63–73.

Kanowski S (1991) Klinischer Wirksamkeitsnachweis bei Nootropika. Münch Med Wschr 133: 5–8.

Kanowski S, Herrmann WM, Stephan K, Wierich W, Hörr R (1996) Proof of efficacy of the Ginkgo biloba special extract EGb 761 in outpatients suffering from mild to moderate primary degenerative dementia of the Alzheimer type or multi-infarct dementia. Pharmacopsychiatry 29: 47–56.

Kleijnen J, Knipschild P (1992a) Ginkgo biloba for cerebral insuffficiency. Br J Clin Pharmac 34: 352–358.

Kleijnen J, Knipschild P (1992b) Ginkgo biloba. Lancet: 1136–1139.

Koalik F et al (1992) Kombinierte Anwendung von nootroper Therapie und kognitivem Training bei chronischen organischen Psychosyndromen. Neuropsychiatrie 6: 47–52.

Krieglstein J, Ausmeier F, El-Abhar H, Lippert K, Welsch M, Rupalla, K, Heinrich-Noack P (1995) Eur J Pharm Sci 3: 39–48.

Kurz A (1995) Ginkgo biloba bei Demenzerkrankungen. In: Loew D, Rietbrock N (eds) Phytopharmaka. Steinkopff Verlag, Darmstadt, pp 145–149.

Nieder M (1991) Pharmakokinetik der Ginkgo-Flavonole im Plasma. Münch Med Wschr 133: 61–62.

Oberpichler-Schwenk H, Krieglstein J (1992) Pharmakologische Wirkungen von Ginkgo-biloba-Extrakt und -Inhaltsstoffen. Pharmazie in unserer Zeit 21: 224–235.

Riederer P, Laux G, Pöldinger W (eds) (1992) Neuropsychopharmaka. Vol.5: Parkinsonmittel und Nootropika. Springer Verlag, Vienna New York: 161–324.

Rupalla K, Oberpichler-Schwenk H, Krieglstein J (1995) Neuroprotektive Wirkungen des Ginkgo-biloba-Extrakts und seiner Inhaltsstoffe. In: Loew D, Rietbrock N (eds) Phytopharmaka in Forschung und klinischer Anwendung. Steinkopff Verlag, Darmstadt, pp 17–27.

Schmid M, Schmoll H (eds) (1994) Ginkgo. Wissenschaftliche Verlagsgesellschaft mbH Stuttgart.

Schwabe U, Paffrath D (eds) (1995) Arzneiverordnungsreport '95. Gustav Fischer Verlag, Stuttgart Jena, pp 214–224, 373–374.

Sticher O (1993) Ginkgo biloba – Ein modernes pflanzliches Arzneimittel. Vierteljahresschrift der Naturforschenden Gesellschaft in Zürich 138/3: 125–168.
Vesper J, Hänsgen KD (1994) Efficacy of Ginkgo biloba in 90 outpatients with cerebral insufficiency caused by old age. Phytomedicine 1: 9–16.
Volz HP, Hänsel R (1994) Ginkgo biloba – Grundlagen und Anwendung in der Psychiatrie. Psychopharmakotherapie 1: 70–76.
Vorberg G, Schenk N, Schmidt U (1989) Wirksamkeit eines neuen Ginkgo-biloba-Extraktes bei 100 Patienten mit zerebraler Insuffizienz. Herz + Gefäße 9: 396–401.

2.2
St. John's Wort as an Antidepressant

2.2.1
Introduction

St. John's wort (Fig. 2.7) has been used in herbal healing for more than 2000 years. Paracelsus may have known about its use in the treatment of psychiatric disorders (Czygan, 1993). The German poet-physician Justinus Kerner (1786–1862) reported on the use of St. John's wort in the treatment of mood disorders in the early nineteenth century (Engelhardt, 1962).

With the rise of scientifically oriented medicine, St. John's wort was all but forgotten as a psychotropic drug. A full century passed before reports were again published on the successful use of St. John's wort in the treatment of depression (Daniel, 1939).

A treatise on the St. John's wort was one of the first herbal monographs published by Commission E during its 12 years of activity in the former German Federal Health Agency. The monograph was published in the Bundesanzeiger on December 5, 1984, and will be published by the American Botanical Council (Blumenthal et al., in press). Based on information available at the time, the Commission cited depressed mood as the indication for St. John's wort, making specific reference to psychoautonomic disturbances and anxiety and/or nervous unrest. During the next 10 years, definitive clinical and pharmacologic studies were conducted that enabled the indications for St. John's wort to be defined more precisely. Today, alcoholic extracts of the botanical are placed in the category of herbal antidepressants. The example of St. John's wort offers convincing proof that modern, orthodox methods of medical research are both necessary and effective in advancing the development of traditional herbal remedies.

2.2.2
Botanical Description

The genus Hypericum occurs throughout the world and encompasses 378 known species. The 1986 *Deutscher Arzneimittel-Codex* (German Drug Codex) identifies *Hypericum perforatum* as the species from which the crude drug is obtained. St. John's wort is an herbaceous plant that grows to a height of about 60 cm. It has yellow, star-shaped flowers with numerous long stamens and opposing leaves studded with translucent glandular dots. The stem bears two characteristic longitudinal ridges

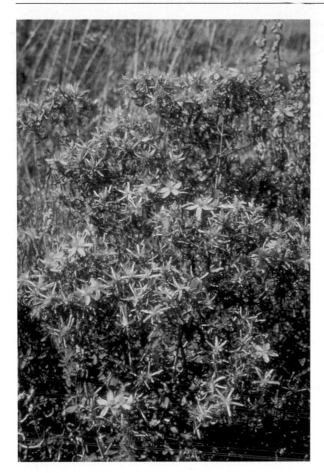

Fig. 2.7.
St. John's wort *(Hypericum perforatum).*

that distinguish the plant from other Hypericum species. St. John's wort grows wild throughout much of Europe, Asia, North America, and South America, showing a preference for dry, sunny locations. It is found on roadsides, railway embankments, and in clearings. The mesophyll of the leaves contains spherical glands filled with a highly refractive volatile oil that is secreted by the plant. Holding a leaf against the light displays numerous translucent dots that give it a perforated appearance, hence the botanical name perforatum (Hänsel et al., 1993).

2.2.3
Crude Drug and Extract

In years past, St. John's wort was mainly gathered in the wild, but now much of the herb is obtained by controlled cultivation (in Germany, Poland, and South America). Herbs for medicinal use should be gathered when the flowers start to open.

The harvested material should be dried rapidly but carefully to preserve the content of the secretory glands. The drying temperature should not exceed 30–40 °C. The key constituents of St. John's wort (see Sect. 2.2.4) are most concentrated in the buds, flowers, and distal leaves, so the pharmaceutical and therapeutic quality of the extracts is highly dependent on the quality of the original herbal material. Quality testing in drug manufacture is accomplished by quantitative measurement of the hypericins contained in the crude drug or extracts; poorer grades are identified and discarded.

All antidepressant medications made from St. John's wort are based on alcoholic extracts, generally with an herb-to-extract ratio in the range of 4:1 to 7:1. So far, the only clinical proof of therapeutic efficacy for depression and other symptoms has been furnished for products that use methanol or ethanol as the solvent. Evidence to date shows that the highest yield of active principles is obtained by extracting the dried herb with aqueous methanol containing 20–40 % water. The extraction must be performed in darkness with temperatures raised only briefly to 60–80 °C (Niesel, 1992; Wagner and Bladt, 1993). The best clinical trials to date used a hypericum extract designated in the technical literature as LI 160 (Harrer et al., 1993; Jenike, 1994; Müller and Kasper, 1997).

2.2.4
Key Constituents, Analysis, Pharmacokinetics

Rubbing a bud or flower from the St. John's wort between the fingers immediately produces a purple stain caused by characteristic constituents of the plant – hypericin, pseudohypericin, protohypericin, protopseudohypericin, and cyclopseudohypericin, all belonging to the group of naphthodianthrones. The dried plant parts contain an average of about 0.1 % of these compounds; standardized extracts may contain several times that amount. High-performance liquid chromatography (HPLC) or photometric analysis is used for the qualitative and quantitative analysis of the hypericin compounds as described in the German Drug Codex (DAC 1986).

Besides these species-specific components, the dried herb and ist extracts also contain significant amounts of hyperforin, and some very common plant constituents: flavonoids and flavonoid derivatives (e. g., rutin and hyperin), xanthone derivatives, amentoflavone, biapigenin, and a volatile oil (Nahrstedt and Butterweck, 1997). The dried herb contains no more than about 1 % of the volatile oil, which is isolated by steam distillation. Hypericum oil is made by macerating the ground fresh flowers of St. John's wort in olive oil (25:100 ratio) in a sealed vessel. Hypericum oil is a traditional topical remedy for use on wounds and burns (see Chap. 8).

The pharmacokinetics (absorption and elimination) of hypericin and pseudohypericin have been well researched for the therapeutic use of hypericum extract LI 160 in humans. Figure 2.8 shows the progression and dose-dependence of the plasma concentrations of hypericin. The ingestion of 300, 900, and 1800 mg of raw whole extract led to respective maximum plasma levels of 1.3, 17.3, and 66.3 ng/mL for hypericin and 7.1, 28.4, and 48.0 ng/mL for pseudohypericin. The elimination half-life was dose-dependent, averaging 24–48 h for hypericin and 18–24 h for pseu-

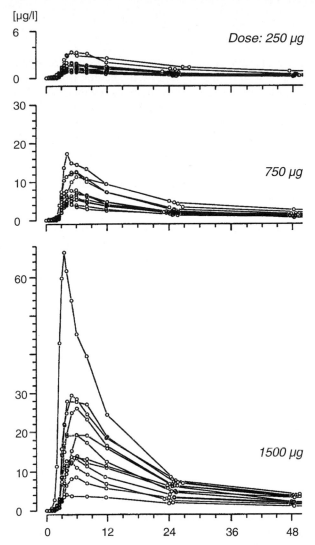

Fig. 2.8. Plasma concentrations of Hypericin in twelve healthy subjects after intake of 300 mg, 900 mg and 1800 mg St. John's Wort extract according to 250 μg, 750 μg and 900 μg Hypericin per dosage (Kerb et al., 1996).

dohypericin. Plasma levels of hypericin were measurable 2–3 h after ingestion and plasma levels of pseudohypericin in just 15–30 min. The cumulative rise in plasma levels was measured during the first three days of a regimen that was continued for several weeks (Kerb et al., 1996).

2.2.5
Pharmacology

Most currently known antidepressants inhibit the active, energy-dependent reuptake of monoamines (norepinephrine, serotonin, dopamine) into the neuron from the synaptic gap. The inhibition of monoamine uptake forms the basis for the classic hypotheses on the pathophysiology of depression and the mechanism of action of antidepressant drugs, which are classified accordingly as norepinephrine-reuptake inhibitors, selective serotonin-reuptake inhibitors, MAO inhibitors, and receptor antagonists. Not all substances with clinically documented antidepressant activity can be classified according to these criteria, however. Substances that do not act primarily on noradrenergic and/or serotoninergic neurotransmitters are classified as atypical antidepressants – a category that includes hypericum extract (Cott, 1997; Müller et al., 1997).

When antidepressants are administered to laboratory animals in relatively high doses, their main effects are an inhibition of spontaneous behavior and exploratory activity and a suppression of the arousal response in the EEG. Antidepressants have varying effects on the actions of neuroleptics, hypnotics, and sedatives; frequently they attenuate these drug actions after several doses have been administered. It can be misleading, however, to apply the findings in animal studies to therapeutic effects in human patients. The best approach is to evaluate the results obtained from various animal models simultaneously. One such model, the forced swimming test of Porsolt, has proven fairly specific for testing antidepressant activity. Antidepressants significantly shorten the duration of immobility in this test, an effect that is believed to correlate well with clinical efficacy (Borsini et al., 1988; Thiebot et al., 1992; Willner, 1984; Winterhoff et al., 1993, Butterweck et al., 1997).

Table 2.4 reviews nine pharmacologic studies using a standardized hypericum extract (LI 160, extracted with 80 % v/v methanol, herb-to-extract ratio 4–7:1). The "Test medium" column in the table shows that seven of these studies used in vitro receptor models and two used live animals. Based on the results of previous studies with hypericum extract or hypericin, the mechanism of the antidepressant action of St. John's wort was presumed to involve monoaminooxidase inhibition (Suzuki et al., 1984). The studies of Thiede et al. (1994) and Bladt et al. (1994) were unable to confirm this mechanism, at least for pharmacologically active concentrations in an experimental setting. The same applies to the inhibition of catechol-O-methyltransferase (Thiede et al., 1994). However, one group of authors found evidence for a relatively strong inhibitory effect of the hypericum extract LI 160 on the synaptosomal uptake of norepinephrine and serotonin in mouse brain preparations (Müller, 1997). Similar studies in rat brain preparations confirmed these results for the inhibition of synaptosomal serotonin uptake. A concentration of 6.2 µg/mL of the extract LI 160 caused 50 % inhibition (IC_{50} value). This is considered the pharmacologically active concentration and is consistent with the dose of 900 mg/day usually prescribed in human patients (Perovic et al., 1995). Two studies of LI 160 have shown evidence of neurohormonal actions (Butterweck et al., 1997) and neuroimmunologic actions (Thiele et al., 1994). Another study (Müller et al., 1994) demonstrated a down-regulation of serotonin receptors in cultured rat neuroblastoma cells. Experiments in mice and rats showed evidence of reserpine antagonism, with a shortened duration of anesthesia and a

Table 2.4. Pharmacologic tests with the methanol extract of St. John's wort (test designation LI 160).

Author/Investigator	Test medium	Parameters tested
Winterhoff (1993)	Wistar rats	Reserpine antagonism, duration of general anesthesia, neurotransmitter concentrations in the brain
Thiele (1994)	Human blood in vitro	Cytokine expression
Müller (1994)	Neuroblastoma cells	Expression of serotonin receptors
Thiede (1994)	Enzyme homogenate from porcine liver	MAO and COMT inhibition
Bladt (1994)	Enzyme homogenate from rat liver and brain	MAO inhibition
Perovic (1995)	Cell cultures of neurons from embryonic rat brains	Postsynaptic serotonin reuptake
Butterweck (1997)	NMRI mice, Wistar rats	Body temperature, duration of general anesthesia, open-field mobility, forced swimming test (Porsolt), neurotransmitter concentrations in the brain; serum levels of TSH, cortisol, and prolactin
Cott (1997)	Test program in vitro	Screening with 39 receptor types
Müller (1997)	Synaptosome homogenates from mouse brains	Binding to muscarinic, α_1, α_2, β, 5-HT$_2$, 5-HT$_{1A}$ and imipramine receptors; synaptosomal norepinephrine and serotonin reuptake, β-down regulation

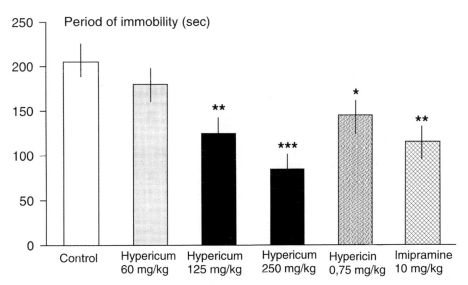

Fig. 2.9. Pharmacologic activity of a standardized St. John's wort extract (hypericum) compared with pure hypericin (0.75 mg = amount contained in 250 mg extract) and the standard antidepressant drug imipramine as measured by the Porsolt swimming test. The whole extract was significantly more active than the equivalent amount of hypericin. Imipramine was about 10 times more active than the whole extract, reflecting the approximate dose relationship of both substances when used therapeutically in human patients (Butterweck et al., 1997).

shortened period of immobility in the forced swimming test (Winterhoff et al., 1993, Butterweck et al., 1997). The swimming test indicated about a 10:1 active dosage ratio between the hypericum extract and imipramine, consistent with the ratio of therapeutic doses that has been established in the practical treatment of depressed patients (900 mg/day hypericum extract versus 50–150 mg/day imipramine) (Fig. 2.9).

Based on pharmacologic data presently available, it is appropriate to classify the hypericum extract as an atypical antidepressant. However, its mechanism of action could be based partly on the inhibition of the neuronal reuptake of serotonin (Perovic et al., 1995) as well as the down-regulation of serotonin receptors (Müller et al., 1994) and neurohormonal mechanisms (Thiele et al., 1994; Butterweck et al., 1997). Since hypericum extract, unlike synthetic chemical antidepressants, represents a natural mixture of the constituents of St. John's wort, it is not surprising that the herb could have various potential mechanisms of action.

2.2.6
Toxicology

The toxicologic properties of hypericum extract LI 160 have been tested both acutely and over a period of 26 weeks in mice, rats, and dogs. The maximum test dose was 5000 mg/kg. The first intolerance reactions appeared at 900 mg/kg/day, and the LD_{50} was greater than the maximum dose. None of the tests showed evidence of genotoxic or mutagenic effects (Leuschner, 1995).

Photosensitization and even phototoxic reactions (hypericism) are known to occur in grazing animals, especially sheep and cattle, that have consumed large amounts of St. John's wort (Araya and Ford, 1981; Giese, 1980). Phototoxic reactions also developed in AIDS patients given intravenous injections of 30–40 mg hypericin to test its antiviral activity (equal to the total amount of hypericin and pseudohypericin in about 50–70 tablets of the highest-dose St. John's wort product, see Sect. 2.2.10) (NN, 1995). This suggests that, at least when excessive doses are administered, there is a significant risk of phototoxic skin reactions from hypericum preparations.

Studies have been done in human subjects to determine the threshold dose at which initial signs of photosensitization occur. In one placebo-controlled crossover study, 13 healthy male subjects took 900, 1800, and 3600 mg of hypericum extract once a day. The lowest dose, 900 mg/day, has been established as the effective daily dose by most clinical studies. In another study, 50 healthy subjects of both sexes took 600 mg 3 times daily (t.i.d.) for 15 days. In both tests the subjects were exposed on days 1 and 15 to UV-A and UV-B irradiation of standard duration and intensity 4h after taking the morning dose. The skin reactions were assessed at 5h, 20h, and 7 days after the UV exposures as the minimum erythematous dose (MED) in one study and as the minimum pigmentation dose (MPD) in the other.

A significant decrease in the MPD (approximately 20%) was noted in hypericum-treated subjects who had been exposed to UV-A light on day 15 of treatment. This lowering of the threshold for a pigmentation response was more pronounced in subjects with light-sensitive skin (skin type < 2, approximately 30% reduction) than in subjects with a skin type > 2 (insignificant decrease of about 10%). A correlation was established between the lowering of the MPD threshold and the skin type of the subjects. Exposure to UV-B light on day 15 tended to decrease the MED by a maximum of about 10 % relative to the response on day 1. Based on these results, it has been recommended that no more than 1800 mg of the tested hypericum extract (equivalent to 6 tablets of the product Jarsin 300) be taken daily for antidepressant therapy (Brockmöller et al., 1997).

2.2.7
Clinical Efficacy in Depressed Patients

Traditionally, St. John's wort has been taken medicinally in the form of a tea. Such a preparation delivers a single dose equivalent to an aqueous extract of 2–3 g of the dried herb. Dividing the minimum dose of 2 g of the dried herb by 7 (based on the usual herb-to-extract ratio, see Sect. 1.3.2.2) gives a minimum single dose equivalent to approximately 300 mg for the dry extract. This may be considered a reasonable standard dose by the physician who relies on empirical principles in the practice of phytotherapy and believes that they will yield positive therapeutic results.

Studies on the therapeutic efficacy of St. John's wort preparations have also disclosed the key importance of communication between the physician and the patient seeking treatment for depression. The office consultation serves a function that goes beyond diagnostic assessment; it also initiates the therapeutic process. An associated finding in nearly all placebo-controlled double-blind studies has been that

Table 2.5. Controlled studies with the methanol hypericum extract LI 160 (brand name Jarsin 300) and a related product (Jarsin, marked with * under "Daily dose", contains up to 50 % excipients, so the daily dose in these 4 studies was up to 50 % lower compared to the crude extract) (References from Harrer and Schulz, 1993; Linde et al., 1996; and Volz, 1997).

First author, year	Number of cases	Daily dose	Duration (days)	Reference therapy	Significant parameters
Halama, 1991	50	900 mg*	28	Placebo	HAMD, B-L, CGI
Johnson, 1992	12	900 mg*	42	Placebo	Drug-induced EEG changes
Lehrl, 1993	50	900 mg*	28	Placebo	HAMD, KAI
Schmidt, 1993	32	900 mg	7	Placebo	Interactions with alcohol use
Sommer, 1994	105	900 mg*	28	Placebo	HAMD
Johnson, 1994	24	900 mg	42	Maprotiline	Drug-induced EEG changes, Bf-S
Harrer, 1994	102	900 mg	28	Maprotiline	HAMD, D-S, CGI
Hübner, 1994	39	900 mg	28	Placebo	HAMD, B-L, CGI
Martinez, 1994	20	900 mg	35	Phototherapy	HAMD (SAD patients)
Schulz, 1994	12	900 mg	28	Placebo	Sleep EEG, D-S, Bf-S
Vorbach, 1994	130	900 mg	42	Imipramine	HAMD, D-S, CGI
Hänsgen, 1996	101	900 mg	42	Placebo	HAMD, D-S, BEB, CGI
Kerb, 1996	12	300–1800 mg	1–14	Placebo	Pharmacokinetics
Wheatley, 1997	149	900 mg	42	Amitriptyline	HAMD, MADRS, CGI
Vorbach, 1997	209	1800 mg	42	Imipramine	HAMD, D-S, CGI

Abbreviations: HAMD = Hamilton Depression Scale; HAMA = Hamilton Anxiety Scale; CGI = Clinical Global Impressions Scale; B-L = von Zerssen complaint list; D-S = von Zerssen depression scale; Bf-S = von Zerssen mood scale; DSI = Zung depression scale; BEB = Hänsgen complaint inventory; KAI = Lehrl brief test of general information processing; SAD = patients with seasonal affective disorder; MADRS = Montgomery Asberg Depression Rating Scale.

sensitive and empathic guidance by the physician can, in itself, lead to significant improvement in 10–40% of all patients as measured by the Hamilton Depression Rating Scale (see paragraph below). The addition of pharmacotherapy can increase this success rate to 60–80%. This casts doubt on the validity of clinical studies that are conducted without benefit of double-blind control groups.

It is only during the past decade that therapeutic studies conforming to this standard have been conducted on preparations of St. John's wort, and most have been completed during the past 5 years (Tables 2.5 and 2.6). The results of 26 controlled studies involving a total of about 1700 patients have been published thus far (surveys in Harrer et al., 1993; Jenike, 1994; Ernst, 1995; Volz and Hänsel, 1995; Linde et al., 1996; Volz, 1997). Fourteen of these studies (Table 2.5) employed a specific methanol dry extract; 12 other studies used various ethanol-extracted preparations, in some

Table 2.6. Controlled studies with ethanolic hypericum extracts. A solids content of 10–15% was assumed in calculating the dose in mg of the liquid products Hyperforat and Psychotonin M. Sedariston (*) is a combination product containing valerian extract in addition to hypericum. (References from Harrer and Schulz, 1993; Linde et al., 1996; and Volz, 1997).

First author, year	Number of cases	Daily dose	Duration (days)	Product name	Reference therapy	Significant parameters
Hoffmann, 1979	60	4.5 mL (450–675 mg)	42	Hyperforat	Placebo	Hoffmann's own scale
Panijel, 1985	100	200–400 mg	14	*Sedariston	Diazepam	CGI, B-L, STAI
Steger, 1985	93	400–600 mg	42	*Sedariston	Desipramine	CGI, D-S, B-L
Schlich, 1987	49	3 mL (300–450 mg)	28	Psychotonin M	Placebo	HAMD, STAI
Kniebel, 1988	130	300–600 mg	42	*Sedariston	Amitriptyline	HAMD, CGI, Bf-S
Schmidt, 1989	40	4.5 mL (450–675 mg)	28	Psychotonin M	Placebo	HAMD
Werth, 1989	30	4.5 mL (450–675 mg)	23	Psychotonin M	Imipramine	HAMD
Kugler, 1990	80	4.5 mL (450–675 mg)	28	Psychotonin M	Bromazepam	DSI, STAI
Harrer, 1991	116	3 mL (300–450 mg)	42	Psychotonin M	Placebo	HAMD, HAMA, D-S
Osterhelder, 1992	46	?	?	Psychotonin M	Placebo	HAMD, HAMA, CGI
Bergmann, 1993	80	?	42	Esbericum	Amitriptyline	HAMD, Bf-S
Quandt, 1993	88	4.5 mL (450–675 mg)	28	Psychotonin M	Placebo	HAMD

Abbreviations: HAMD = Hamilton Depression Scale, CGI = Clinical Global Impressions Scale, B-L = von Zerssen complaint list, KAI = Lehrl brief test of general information processing, SAD = patients with seasonal affective disorder, D-S = von Zerssen depression scale, Bf-S = von Zerssen mood scale, STAI = State Trait Anxiety Inventory.

cases combined with other active ingredients (Table 2.6). Sixteen of the studies compared hypericum therapy with a placebo, and 10 compared it with standard synthetic drug products. The Hamilton Depression Rating Scale (HAMD) was the primary instrument used in patient assessment.

The HAMD is an observer rating scale used to evaluate degree of depression. The physician interviews the patient and assigns a score based on the severity of 17 or 21 items. The criterion for therapeutic success is a 50% reduction in the total HAMD score or a total score less than 10. To date, the HAMD scale has been the instrument of choice in most clinical trials of antidepressant drug efficacy. Its reliability is internationally recognized. In addition to the HAMD scale, most hypericum studies have used other validated scales for the assessment of depression and mood (Tables 2.5 and 2.6, last column).

Most of the studies in Table 2.6 predate those in Table 2.5 and used a more heterogeneous range of extracts and dosages. Eight of the 12 studies in Table 2.6 used liquid extract preparations; experience has shown that it is difficult or impossible to "blind" the treatment groups when this type of preparation is used. Also, the published data allow only an approximate dose estimation in terms of the total amount of dry extract administered. As column 3 in Table 2.6 indicates, the average daily

Table 2.7. Results of the controlled treatment studies (Extract LI 160) with depressive patients measured by the (responder) criteria of the Hamilton Depression Scale (HAMD). The average score with hypericum preparations was between 42 and 79%, which corresponds favorably to the results obtained with synthetic antidepressant drugs.

First author, year	Evaluable protocols	HAMD total score		HAMD responders
		Initial	Endpoint	
Halama, 1991	25 LI 160	18.3^2	10.9	50%
	25 Placebo	18.0^2	18.2	0%
Sommer, 1994	42 LI 160	15.8^2	11.3	67%
	47 Placebo	15.8^2	7.2	28%
Lehrl, 1993	25 LI 160	23.7^2	17.4	42%
	25 Placebo	21.6^2	16.8	25%
Hübner, 1994	20 LI 160	12.6^2	5.6	70%
	19 Placebo	12.4^2	10.3	47%
Hänsgen, 1996	51 LI 160	21.0^2	8.9	70% (79%)*
	50 Placebo	20.4^2	14.4	24%
Martinez, 1994	10/10 LI 160	21.9^2	6.1	–
	with/without phototherapy	20.6^2	8.2	–
Harrer, 1994	51 LI 160	20.5^1	12.2	61%
	51 Maprotiline	21.5^1	10.5	67%
Vorbach, 1994	66 LI 160	20.2^1	8.8	64%
	64 Imipramine	19.4^1	10.7	58%
Wheatley, 1997	82 LI 160	20.6^1	9.9	60%
	67 Amitriptyline	20.8^1	7.1	78%
Vorbach, 1997	107 LI 160	25.3^1	14.6	35%
	102 Imipramine	26.1^1	13.6	41%

* Results after 6 weeks' therapy, [1] 17-Item scale, [2] 21-Item scale

doses in these studies ranged from 200 to 700 mg/day of hypericum dry extract. It is still noteworthy that most of these studies demonstrated significant effects that support the efficacy of the preparations and dosages in the treatment of depression or at least certain of its symptoms.

The results of the 14 studies in Table 2.5 allow for an even more confident interpretation. In four of five placebo-controlled studies, statistical analysis showed significant differences between the hypericum extract and the placebo in terms of total Hamilton depression scores (Table 2.7). One study showed no significant differences in HAMD scores between the treatment groups. In the two studies comparing hypericum with a reference therapy, the HAMD scores showed significant improvement in all treatment groups. However, there were no significant differences between treatment with the hypericum extract and treatment with maprotiline or imipramine. Overall, the responder rates based on the HAMD scale items (at least a 50 % score reduction or a total score less than 10) ranged from 42 % to 79 % – equivalent to the rates achieved with high-potency synthetic antidepressant drugs (Laux et al., 1995). We may conclude, therefore, that a daily dose of 900 mg of an extract of St. John's wort adjusted to 0.3 % total hypericin should provide therapeutic efficacy similar to that achieved with modern synthetic antidepressants. If we also consider the studies in Table 2.6, their results indicate that the threshold of efficacy for certain symptoms and complaints that accompany depressive disorders is approximately 300 mg of extract daily, while a dose of 450–700 mg/day appears to be effective for a mild to moderate degree of depression in at least the majority of patients treated.

As an example, Fig. 2.10 shows the results of a placebo-controlled double-blind study in 101 outpatients with moderately severe depression (meeting the criteria for major depression according to the Diagnostic and Statistical Manual [DSM] III-R).

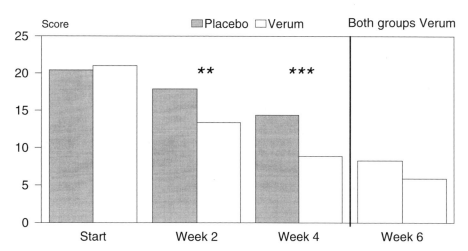

Fig. 2.10. Mean scores in the Hamilton Depression Scale (HAMD). Placebo-controlled double-blind study in 101 depressed patients treated with 900 mg hypericum extract daily compared with a placebo. A parallel group design was followed until week 4; thereafter both groups received the hypericum extract. Scores recorded in weeks 2 and 4 showed statistically significant differences between hypericum and placebo (*** = $p < 0.001$). Scores in weeks 5 and 6, when both groups received hypericum, showed marked improvement in the original placebo group (Hänsgen et al., 1996).

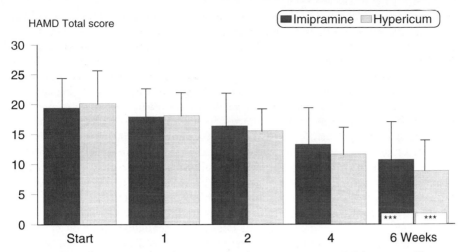

Fig. 2.11. Mean values and standard deviations of total HAMD scores recorded during 6 week's treatment with 900 mg/day hypericum extract (67 patients) compared with 75 mg/day imipramine (68 patients). Statistical analysis showed that both medications were equally effective (Vorbach et al., 1994).

The patients received either 300 mg of hypericum extract or a placebo t.i.d. for 4 weeks. Both groups then received the hypericum extract for an additional 2 weeks. With allowance for typical placebo effects, the results at 4 weeks showed a statistically highly significant difference in favor of the group treated with the hypericum extract. As expected, a smaller difference was seen after both groups had taken the hypericum extract for an additional 2 weeks.

Figure 2.11 shows the results of a study comparing St. John's wort with a standard therapy in 135 depressed patients. As in the previous trial, the patients had been selected according to the criteria in the Diagnostic and Statistical Manual (DSM-III-R). For 6 weeks the patients received either 300 mg of hypericum extract t.i.d. or 25 mg of imipramine t.i.d. All drugs were administered in the form of look-alike coated tablets. Response was evaluated by the HAMD rating scale as well as two other validated observer- and self-rating scales. The HAMD scores showed similar declines in both treatment groups, decreasing from 20.2 to 8.8 in the hypericum-treated patients and from 19.4 to 10.7 in the patients treated with imipramine. It is noteworthy that a subgroup of 51 patients with severe depression (average Hamilton score of 26) responded as well to the hypericum therapy as to imipramine, justifying the use of hypericum even in severely depressed patients.

2.2.8
Indications, Dosages, Risks, and Contraindications

The monograph on the St. John's wort published by Commission E of the German Fedral Health Agency on December 5, 1984, cites the following indications for hypericum preparations: psychoautonomic disturbances, depressive mood disorders, anxiety and/or nervous unrest.

Considering that only 1 of the 27 controlled clinical studies in Tables 2.5 and 2.6 had been published at the time this monograph was issued, we must credit the Commission with making a fairly accurate appraisal of the herb's therapeutic applications. In the light of what is known today, however, medications made from St. John's wort should be classified strictly as antidepressants when administered in the proper form and dosage. St. John's wort may benefit psychoautonomic disturbances and anxiety and/or nervous unrest only within the context of its overall antidepressant activity. Generally, though, marked improvement cannot be expected until the patient has taken the product for several weeks. Preparations of St. John's wort do not produce acute effects, so they are not suitable for use as daily sedatives or sleep aids.

The Commission E monograph gives the following average daily dose: 2–4 g of crude drug or 0.2–1 mg of total hypericin. The recommended dose of the dried herb not only corresponds to traditional empirical medicine but is consistent with the quantities of extract shown to have therapeutic efficacy in controlled clinical studies (Tables 2.5 and 2.6). In contrast, the dose recommendation based on hypericin is no longer tenable in the light of current knowledge and recently was rescinded by the Federal Institute for Drugs and Medical Products in Germany. Current dose recommendations are no longer based on total hypericin but strictly on the total amount of extract contained in the drug product. For the reasons stated in the preceding sections, an initial daily dose of 900 mg of a high-quality extract should be prescribed in depressed patients. If maintenance therapy is indicated following a positive response or if only certain symptoms require treatment in milder cases, daily doses of 300–600 mg of total extract may be sufficient.

Even the 1984 monograph mentioned photosensitization as a possible side effect of St. John's wort. It is caused by hypericins that are absorbed and reach plasma concentrations higher than about 50 µg/mL (Brockmöller et al., 1997). Animal experiments and human pharmacologic studies (Araya and Ford, 1981; Brockmöller et al., 1997) have shown that photosensitization is extremely unlikely to occur at the therapeutic doses recommended above. So far, there have been no reported instances of photosensitization from the therapeutic use of hypericum products. Based on experimental studies in animals and human subjects, however, it is reasonable to assume that 30–50 times the recommended daily dose taken at one time could lead to severe phototoxic reactions in humans. If such an amount were ingested (e. g., in a suicide attempt), the patient would have to be shielded from all sunlight and other UV light for one week due to the long elimination half-life of hypericins. If this important precaution is followed, even a massive overdose should not cause serious complications.

2.2.9
Therapeutic Significance

Depression is the most common psychiatric disorder. Epidemiologic studies indicate a 13–20 % prevalence of depressive symptoms in the population as a whole, with a 2–5 % prevalence of severe depression. Thus, adjustment disorders with depressed mood, brief depressive reactions, and mild depressive episodes are about 5–10 times more prevalent in the general population than full-blown depression. The lifetime prevalence of depressive disorders requiring treatment is about 10–20 %, because depressive disorders have a high rate of recurrence and mood disturbances may progress to depression. Untreated episodes of depression usually last from 6 to 9 months; antidepressant medication prescribed by a private physician is generally continued for 1–3 months. Depression can occur at any age but shows a statistical peak around age 50 (Riederer, 1993; Smith, 1992).

Epidemiologic data show that most patients with depression are not treated by a specialist in neurology or psychiatry, and very few are hospitalized for treatment. Most depressed patients are treated by their family doctors on an outpatient basis. Important criteria for selecting an antidepressant medication in this setting are lack of side effects and acceptable cost.

Approximately 20–50 % of patients experience adverse drug effects while on treatment with tricyclic antidepressants. Generally these occur within a few days after the drug is started so they precede the onset of a therapeutic response. Working patients in particular may find these side effects so objectionable (sedation!) that they discontinue the medication on their own, depriving themselves of any further therapeutic benefits.

As noted in the previous sections, preparations of St. John's wort are no more effective than conventional synthetic antidepressants. Their advantage, especially in the ambulatory setting, is that they are extremely well tolerated by patients. As observational studies in 3250 treatment cases have shown, there is about a 3 % incidence of relatively harmless side effects. This rate is far lower than that associated with even the modern non-tricyclic antidepressants (10–25 %).

According to statistical data in the 1996 Drug Report (Schwabe and Paffrath, 1996), the daily treatment costs in Germany average about $ .75 for tricyclic antidepressants (which cause numerous side effects) and about $ 2.25 for non-tricyclic antidepressants (which have fewer side effects). Treatment with the highest-dose and best-documented commercial product made from St. John's wort has an average daily cost of about $ .80.

2.2.10
Drug Products

The *Rote Liste 1995* identifies 18 single-herb hypericum products that are marketed in Germany. For the reasons stated earlier, the dose of the active ingredients is based on the total amount of extract in the product (stated in mg). The total hypericin content (stated in µg) must also be considered because, as a marker compound, it provides an index for evaluating the pharmaceutical quality of the original dried herb or extract.

The most widely studied product (the hypericum extract LI 160, marketed as Jarsin 300) is supplied in coated tablets. Each tablet contains 300 mg of extract, standardized to 900 µg total hypericin, as the active ingredient.

References

Araya OS, Ford EJH (1981) An investigation of the type of photosensitization caused by the ingestion of St. John's wort (Hypericum perforatum) by calves. J Comp Pathol 91: 135–141.
Bladt S, Wagner H (1994) Inhibition of MAO by fractions and constituents of hypericum extract. J Geriatr Psychiatry Neurol 7 (Suppl 1): 57–59.

Blumenthal M, Hall T, Rister RS (eds) German Commission E Monographs. Therapeutic Monographs on Medicinal Plants for Human Use by Commission E – a Special Expert Committee of the German Federal Health Agency. American Botanical Council, Austin, TX, in press.

Borsini F, Meli A (1988) Is the forced swimming test a suitable model for revealing antidepressant activity? Psychopharmacology 94: 147–160.

Brockmöller J, Reum T, Bauer S, Kerb R, Hübner WD, Roots I (1997) Hypericin and Pseudohypericin: Pharmacokinetics and Effects on Photosensitivity in Humans. Pharmacopsychiatry (Suppl 2) 30: 94–101.

Butterweck V, Wall A, Liefländer-Wulf U, Winterhoff H, Nahrstedt A (1997) Effects of the Total Extract and Fractions of Hypericum perforatum in Animal Assays for Antidepressant Activity. Pharmacopsychiatry (Suppl 2) 30: 117–124.

Cott JM (1997) In vitro receptor binding and enzyme inhibition by Hypericum perforatum extract. Pharmacopsychiatry (Suppl 2) 30: 108–112.

Czygan FC (1993) Kulturgeschichte und Mystik des Johanniskrautes. Z Phytother 14: 276–281.

Daniel K (1939) Inhaltsstoffe und Prüfmethoden homöopathisch verwendeter Arzneipflanzen. Hippokrates 10: 5–6.

Engelhardt A (1962) Justinus Kerner und das Johanniskraut. Apotheker-Dienst Roche 3: 51–55.

Ernst E (1995) St. John's wort, an antidepressant? A systematic, criteria-based overview. Phytomedicine 2: 67–71.

Giese AC (1980) Hypericism. Photochem Photobiol Rev 5: 229–255.

Halama P (1991) Wirksamkeit des Johanniskrautextraktes LI 160 bei depressiver Verstimmung. Nervenheilkunde 10: 250–253.

Hänsel R, Keller K, Rimpler H, Schneider G (eds) (1993) Hagers Handbuch der Pharmazeutischen Praxis, 5th Edition, Drogen E–O. Springer Verlag, Berlin Heidelberg New York, pp 268–292.

Hänsgen KD, Vesper J, Ploch M (1994) Multicenter Double-Blind Study Examining the Antidepressant Effectiveness of the Hypericum Extract LI 160. J Geriatr Psychiatry Neurol 7 (Suppl 1): 15–18.

Hänsgen KD, Vesper J (1996) Antidepressive Wirksamkeit eines hochdosierten Hypericum-Extraktes. Münch Med Wschr 138: 29–33.

Harrer G, Schulz V (1994) Clinical investigation of the antidepressant effectiveness of hypericum. J Geriatr Psychiatry Neurol 7 (Suppl 1): 6–8.

Harrer G, Hübner WD, Podzuweit H (1994) Effectiveness and Tolerance of the Hypericum Extract LI 160 Compared to Maprotiline: A Multicenter Double-Blind Study. J Geriatr Psychiatry Neurol 7 (Suppl 1): 28–28.

Hübner WD, Lande S, Podzuweit H (1994) Hypericum Treatment of Mild Depressions with Somatic Symptoms. J Geriatr Psychiatry Neurol 7 (Suppl 1): 12–14.

Jenike MA (ed) (1994) Hypericum: a novel antidepressant. J Geriatr Psychiatry Neurol 7: S 1–S 68.

Johnson D, Siebenhüner G, Hofer E, Sauerwein-Giese E, Frauendorf A (1992) Einfluss von Johanniskraut auf die ZNS-Aktivität. Neurol Psychiatr 6: 436–444.

Johnson D, Ksciuk H, Woelk H, Sauerwein-Giese E, Frauendorf A (1994) Effects of Hypericum Extract Compared with Maprotiline on Resting EEG and Evoked Potentials in 24 Volunteers. J Geriatr Psychiatry Neurol 7 (Suppl 1): 44–46.

Kerb R, Brockmöller J, Staffeldt B, Ploch M, Roots I (1996) Single-dose and steady-state pharmacokinetics of hypericin and pseudohypericin. J Clin Pharmacol Therapeutics 40: 2087–2093.

Laux G (1995) Kontrollierte Vergleichsstudien mit Moclobemid in der Depressionsbehandlung. Münch Med Wschr 137: 296–300.

Lehrl S, Willemsen A, Papp R, Woelk H (1993) Ergebnisse von Messungen der kognitiven Leistungsfähigkeit bei Patienten unter der Therapie mit Johanniskraut-Extrakt. Nervenheilkunde 12: 281–284.

Leuschner J (1995) Gutachten zur experimentellen Toxikologie von Hypericum-Extrakt Ll 160. Lichtwer Pharma GmbH, Berlin.

Linde K, Ramirez G, Mulrow CD, Pauls M, Weidenhammer W, Melchart D (1996) St. John's wort for depression – an overview and meta-analysis of randomized clinical trials. Br Med J 313: 253–258.

Martinez B, Kasper S, Ruhrmann S, Möller HJ (1994) Hypericum in the Treatment of Seasonal Affective Disorders. J Geriatr Psychiatry Neurol 7 (Suppl 1): 29–33.

Müller WEG, Rossol R (1994) Effects of hypericum extract on the expression of serotonin receptors. J Geriatr Psychiatry Neurol 7 (Suppl 1): 63–64.

Müller WE, Kasper S (ed) (1997) Hypericum Extract (LI 160) as a Herbal Antidepressant. Pharmacopsychiatry (Suppl 2) 30: 71–134.

Müller WE, Roli M, Schäfer C, Hafner U (1997) Effects of Hypericum Extract (LI 160) on Biochemical Models of Antidepressant Activity. Pharmacopsychiatry (Suppl 2) 30: 102–107.

Nahrstedt A, Butterweck V (1997) Biologically active and other chemical constituents of the herb of Hypericum perforatum L. Pharmacopsychiatry (Suppl 2) 30: 129–134.

Niesel S (1992) Untersuchungen zum Freisetzungsverhalten und zur Stabilität ausgewählter wertbestimmender Pflanzeninhaltsstoffe unter besonderer Berücksichtigung moderner phytochemischer Analysenverfahren. Inaugural-Dissertation. Freie Universität Berlin.

NN (1995) Hypericin (VIMRxyn®), a promising new antiviral agent. Scientific report. VIMRx Pharmaceuticals Inc., Stanford, USA.

Perovic S, Müller WEG (1995) Pharmacological profile of hypericum extract: effect on serotonine uptake by postsynaptic receptors. Arzneimittelforschung/Drug Res 45: 1145–1148.

Riederer P, Laux G, Pöldinger W (1993) Neuro-Psychopharmaka. Ein Therapie-Handbuch, Vol. 3: Antidepressiva und Phasenprophylaktika. Springer-Verlag Vienna New York, pp 1–10.

Schmidt U, Harrer G, Kuhn U, Berger-Deinert W, Luther D (1993) Wechselwirkungen von Hypericum-Extrakt mit Alkohol. Nervenheilkunde 12: 314–319.

Schulz H, Jobert M (1994) Effects of Hypericum Extract on the Sleep EEG in Older Volunteers. J Geriatr Psychiatry Neurol 7 (Suppl 1): 39–43.

Schwabe U, Paffrath D (eds) (1996) Arzneiverordnungsreport '96. Gustav Fischer Verlag, Stuttgart Jena.

Smith AL, Weissmann MM (1992) Epidemiology. In: Paykel ES (ed) Handbook of Affective Disorders. Churchill Livinstone, 2nd Edition, pp 111–129.

Sommer H, Harrer G (1994) Placebo-Controlled Double-Blind Study Examining the Effectiveness of a Hypericum Preparation in 105 Mildly Depressed Patients. J Geriatr Psychiatry Neurol 7 (Suppl 1): 9–11.

Staffeldt B, Kerb R, Brockmöller J, Ploch M, Roots I (1993) Pharmakokinetik von Hypericin und Pseudohypericin nach oraler Einnahme des Johanniskraut-Extraktes LI 160 bei gesunden Probanden. Nervenheilkunde 12: 331–338.

Suzuki O, Katsumata Y, Oya M, Bladt S, Wagner H (1984) Inhibition of monoamine oxidase by hypericin. Planta Med 50: 272–274

Thiebot M, Martin P, Puech AJ (1992) Animal behavioral studies in the evaluation of antidepressant drugs. Brit J Psych 160 (Suppl. 15): 44–50.

Thiede HM, Walper A (1994) Inhibition of MAO and COMT by hypericum extracts and hypericin. J Geriatr Psychiatry Neurol 7 (Suppl 1): 54–56.

Thiele B, Brink I, Ploch M (1993) Modulation of cytokine expression by hypericum extract. J Geriatr Psychiatry Neurol 7 (Suppl 1): 60–62.

Volz HP, Hänsel R (1995) Hypericum (Johanniskraut) als pflanzliches Antidepressivum. Psychopharmakotherapie 2: 1–9.

Volz HP (1997) Controlled clinical trials of hypericum extracts in depressed patients – an overview. Pharmacopsychiatry (Suppl 2) 30: 72–76.

Vorbach EU, Hübner WD, Arnoldt KH (1994) Effectiveness and Tolerance of the Hypericum Extract LI 160 in Comparison with Imipramine: Randomized Double-Blind Study with 135 Outpatients. J Geriatr Psychiatry Neurol 7 (Suppl 1): 19–23.

Vorbach EU, Arnoldt KH, Hübner WD (1997) Efficacy and tolerability of St. John's wort extract LI 160 versus imipramine in patients with severe depressive episodes according to ICD-10. Pharmacopsychiatry (Suppl 2) 30: 81–85.

Wagner H, Bladt S (1994) Pharmaceutical quality of hypericum extracts. J Geriatr Psychiatr Neurol 7 (Suppl 1): 65–68.

Wheatley D (1997) LI 160, an Extract of St. John's Wort, Versus Amitriptyline in Mildly to Moderately Depressed Outpatients – A Controlled 6-week Clinical Trial. Pharmacopsychiatry (Suppl 2) 30: 77–80.

Willner P (1984) The validity of animal models of depression. Psychopharmacology 83: 1–16.

Winterhoff H, Hambrügge M, Vahlensieck W (1993) Testung von Hypericum perforatum L. im Tierexperiment. Nervenheilkunde 12: 341–345.

Woelk H, Burkard G, Grünwald J (1994) Benefits and Risks of the Hypericum Extract LI 160: Drug Monitoring Study with 3250 Patients. J Geriatr Psychiatry Neurol 7 (Suppl 1): 34–38.

2.3
Kava as an Anxiolytic

2.3.1
Introduction

When Europeans discovered the island world of Oceania in the 18th century, they learned about the custom of kava drinking. Natives of Polynesia, Melanesia, and Micronesia harvested the large rhizome of the kava shrub *(Piper methysticum)*, masticated it, and mixed it with water and coconut milk to make a beverage that produced a calming, relaxing effect without altering consciousness. Published reports on kava quickly led to studies aimed at isolating the psychotropic active principle and elucidating its chemical structure. It was not until 1966 that the German pharmacologist H. J. Meyer proved that the characteristic effects of the kava beverage were due to kavapyrones (kavalactones). These compounds are poorly water-soluble and, to become bioavailable, must be converted to a finely divided form. The first kava product to appear on the drug market contained synthetic kawain. Most subsequent kava products have contained extracts from the kava rhizome; only the extract-based products are considered true phytomedicines. The pharmacy, pharmacology, and clinical characteristics of kava preparations are reviewed in Hänsel and Woelk (1995).

2.3.2 Botanical Description

The kava shrub *(Piper methysticum)* grows to a height of 2–3 m. It has large, hard-shaped leaves and bears numerous small flowers arranged in clusters shaped like ears of corn. The crude drug is obtained from the large, branched, juicy rhizome which can weigh up to 10 kg (Fig. 2.12). The actual home of the kava plant is unknown but may have been Vanuatu (formerly New Hebrides). As Polynesians settled the surrounding Pacific islands, the shrub became naturalized to areas as far east as Hawaii. Today kava is cultivated commercially, and no longer grows in the wild.

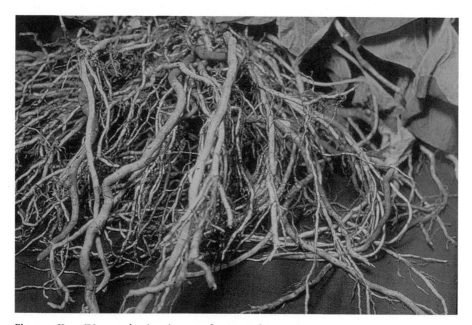

Fig. 2.12. Kava *(Piper methysticum):* roots of a young plant.

2.3.3
Crude Drug and Extract

The crude drug consists of the dried rhizome. It has a faintly aromatic odor and a slightly bitter, soapy, acrid taste. Chewing a piece of kava rhizome causes prolonged numbness of the tongue and stimulates salivation.

The kava beverage is made by chewing or grinding the dried rhizome, macerating it in cold water, and straining off the liquid. Medicinal extracts are prepared by extracting the dried herb with an ethanol-water mixture (for extracts containing about 30 % kavapyrones) or with an acetone-water mixture (for extracts containing about 70 % kavapyrones). The herb-to-extract ratio is about 12–20:1 in both preparations. Kavapyrones are very poorly soluble in water, so for medicinal use they must be placed in colloidal solution or at least converted to a finely divided form to promote absorption from the gastrointestinal tract.

2.3.4
Key Constituents, Analysis, Pharmacokinetics

The kava rhizome is among the few phytomedicines whose key active constituents (see Sect. 1.2) are known. They are the kavapyrones, including kawain (1–2 % in the crude drug), dihydrokawain (0.6–1%), methysticin (1.2–2%), and dihydromethysticin (0.5–0.8%). The dried herb should contain at least 3.5 % kavapyrones, calculated as kawain. Quantitative analysis of the kawains is accomplished by photometric assay of the total fraction or of its individual components following separation by HPLC. Despite their low water solubility, kawain and dihydrokawain were shown to be readily absorbed from the gastrointestinal tract. In experiments with mice, plasma levels of approximately 2 μg/mL kawain were measured 30 min after the oral administration of 100 mg/kg b.w. of a kava extract containing 70 % kavapyrones. Kawain levels in the brain tissue were approximately the same and paralleled the time course of the plasma levels. The kavapyrones have a plasma half-life ranging from 90 min to several hours. Bioavailability depends strongly on the galenic formulation and can vary 10-fold among different preparations (Hänsel et al., 1994).

2.3.5
Pharmacology and Toxicology

The four pyrones of the kawain-methysticin type act centrally as muscle relaxants and anticonvulsants; their actions are comparable to those of mephenesin. They exert a strong protective effect against experimental strychnine poisoning and are superior in this regard to all previously known, non-narcotic strychnine antagonists. The kawains and methysticins reduce the excitability of the limbic system as measured by electrical stimulation of corresponding brain areas in rabbits; this is analogous to the effect produced by benzodiazepine. Methysticin and dihydromethysticin show marked neuroprotective properties in mice and rats, significantly reducing the volume of an ischemic infarction induced by ligation of the middle cerebral artery. The two methysticins have the same potency as memantine in this infarction model. Peripherally, the kawains act as local anesthetics comparable in potency to the topical anesthetics cocaine and benzocaine (Jamieson et al., 1989; Backhaus and Krieglstein, 1992).

A kava extract containing 70 % kavapyrones was tested for toxic effects in rats and dogs over a 26-week period. The maximum dose was 320 mg/kg (rats) or 60 mg/kg (dogs). The highest doses were associated with mild histopathologic changes in liver and kidney tissues. The dogs tolerated 24 mg/kg/day and the rats 20 mg/kg/day with no adverse reactions. Testing of the same extract in corresponding in vitro models showed no evidence of mutagenic potential. Only dihydromethysticin has been tested for genotoxicity, and no teratogenic effects were observed (Hänsel et al., 1994).

There have been reports from Australia and the South Sea region of toxic reactions in humans following the consumption of kava beverages. The following symptoms were observed after the ingestion of up to 13 liters/day, equivalent to 300–400 g of dried rhizome powder per week: ataxia, skin rash, hair loss, yellowing of the skin and scleras, redness of the eyes, visual accommodation difficulties, respiratory problems, and loss of appetite. It should be noted that these dose levels are at least 100 times higher than the clinically tested and recommended therapeutic doses (Hänsel et al., 1994).

2.3.6
Clinical Efficacy

The therapeutic efficacy of an anxiolytic drug can be documented only by therapeutic trials in patients; studies in healthy subjects are of no value. Human pharmacologic studies are nevertheless useful in that they can provide evidence of possible mechanisms of action, associated effects, and side effects. A kava extract containing 70 % kavapyrones (designated in the literature as WS 1490, brand name Laitan) was investigated in four human pharmacologic studies (Johnson et al., 1991; Emser and Bartylla, 1991; Herberg, 1991; Münte et al, 1993). The first two studies were open, and the last two were double-blinded and placebo-controlled. The key parameters were drug-induced EEG changes and psychometric tests of intellectual and motor functioning. According to the authors, the observed EEG changes and (partial) psychometric test results showed no evidence of a decline in vigilance or responsiveness in subjects who took the extract for up to 14 days at doses equivalent to 105 mg, 210 mg, or 420 mg of kavapyrones daily. The author of one study (Herberg, 1991) concluded that use of the kava extract did not impair the ability to drive a motor vehicle. In another human pharmacologic study using a crossover design, a kava extract standardized to 30 % kavapyrones (brand name Antares 120, equivalent to 120 mg/day kavalactones) was compared to a placebo over a treatment period of 7 days. The results, based on quantitative EEG studies and psychometric testing, were similar to those of the studies described above (Gessner and Cnota, 1994).

To date, a total of six controlled double-blind studies have been published on the therapeutic efficacy of kava kava in patients. Two of the studies were done with an extract standardized to 15 % kavapyrones (Bhate et al., 1989; Warnecke et al., 1990) and four with an extract standardized to 70 % kavapyrones (WS 1490, brand name Laitan). Details on the studies are shown in Table 2.8. The results of the study by

Table 2.8. Controlled double-blind studies with kava extract preparations. The first two studies used standardized extracts containing 15% kavapyrones; the next four used a standardized extract containing 70% kavapyrones. Dosage figures are based on the kavapyrones.

First author, year	Cases (n)	Dose (mg/day)	Duration (days)	Indications, key parameters, and results
Bhate, 1989	59	60	2	Improvement in perioperative mood, questionable clinical relevance
Warnecke, 1990	40	30–60	56–84	Climacteric symptoms, Kuppermann index and ASI scale significant vs. placebo
Warnecke, 1991	40	210	56	Climacteric symptoms, HAMA, DSI and Kuppermann index significant vs. placebo
Kinzler, 1991	58	210	28	Anxiety syndrome, HAMA, EWL, CGI, FSUCL index significant vs. placebo
Woelk, 1993	172	210	42	Anxiety syndrome, HAMA, CGI, KEPS and EAAS not significant vs. oxazepam and bromazepam
Volz, 1995	100	210	168	HAMA, CGI, Bf-S

Abbreviations: ASI = Anxiety Status Inventory; HAMA = Hamilton Anxiety Scale; DSI = Depression Status Inventory; CGI = Clinical Global Impressions; Bf-S = von Zerssen mood scale; EWL = adjective list; FSUCL = Fischer Somatic Symptoms or Undesired Effects Checklist; KEPS = brief test for evaluating personality structure; EAAS = Erlanger scale for anxiety, aggression, and tension.

Bhate et al. are of dubious clinical relevance due to the brief duration of treatment (2 doses of 60 mg kavapyrones) and the nature of the results (nonstandard scoring scale, relatively small numerical differences between the treatment groups).

Warnecke et al. (1990, 1991) conducted two placebo-controlled therapeutic studies, each involving 40 women with menopausal symptoms. Each of the studies used different preparations and dosages (see Table 2.8). The duration of treatment was at least 56 days in both studies. In the second study, the total score on the Hamilton Anxiety Rating Scale (HAMA) was used as the confirmatory parameter, and three other scales were used as adjuncts. The total HAMA score showed significant improvement after just 1 week on the kava extract and reached a plateau after 4 weeks' therapy (Fig. 2.13). Overall, the therapeutic response was highly significant in relation to the placebo ($p < 0.001$).

In the study of Kinzler et al. (1991), 58 patients from 18 to 60 years of age with symptoms of anxiety, tension, or agitation of nonpsychotic origin were tested against a placebo in a 4-week double-blind comparative study. Again, the confirmatory parameter was the total score on the Hamilton Anxiety Rating Scale. A comparison of the groups after 1 week's therapy already showed a significant disparity in total scores. This difference continued to increase over the next 3 weeks. The results of the adjunctive rating scales correlated with the HAMA scores. Surprisingly, no unpleasant or adverse side effects were observed in patients taking the medication.

In a study by Woelk et al. (1993), the effect of a daily dose equivalent to 210 mg of kavapyrones was compared with that of 15 mg/day oxazepam or 9 mg/day bromazepam in a double-blind study lasting 6 weeks. The main study criterion was a decline

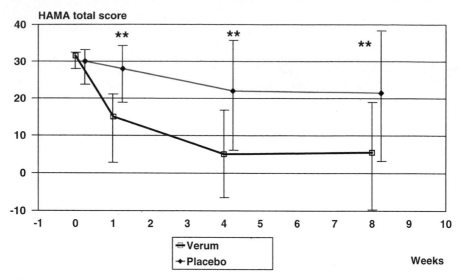

Fig. 2.13. Progression of Hamilton anxiety scores (HAMA) during 8 weeks' treatment with a kava extract equivalent to a dose of 210 mg/day kava pyrones. ** = p < 0.01 (Warnecke et al., 1991).

in total score on the HAMA rating scale. When a total of 164 treatment protocols had been completed, the improvement in symptoms was approximately the same in all three treatment groups (Fig. 2.14). Because the statistical analysis focused on the degree of difference rather than the demonstration of equivalence, however, we cannot conclude that the drugs are equally effective in the strict sense.

One criticism that has been leveled at all therapeutic studies with kava extracts is that the inclusion criteria were not sufficiently rigorous and allowed the inclusion of a heterogeneous population (depression with anxious features, panic disorders, phobias, somatoform disorders, and generalized anxiety disorders) (Volz and Hänsel, 1994).

In a randomized, placebo-controlled, double-blind multi-center study based on Good Clinical Practice (GCP) guidelines and lasting 6 months, the efficacy and tolerance of the kava extract WS 1490 were tested in 100 outpatients with nervous conditions involving states of anxiety, tension, and unrest. The daily dose was 300 mg of extract, equivalent to 210 mg of kavapyrones. The main criterion was the change in total HAMA scores from the start of therapy to its termination (week 24). A comparison of the change in total HAMA scores showed a significant (p = 0.015) superiority of the kava extract over the placebo. The difference between the treatment groups was significant after just 8 weeks (p = 0.05). The kava extract was very well tolerated, with 5 reports of unpleasant side effects versus 15 reports from patients taking the placebo (Volz, 1995).

Besides the six double-blind therapeutic studies with kava extracts, a total of nine double-blind studies have been done with the isolated compound DL-kawain. Two of the studies compared kawain with reference drugs and seven compared it with a placebo. The therapeutic results achieved with doses of 200–600 mg/day in these studies were similar to the results of studies using extracts, but they were also similar

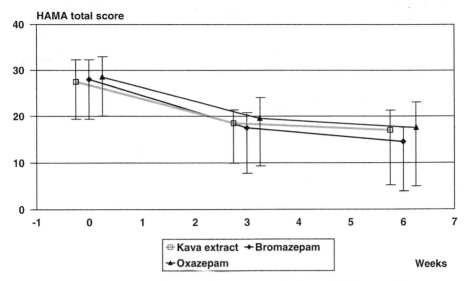

Fig. 2.14. Progression of scores of the Hamilton Anxiety Scale (HAMA) during 6 weeks' treatment with a kava extract equivalent to 210 mg/day kavapyrones compared with 15 mg/day oxazepam and 9 mg/day bromazepam. There were no statistically significant differences in the degree of improvement achieved in the three treatment groups (Woelk et al., 1993).

with regard to deficiences noted in the study methodologies (Volz and Hänsel, 1994). Nevertheless, the placebo-controlled studies in particular allow us to apply the results obtained with extracts to pure compounds and vice-versa to a certain degree, although treatment with isolated compounds is, by definition, outside the bounds of phytotherapy (Sect. 1.2).

2.3.7
Side Effects and Risks

In an observation study of 4049 patients who took 105 mg/day of an extract standardized to 70 % kavapyrones for 7 weeks, objectionable side effects were documented in 61 patients, representing an incidence of 1.5 %. The side effects were mild in nature and reversible. Most consisted of gastrointestinal complaints or allergic skin reactions. A 4-week study in 3029 patients who took 800 mg/day of an extract standardized to 30 % kavapyrones (= 240 mg kavapyrones) showed a 2.3 % incidence of unpleasant side effects. All these effects were mild, consisting of 9 cases of allergic reactions, 31 cases of gastrointestinal discomfort, and 22 cases of headache or dizziness (Hänsel et al., 1994; Hoffmann and Winter, 1993).

The prolonged use of kava can cause a transient yellowish discoloration of the skin and its appendages; the product should be discontinued if this occurs. Allergic skin reactions can occur in rare cases. There have also been reports of impaired visual accommodation, pupillary dilation, and disturbances of oculomotor equilibrium. Twenty-nine of 200 chronic kava drinkers from Polynesia had pellagra-like skin changes that did not respond to 4 weeks' treatment with 100 mg niacinamide (Ruze, 1990). Chronic abuse of kava preparations has been associated with even more serious toxic effects (Siegel, 1976).

2.3.8
Indications and Dosages

The results of clinical studies indicate that mild anxiety states due to various causes are the primary indication for the use of kava preparations. Commission E defined the indications as "states of nervous anxiety, tension, and agitation" in its 1990 monograph on kava rhizome. The doses of kava extracts used in clinical studies were in the range of 60–120 mg of kavapyrones daily. Generally the duration of use should not exceed 3 months.

2.3.9
Therapeutic Significance

Kava preparations are an herbal alternative to synthetic anxiolytics and tranquilizers, particularly the benzodiazepines. Based on the study of Woelk et al. (1993), suitable kava preparations appear to have an efficacy comparable to that of benzodiazepines in the treatment of anxiety symptoms. In contrast to benzodiazepines, previous experience with the therapeutic use of kava preparations has shown no evidence that there is any potential for physical or psychological dependency (Hänsel et al., 1994). This represents a significant advantage of kava preparations over the benzodiazepines. The daily treatment costs in Germany of approximately $ .60 – $ 1.25 are slightly higher than that of benzodiazepine tranquilizers.

References

Backhaus C, Krieglstein J (1992) Extract of kava and its methysticine constituents protect brain tissue against ischemic damage in rodents. J Pharmacol 215: 265–269.
Bhate H, Gerster G, Gracza E (1989) Orale Prämedikation mit Zubereitungen aus Piper methysticum bei operativen Eingriffen in Epiduralanästhesie. Erfahrungsheilkunde 6: 339–345.
Emser W, Bartylla K (1991) Verbesserung der Schlafqualität. TW Neurol Psychiatr 5: 636–642.
Gessner B, Cnota P (1994) Untersuchung der Vigilanz nach Applikation von Kava-Kava-Extrakt, Diazepam oder Placebo. Z Phytother 15: 30–37.
Hänsel R, Keller K, Rimpler H, Schneider G (eds) (1994) Hagers Handbuch der Pharmazeutischen Praxis, 6th Edition, Drogen E–O. Springer Verlag, Berlin Heidelberg New York, pp 201–221.
Hänsel R, Woelk H (1995) Spektrum Kava-Kava. 2nd Edition. Aesopus Verlag GmbH, Basel.
Herberg KW (1991) Fahrtüchtigkeit nach Einnahme von Kava-Spezial-Extrakt WS 1490. Z Allg Med 67: 842–846.
Hofmann R, Winter U (1993) Therapeutische Möglichkeiten mit einem hochdosierten standardisierten Kava-Kava-Präparat (Antares 120) bei Angsterkrankungen. V. Phytotherapiekongress; Bonn Nov. 3–5.
Jamieson DD, Duffield PH, Cheng D, Duffield AM (1989) Comparison of the central nervous system activity of the aqueous and lipid extract of kava (Piper methysticum). Arch Int Pharmacodyn 301: 66–80.

Johnson E, Frauendorf A, Stecker K, Stein U (1991) Neurophysiologisches Wirkprofil und Verträg-lichkeit von Kava-Extrakt WS 1490. TW Neurol Psychiatr 5: 349–354.
Kinzler E, Krömer J, Lehmann (1991) Wirksamkeit eines Kava-Spezial-Extraktes bei Patienten mit Angst-, Spannungs- und Erregungszuständen nicht-psychotischer Genese. Arzneim Forsch/Drug Res 41: 584–588.
Münte TF, Heinze HJ, Matzke M, Steitz J (1993) Effects of oxacepam and an extract of kava roots (Piper methysticum) on event-related potentials in a word recognition task. Neuropsychobiology 27: 46–53.
Ruze P (Iggo) Kava-induced dermopathy: a niacin deficiency? Lancet: 1442–1445.
Siegel RK (1976) Herbal intoxication. Psychoactive effects from herbal cigarettes, tea and capsules. JAMA 236: 473–476.
Volz HP, Hänsel R (1994) Kava-Kava und Kavain in der Psychopharmakotherapie. Psychopharmako-therapie 1: 33–39.
Volz HP (1995) Die anxiolytische Wirksamkeit von Kava-Spezialextrakt WS 1490 unter Langzeitthe-rapie – eine randomisierte Doppelblindstudie. Z Phytother Abstractband, p 9.
Warnecke G, Pfaender H, Gerster G, Gracza E (1990) Wirksamkeit von Kawa-Kawa-Extrakt beim kli-makterischen Syndrom. Z Phytother 11: 81–86.
Woelk H, Kapoula O, Lehrl S, Schröter K, Weinholz P (1993) Behandlung von Angst-Patienten, Z Allg Med 69: 271–277.

2.4
Restlessness and Sleep Disturbances

States of nervous unrest and sleep disturbances are considered traditional indica-tions for the use of preparations made from valerian, hops, lemon balm, and passion flower. These are gentle herbs that do not produce strong sedative or hypnotic ef-fects. It is true that several constituents have been isolated that appear to have seda-tive effects in some experimental settings, such as valepotriates and valerenic acids isolated from valerian. But the final concentrations of these compounds in medicinal products are so low that they could hardly account for any sedative or tranquilizing effects in human patients.

Valerian is somewhat unique in that its actions and efficacy have been better documented (for selected valerian extracts) than for the other three herbs men-tioned above. Moreover, valerian is a widely known herb both in Germany and abroad, so a separate section will be devoted to its discussion.

2.4.1
Valerian

2.4.1.1
Medicinal Plant
The medicinal valerian used at our latitudes (*Valeriana officinalis*, Fig. 2.15) is but one of approximately 250 valerian species that occur worldwide. Native to Europe and the temperate zones of Asia, it is an erect perennial that reaches a height of about 50–150 cm. It prefers damp, swampy areas and blooms from June to August, developing tiny white to pink flowers that grow in terminal cymes. Valerian for me-dicinal use is cultivated and harvested from September to October. Besides the offi-cial medicinal species, there are other valerian species (V. edulis, V. japonica, V. indi-ca) whose therapeutic uses are not based on the tradition and experience of Eur-

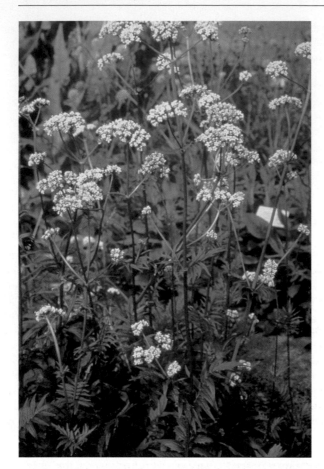

Fig. 2.15.
European valerian *(Valeriana officinalis)*.

opean medicine. Indian valerian and especially the Mexican species *(V. edulis)* are associated with a higher therapeutic risk due to their high content of valepotriates (up to 8 %).

2.4.1.2
Crude Drug and Extract

Only the root of European valerian *(Valeriana officinalis)* is used as an official drug. The characteristic unpleasant odor of valerian, strongly reminiscent of isovaleric (isovalerenic) acid and camphor, appears only after the root has been cut and dried. The cut, dried herb is used in tea preparations. Pharmaceutical products are mainly produced from aqueous or aqueous-alcoholic extracts (70 % ethanol, herb-to-extract ratio 4–7:1). The aqueous and ethanol extracts of valerian root are by no means equivalent in the quality of their actions, however, and they are used in different dosages. The dose for aqueous extracts is based on the traditional tea application, which uses a minimum dose of 2 g of dried herb and a herb-to-extract ratio of 5:1 to yield a single dose of approximately 400 mg. The dose for alcoholic dry extracts is not easily derived from traditional applications, and clinical studies with specific extracts are needed to gain better information on proper dosing.

2.4.1.3
Key Compounds, Analysis, and Pharmacokinetics

The dried root contains, on average, 0.3–0.8 % volatile oil. The characteristic odor is caused by small amounts of isovaleric acid, which is formed by the breakdown of valepotriates. More than 100 constituents have been identified to date, but it is unknown which of them is responsible for the characteristic medicinal actions of the root. Medicinal valerian contains 0.1–0.3 % of the two sesquiterpenes valerenic acid and acetoxyvalerenic acid. These characteristic constituents do not occur in species that grow outside Europe. Thus, both compounds make suitable marker compounds for testing the pharmaceutical quality of valerian extracts.

The carefully dried root also contains up to 1 % valepotriates (up to 8 % in Mexican valerian). Chemically, these compounds are esters of lower fatty acids, i. e., of acetic acid, isovaleric acid, and β-acetoxyisovaleric acid, with a trivalent alcohol. The alcohol component displays the C_{10} carbon skeleton of monoterpenes and contains an epoxy ring, which is mainly responsible for the instability and mutagenic potential of valerian extracts (see Sect. 2.4.1.4). Because the valepotriates are unstable in an acid or alkaline milieu and at higher temperatures, they can be administered only in solid dosage forms (preferably enteric-coated tablets), not in liquid preparations (tinctures).

No data are yet available on the absorption, distribution, and elimination of the components of valerian extracts in humans. Studies on absorption and distribution kinetics in mice have shown that the valepotriates are absorbed by the gastric mucosa, but in small amounts (Hänsel et al., 1994).

2.4.1.4
Pharmacology and Toxicology

Pharmacologic studies have focused on various constituents of the valerian root. Attention was first directed to the volatile oils because it was thought that the action of valerian was mediated by olfactory receptors (Hazelhoff et al., 1984). The volatile oil of valerian consists mainly of valeric acid and isovaleric acid. Other authors tested the valepotriates as possible active principles. Behavioral tests in cats given 10 mg of valepotriate mixture/kg by stomach tube showed a calmative effect manifested by a decrease in restless, fearful, and aggressive behaviors (Eickstedt, 1969). Later studies in rats showed that valepotriates exerted no central nervous system effects in either low or high doses (up to 50 mg/kg) (Grusla, 1987; Krieglstein, 1988).

Experimental studies of valerenic acids in laboratory animals demonstrated sedative and anticonvulsant activity (Hendriks et al., 1985). Riedel, Hänsel, and Ehrke (1982) performed in vitro studies showing that valerenic acid decreased the degradation rate of γ-aminobutyric acid (GABA). The most recent studies (Santos et al., 1994) showed an increased concentration of GABA in the synaptic cleft after the administration of valerian. These authors used a valerian extract rather than isolated valerenic acid. They found that this extract increased the secretion of GABA from the synaptosomes and inhibited its reuptake. GABA is considered an important inhibitory neurotransmitter that plays a key role in stress and anxiety. Thus, these results are highly promising and could partly explain the therapeutic actions of valerian extract. Other animal studies have shown that the whole extract has central calmative effects that are not referable to valeric acids, valepotriates, or the volatile oil fraction (Krieglstein, 1988). On the whole, the results of pharmacologic studies give an inconsistent picture, and we cannot yet draw definite conclusions on the specific constituents that underlie the therapeutic properties of valerian extracts.

No animal studies have yet been done on the toxicity of valerian extracts. The constituent valeranone showed very low toxicity in experiments on mice and rats (Rücker et al., 1978). The valepotriates have shown alkylating, cytotoxic, and mutagenic properties in vitro (Braun et al., 1982, 1985), but these effects were not from the valepotriates themselves but from their metabolites baldrinal and homobaldrinal. Baldrinals form in the gastrointestinal tract, are almost quantitatively absorbed, and are subject to a strong first-pass effect. Glucuronidation of these metabolites yields esters that are no longer genotoxic. At most, then, the administration of valepotriates may pose some genotoxic risk to the gastrointestinal tract and liver.

2.4.1.5
Pharmacologic Effects in Humans and Clinical Efficacy in Patients

Table 2.9 reviews ten controlled clinical studies dealing with valerian preparations containing no other herbal extracts. However the doses stated in column 3 refer to various types of extract. The study by Jansen (1977) did not specify the nature of the extract. The next four studies (Leathwood and Chauffard, 1983, 1984; Kamm-Kohl et al., 1984; Balderer and Borbely, 1985) used freeze-dried aqueous valerian extracts (with a 3–6:1 ratio of dried herb to extract). Schulz (1994, 1995) and Vorbach (1996) used ethanol extracts. The doses indicated for the two most recent studies refer to a standardized ethanol extract (70 % v/v, herb-to-extract ratio 4–7:1, valerenic acid content 0.4–0.6 %).

Three of the studies (Leathwood and Chauffard, 1983, 1984; Balderer and Borbely, 1985) were done in healthy subjects. The other five studies in Table 2.9 were conducted in patients with sleep disorders.

Leathwood reported in 1983 and 1984 on the results of studies in three groups of healthy subjects. In each case the test dose was taken only once. Two groups consisting of 128 and 8 subjects evaluated their subjective sleep parameters by filling out a self-rating scale the morning after taking the medication. Both studies by Leathwood showed a significant reduction in latency to sleep onset compared with a placebo. The quality of sleep was also improved in one of the three studies. Comparison of the response to 450 mg and 900 mg showed no sign that the measured effects were dose-dependent. In a separate group of 29 subjects, EEG traces recorded in a sleep laboratory showed no significant differences in comparison to placebo.

Balderer and Borbely (1985) reported similar results in a study of healthy subjects. A self-rating scale in 10 subjects indicated a significant decrease in latency to sleep onset and nocturnal awakening, but the sleep EEG's showed no objective evidence of significant effects.

Two other pharmacodynamic studies (Schulz et al., 1994; Schulz and Jobert, 1995) dealt with the effects of ethanol extracts in patients with sleep disorders. The second study (1995) used a randomized crossover design to compare valerian extract

Table 2.9. Controlled clinical studies with valerian extract preparations. The study of Jansen (1977) does not specify the extraction medium. Leathwood (1983, 1984), Kamm-Kohl (1984), and Balderer (1985) used aqueous extracts, while Schulz (1994, 1995) and Vorbach (1996) used an ethanol and water extract (70 % v/v).

First author, year, design, extract	Cases (n)	Dose (mg/day)	Duration (days)	Methods	Results
Jansen, 1977, PDB, type of extract not indicated	150	300	30	Observer rating scale (using 10 psychological symptoms and 8 somatic)	Progressive decrease in intensity of almost all symptoms over a 30-day period in sleep-disturbed patients in a geriatric hospital; no statistical evaluation.
Leathwood, 1983, PDB, aqueous	128	400	1	Self-rating scale	Sleep latency reduced ($p < 0.05$), sleep quality improved ($p < 0.05$);
	29	400	1	Sleep EEG	no significant effects on EEG.
Leathwood, 1984, PDB, aqueous	8	450 900	1	Self-rating scale	Sleep latency reduced ($p < 0.01$), but response was not dose-dependent.
Kamm-Kohl, 1984, PDB, aqueous	80	270	14	von Zerssen mood scale, NOSIE scale, sleep score	Significant improvements ($p < 0.01$) in mood (von Zerssen), behavioral disturbances (NOSIE), and difficulties falling asleep and staying asleep in geriatric hospital patients.
Balderer, 1985, PDB crossover, aqueous	10	450 900	1	Self-rating scale	Significant, dose-dependent decrease in sleep latency ($p < 0.01$) and awakening time ($p < 0.05$).
	8	900	1	Sleep EEG	No significant effects.
Schulz, 1994, PBD crossover, 70 % ethanol	14	405	1 7	Sleep EEG, self-rating scale	Increase in slow-wave sleep and density of K complexes; stage 1 sleep, sleep latency, awakening time, and sleep quality showed no significant changes.
Schulz, 1995, PBD crossover, 70 % ethanol	12	1200	1	Drug-induced EEG changes, flicker fusion frequency (CFF)	EEG: characteristic waveform changes compared with placebo and diazepam. CFF showed no decrease in vigilance.
Vorbach, 1996, PDB, 70 % ethanol	121	600	28	HAMD, CGI scale, Bf-S, SF-B, SRA	Statistically significant effects in 2 scales after 14 days and in 4 scales after 28 days; initially no acute effects on sleep, but progressive improvement in daily mood.

Abbreviations: PDB = placebo-controlled double-blind study; EEG = electroencephalogram; CFF = flicker fusion frequency; Bf-S = von Zerssen mood scale; NOSIE = Nursel9s Observation Scale for Inpatient Evaluation; HAMD = Hamilton Depression Scale; CGI = Clinical Global Impressions; SF-B = sleep questionnaire of Görtelmayer; SRA = sleep rating by physician.

(1200 mg) with diazepam (10 mg), lavender extract (1200 mg), passion flower extract (1200 mg), kava extract (600 mg), and a placebo. All these substances were associated with distinctive patterns of quantitative EEG responses. The herbal extracts, unlike diazepam, caused a relative increase of amplitudes in the theta band of EEG frequencies. The herbs also differed from diazepam in that none of the extracts caused a relative amplitude increase in the beta frequency band. Instead, they tended to cause a reduction in this range that was especially marked with valerian and lavender. The herbal extracts showed varying patterns of effects in the long-wave delta frequency range. Marked increases were observed with lavender extract, moderate increases with valerian and passion flower extract, and decreases with kava extract.

There are, however, two problems with human pharmacodynamic studies based on quantitative EEG analysis. One involves the large range of variation and the poor reproducibility of results when different studies are compared. The second involves the therapeutic interpretation of the data. In themselves, drug-induced EEG changes do not prove therapeutic efficacy. Only controlled therapeutic studies in suitable patient groups can furnish this type of proof. Only three such studies have been conducted to date, one of which (Jansen, 1977) fails to meet current standards because it cannot be statistically evaluated. One of the remaining two studies used an aqueous valerian extract (Kamm-Kohl et al., 1984), and the second used the ethanol extract described above.

Kamm-Kohl et al. (1984) studied the effects of valerian in sleep-disturbed patients from geriatric hospitals. The study involved 150 patients treated for 30 days and 80 patients treated for 14 days, using two standard observer rating scales and a scoring system for rating difficulties falling asleep and staying asleep. The results after 14 days' treatment showed statistically significant improvements in mood (von Zerssen mood scale), behavioral disturbance (NOSIE), and difficulties falling and staying asleep (sleep score).

The results of a recently concluded placebo-controlled double-blind study by Vorbach et al. (1996) are even more impressive. This study involved 121 patients who had experienced significant sleep disturbance for a period of at least 4 weeks. Patients with depression (HAMD > 16) and patients who were taking or had taken medication that could affect sleep were excluded from the study. Therapeutic efficacy was evaluated by four standard rating scales: a physician-rated sleep scale (SRA), the Görtelmayer sleep questionnaire (SF-B), the von Zerssen mood scale (Bf-S), and the Clinical Global Impressions (CGI) scale. All rating scales were administered before the start of treatment, at 14 days, and at 28 days.

The results of this study are shown graphically in Figs. 2.16–2.18. It is noteworthy that the patients observed virtually no acute effects during the initial days of treatment. All the rating scales showed marked placebo effects over the 4-week course of treatment, with the result that the physician-rated sleep scale (SRA) showed no statistically significant differences between the valerian extract and the placebo. The Görtelmayer sleep questionnaire (SF-B) showed no difference at 14 days, but by 28 days there was a significant difference favoring the valerian-treated group (Fig. 2.16). The von Zerssen mood scale (Bf-S) also showed significant intergroup differences after 28 days of treatment (Fig. 2.17). The most pronounced differences were seen with the Clinical Global Impressions (CGI) scale. Ratings by both patient and physician showed very marked differences in favor of the valerian extract, with sta-

SF-B - Feeling rested after sleep

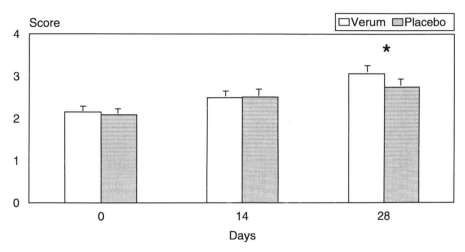

Fig. 2.16. Effect of 4 week's treatment with an ethanol valerian extract (600 mg/day) compared with a placebo. The results were assessed by the Görtelmeyer sleep questionnaire (SF-B) and statistically evaluated. A significant difference between valerian and placebo is seen only after a 4-week course of treatment (Vorbach et al., 1996).

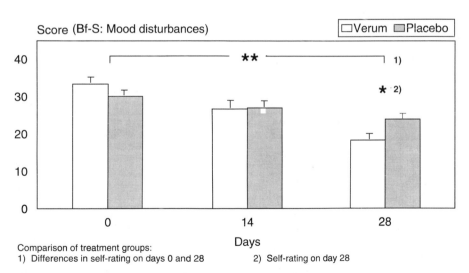

Comparison of treatment groups:
1) Differences in self-rating on days 0 and 28   2) Self-rating on day 28

Fig. 2.17. Same study as in Fig. 2.16, using the von Zerssen scale (Bf-S) for the assessment of daily mood. The valerian and placebo groups show no significant difference after 2 weeks' treatment, but by 4 weeks there is significant improvement with the valerian preparation compared with the placebo.

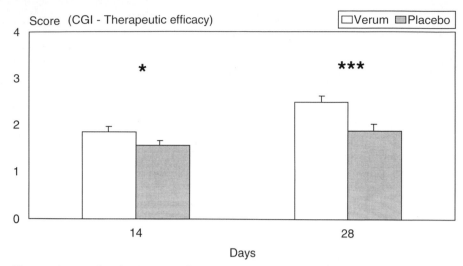

Fig. 2.18. Same study as in Fig. 2.16. Evaluation and statistical analysis of efficacy after 4 weeks' treatment, scored by the physician and patient using Clinical Global Impression (CGI) criteria. Marked intergroup differences are seen at 4 weeks compared with 2 weeks.

tistical analysis indicating a significant difference at 14 days ($p < 0.05$) and a highly significant difference at 28 days ($p < 0.001$; Fig. 2.18).

The results of this study suggest that valerian preparations probably do not produce immediate effects like those of a typical sleep aid, and that 2–4 weeks' therapy is needed to achieve significant improvements, especially in daily mood. The lack of an acute response need not be a disadvantage in sleep-disturbed patients, however, because acute effects can promote dependency and can interfere with necessary psychotherapeutic measures. The delayed onset of action clearly distinguishes valerian from the synthetic hypnotics. Physicians and patients usually associate sleep aids and sedatives with immediate effects, which valerian apparently does not have. Patients should be informed of this at the start of therapy so that they will not discontinue the medication prematurely.

In addition to studies dealing with valerian therapy alone, there are several studies dealing with the combined use of valerian extract and other herbal calmatives. In one double-blind study, a typical combination of valerian and hops extract (150 mg each of valerian extract and hops extract per dose) was compared with flunitrazepam and a placebo in groups of 20 healthy subjects. The test medication was taken in a single morning dose. That afternoon and the following morning, a series of vigilance and reaction tests were administered, and self-assessments were performed using visual analog scales. No impairments were found in the subjects who took the valerian-hops combination, but flunitrazepam was associated with multiple significant impairments based on a decline in vigilance (Gerhard et al., 1996).

2.4.1.6
Indications, Dosages, Risks, and Contraindications

The monograph on valerian root published by Commission E of the former German Health Department in 1985 cites "states of unrest" and "nervous sleep disturbances" as the indications for use. The monograph does not mention contraindications, side effects, or drug-drug interactions. In a recent study, 2 of 61 patients treated with valerian (3.3%) reported side effects consisting of headache and morning grogginess. As for dosage, the monograph recommends taking 2–3 g of the dried herb one to several times daily. Based on the study by Vorbach et al. (1996), it is reasonable to recommend a dose of about 600 mg of the ethanol extract taken 2 h before bedtime.

Objectionable side effects appear to be very rare with products that do not contain valepotriates. There have been occasional reports of headache or gastrointestinal complaints. Products based on Mexican or Indian valerian (which have high concentrations of valepotriates and baldrinals) should not be used due to the mutagenic risk.

2.4.1.7
Therapeutic Significance

As mentioned earlier, valerian is not a suitable agent for the acute treatment of insomnia. Its essential value may lie in its ability to promote natural sleep after several weeks of use, with no risk of dependence or adverse health effects. Thus, valerian offers a gentle alternative to synthetic hypnotics and benzodiazepines in patients with sleep disorders. Due to the lack of an acute response, however, the attending physician must provide suitable counseling, especially at the start of treatment. It is likely that most sleep-disturbed patients have already grown accustomed to the regular use of sleep aids or benzodiazepines. For these patients, it is not enough to change medications; it is also necessary to provide sound, comprehensive management. A suitable valerian preparation can be of substantial benefit in the hands of the family physician.

2.4.2
Hops, Lemon Balm, Passion Flower, and Lavender

Monographs published by Commission E cite restlessness and sleep disturbances as the indications for treatment with hop strobiles, lemon balm leaves, passion flower, and lavender flowers (see Table 2.1). These indications are based on herbal tradition and empirical medicine. There have been no controlled therapeutic studies that can demonstrate efficacy in accordance with current standards. Available pharmacologic data are fragmentary and do not permit a definitive evaluation. Virtually no single-herb products are available for the indications stated above, although the four herbs and their extracts do occur as ingredients in numerous combination products.

2.4.2.1
Hop Strobiles and Hop Glands

While hops have been used in traditional European medicine as a tonic, diuretic, and aromatic bitter, the use of hops as a calmative is a more recent development. The fatigue- and sleep-promoting effects of hops were discovered when it was noticed that hop pickers tired easily, apparently due to the transfer of hop resin from their hands to their mouths (Tyler, 1987). But the assumption that hop resin has a sedative action when administered orally could not be confirmed by experimental studies (Hänsel and Wagener, 1967; Stocker, 1967). Hop-picker fatigue might be caused by inhaling the volatile oil of the hop plant, but ordinary extraction eliminates the volatile oil from the finished product.

Hop strobiles are the female flowers of the cultivated hop plant (*Humulus lupulus,* Fig. 2.19). They contain bitter principles including humulone and lupulone. These principles combine to form hop resin which occurs in 15–30 % concentration in the strobiles and 50–80 % in the hop glands (lupulin). The strobiles also contain up to 1 % volatile oil and up to 4 % tannins. Only the fresh dried herb contains these substances in full concentration. The bitter principles in particular break down rapidly during storage, their concentration decreasing by 50–70 % in 6 months (Hänsel and Schulz, 1986).

Stored hops contain up to 0.15 % methylbutenol, which is too volatile to persist in hop extracts but may form there from bitter acids. In experiments with mice and

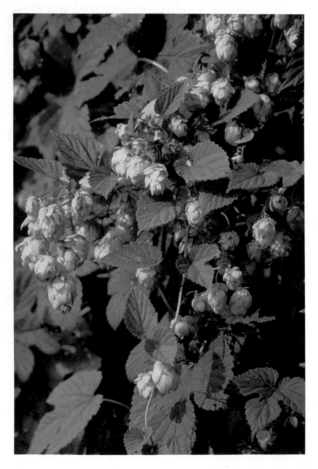

Fig. 2.19.
Hops *(Humulus lupulus).*

rats, methylbutenol was found to have sedative properties when administered in high doses (Wohlfarth et al., 1983). Due to the volatility of methylbutenol, the only preparation that can contain active amounts of this principle is the hops pillow used in traditional folk medicine. Its concentration in extracts is probably much too low to be effective (Wohlfarth, 1983).

When lupulone and ethanol hop extract were tested in four pharmacologic models in mice (motor activity in an exercise wheel, locomotor activity in an exercise box, barbiturate-potentiating effects, tests on a rotating cylinder), oral doses of 10–500 mg/kg were found to have no demonstrable sedative effects (Hänsel and Wagener, 1967). Similar studies in 15 human subjects treated with 250 mg of a lipophilic hop concentrate for 5 days showed no sleep-inducing effects in any of the subjects tested (Stoker, 1967) (see Sect. 7.3).

Based on information currently available, there is no toxicologic risk associated with hops. The LD_{50} for orally administered hop extract or lupulones in mice is in the range of 500–3500 mg/kg (Hänsel et al., 1993).

The Commission E monograph of December 5, 1984, cites "discomfort due to restlessless or anxiety and sleep disturbances" as the indications for hops. The recommended dose is 0.5 g of the dried herb, or its equivalent in extract-based products, taken one to several times daily.

2.4.2.2
Balm Leaves

This herb consists of the dried leaves of the lemon balm plant (Melissa officinalis), which today is cultivated commercially. The leaves emit a fragrant lemony odor when bruised. They contain at least 0.05 % of a volatile oil whose main components are citronellal, geranial, and neral. Balm leaves also contain phenol carboxylic acids, including about 4 % rosemarinic acid. Lemon balm oil is produced by steam distillation from fresh or dried herb gathered at the start of or during the flowering period. Citronellal, geranial, and neral together constitute about 50–75 % of lemon balm oil (Schultze et al., 1995). In the only experimental study to date on possible sedative effects, lemon balm oil was administered in doses of 3–100 mg/kg. Some effects were demonstrated, but the absence of a dose-dependent response suggests that the effects were nonspecific (Wagner and Sprinkmeyer, 1973). Antiviral properties of lemon balm preparations are discussed in Chap. 8.

The Commission E monograph of December 5, 1984, cites "nervous insomnia and functional gastrointestinal complaints" as the indications for balm leaves and preparations made from them. The recommended single dose is 1.5–4.5 g of the dried herb.

2.4.2.3
Passion Flower

Passion flower consists of the dried, leafy aerial parts, which may include the flowers and young fruits, of Passiflora incarnata, a tropical climbing vine native to southern North America. The main constituents of passiflora are flavonoids (up to 2.5 %), coumarin, and umbeliferone. The occurrence of harmala alkaloids, once considered responsible for the effects of the herb, has been disputed (Koch and Steinegger, 1980).

Extracts of passion flower were found to reduce spontaneous locomotor activity in mice and prolong their sleep when administered by the oral and intraperitoneal routes (Speroni and Minghetti, 1988). In one study, an aqueous extract from Passiflora edulis produced a hypnotic sedative effect in human subjects but also showed signs of hepatotoxicity and pancreatotoxicity (Maluf et al., 1991). There have been no controlled therapeutic studies with single-herb preparations based on extracts from Passiflora incarnata. Mayer (1995) recently reviewed the pharmaceutical quality, constituents, and pharmacologic testing of this herb.

Commission E, in its monograph of November 30, 1985, described the indications for passion flower as states of nervous unrest and recommended an average daily dose of 4–8 g of dried herb or its equivalent in passiflora preparations.

2.4.2.4
Lavender

This herb consists of the dried flowers of *Lavendula angustifolia* (Fig. 2.20) gathered just before they are fully open. Lavender flowers contain at least 1.5 % volatile oil, whose main constituents are linalyl acetate, linalool, camphor, β-ocimene, and cineole (eucalyptol). The herb also contains up to 12 % tannins. A low shrub growing to about 60 cm, Lavendula augustifolia is mainly indiginous to the Mediterranean region. Volatile lavender oil is produced from the fresh flowering tops by steam distillation, the main components of the volatile oil being linalyl acetate and linalool.

To date, lavender oil is the only lavendar preparation for which pharmacologic studies in animals and humans have been reported. Intraperitoneal doses of approximately 100–200 mg/kg in mice and rats showed anticonvulsant effects against electric shock, inhibitory effects on spontaneous motor activity, and additive effects

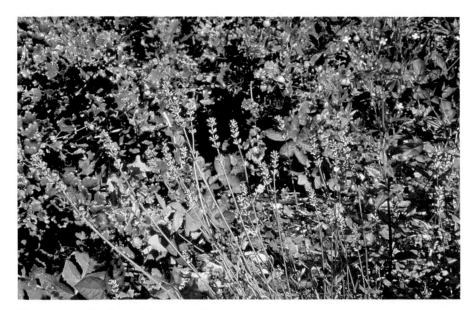

Fig. 2.20. Lavender *(Lavendula angustifolia).*

when combined with several narcotics (Atanassova-Shopova, 1970). Multiple oral doses of 0.4 mg/kg lavender oil in mice followed by the intraperitoneal injection of 40 mg/kg pentobarbital significantly reduced the time of sleep onset and prolonged the duration of sleep relative to a control group (Guillemain, 1989). A significant depression of motor activity was observed in mice exposed to a lavender atmosphere in a dark cage for 30, 60, and 90 min. Linalool and linalyl acetate alone showed similar effects. The plasma levels of linalool rose in proportion to the length of exposure. Lavender oil completely inhibited stimulation by caffeine, and linalool and linalyl acetate inhibited caffeine stimulation by about 50% (Buchbauer et al., 1991).

In another study, seven human subjects who had inhaled lavender oil showed a significant decline in selective EEG potentials (contingent negative variation, CNV) that correlate with vigilance, expectancy, and alertness. Lavender oil was considered to have a sedating and relaxing effect when compared with various other substances. Unlike nitrazepam, however, lavender oil had no effect on heart rate or reaction time (Torii et al., 1991).

In four geriatric patients with sleep disorders who had been taking benzodiazepines and neuroleptics for some time, the synthetic drugs were discontinued for a two-week "washout period" (during which there was a significant decrease in sleep time), and the patients were subjected to aromatherapy with lavender oil. Sleep time increased significantly and reached a level comparable to that previously achieved with the synthetic drugs. The patients reported fewer periods of restlessness during sleep while on treatment with the lavender oil (Hardy et al., 1995).

The calming, relaxing effects of lavender flowers and the oil derived from them are better documented by empirical medicine and experimental studies than the effects of hops, balm, and passion flower. Although it is reasonable to suppose that the actions of lavender are mediated by olfactory receptors, the results of animal studies as well as the high lipid solubility of lavender oil constituents suggest that lavender may act directly on the central nervous system following systemic administration. There is a lack of suitable research in human subjects, and human studies should be conducted as soon as possible.

In its monograph on lavender flowers, Commission E described the indications for internal use as "states of unrest, difficulty falling asleep, and functional upper abdominal complaints," recommending 1–2 teaspoons of dried herb per cup of tea or 1–4 drops of lavender oil (about 20–80 mg) taken with a sugar cube. An extract prepared from 100 g of dried flowers in 2 liters of hot water can be added to bath water for external use.

2.4.3
Sedative Teas

Sedative teas, known also as nerve teas or slumber teas, are most commonly prepared from valerian root, hop strobiles, or balm leaves. Herbs containing volatile oils are frequently used as additives, e.g., chamomile flowers, lavender flowers, orange blossoms, peppermint leaves, and bitter orange peel. Chamomile is widely regarded as a mild calmative and sleep-aid in England and the U.S., where it enjoys almost the same status as valerian does in Germany.

The tea formula listed in the German Pharmacopeia No. 6 contains the bitter leaf bogbean *(Menyanthes trifoliata)* as a major ingredient (40 %). It might be asked how an appetite-stimulating bitter herb could contribute to the efficacy of a sedative tea. For centuries, Europeans have considered bitter-tasting herbs to have general benefical effects on health, almost equating the efficacy of a medicine with its bitterness. This deeply rooted cultural attitude may have heightened the psychological readiness of the user to believe in the hypnogenic potency of the tea. Of course, we cannot rule out the possibility that future clinical trials may confirm that bitter herbs do have a sedative action on the central nervous system.

A handbook issued by the Drug Approval and Pharmacopeia, Commission in France lists the following herbs used in the treatment of nervousness and mild sleep disturbances: valerian root, black horehound *(Ballota foetida),* hop strobiles, corn poppy flowers, lavender flowers, linden flowers, balm leaves, passion flower, bitter orange leaves, bitter orange flowers, woodruff, hawthorn flowers, and lemon verbena leaves *(Aloysia triphylla).*

Tea Formulations

Indications: nervousness, difficulty falling asleep.
Preparation and dosing guidelines: Pour boiling water (about 150 mL) over 1 tablespoon of tea, cover and steep for about 10 min, then pass through a tea strainer. Drink 1 cup of freshly made tea 2 or 3 times during the day and before bedtime.
Directions to patient: One heaping tablespoon per cup (about 150 mL) of tea 2 or 3 times daily and before going to bed.

Nerve tea formula in German Pharmacopeia 6

Rx		
	Bogbean leaves	40.0
	Peppermint leaves	30.0
	Valerian root	30.0
	Prepare tea	
	Directions to patient (see above)	

Nerve tea formula in Swiss Pharmacopeia 6

Rx		
	Valerian root	25.0
	Orange blossoms	20.0
	Passion flower	20.0
	Crushed aniseed	15.0
	Balm leaves	10.0
	Peppermint leaves	10.0

Nerve tea formula in German Pharmacopeia 7

Rx		
	Valerian root	50.0
	Balm leaves	25.0
	Peppermint leaves	25.0

Nerve tea formula in Austrian Pharmacopeia 9

Rx		
	Valerian root	60.0
	Balm leaves	10.0
	Peppermint leaves	10.0
	Orange blossoms	10.0
	Bitter orange peel	10.0

2.4.4
Drug Products

The *Rote Liste 1995* contains a total of 16 single-herb valerian products, 3 single-herb products based on hops, balm, and passion flower, 13 two-herb products containing valerian and hops, and 31 multiherb combination products containing valerian. The herbs most frequently combined with valerian are hops, balm, and passion flower. Based on current information, *Valeriana officinalis* is the only species that should be used in valerian products, which should be produced according to approved standards and whose efficacy should be tested by therapeutic studies. Additionally, products should contain sufficient amounts of the active principle (see Sect. 2.4.1.6). A survey of commercial products reveals a confusing heterogeneity that is compounded by a great many unnamed combination products. Based on current quality criteria for plant species, production methods, and dose, there are very few valerian products now on the market that can be recommended for the physician-guided therapy of sleep disturbances (an example of a satisfactory product is Sedonium, which contains a single dose of 300 mg valerian extract and has a recommended daily dose of 600 mg extract).

References

Atanassova-Shopova S, Roussinov KS (1970) On certain central neurotropic effects of lavender essential oil. Bull Inst Physiol 8: 69–76.

Balderer G, Borbely AA (1985) Effect of valerian on human sleep. Psychopharmacol 87: 406–409.

Bounthanh C, Bergmann C, Beck JP, Haag-Berrurier M, Anton R (1981) Valepotriates, a new class of cytotoxic and antitumor agents. Planta Med 41: 21–28.

Braun R, Dittmar W, von der Hude W, Scheutwinkel-Reich M (1985) Bacterial mutagenicity of the tranquilizing constituents of valerianaceae roots. Naunyn- Schmiedeberg's Arch Pharmacol Suppl 329: R 28.

Braun R, Dittmar W, Machut M, Weickmann S (1982) Valepotriate mit Epoxidstruktur – beachtliche Alkylantien. Dtsch Apoth Z 122: 1109–1113.

Buchbauer G, Jirovet L, Jäger W Dietrich H, Plank C, Karamat E (1991) Aromatherapy: evidence for sedative sffects of the essential oil of lavender after inhalation. Z Naturforsch 46 c: 1067–1072.

Donath F, Roots I (1995) Untersuchung zur Erfassung der Wirkung von Baldrianextrakt (LI 156) auf das Pharmako-EEG bei 16 Probanden. Z Phytother Abstractband, p 10.

Eickstedt KW v, Rahmann R (1969) Psychopharmakologische Wirkungen von Valepotriaten. Arzneim-Forsch 19: 316–319.

Gerhard U, Ninnenbrink N, Georghiadou Ch, Hobi (1996) Effects of two plant-based sleep remedies on vigilance. Schweiz Rsch Med 85: 473–481.

Grusla D (1987) Nachweis der Wirkung eines Baldrianextraktes im Rattenhirn mit der ^{14}C-2-Desoxyglucose-Technik. Dissertation, Phillipps-Universität, Marburg.

Guillemain J, Rousseau A, Delaveau P (1989) Effets neurodepresseurs de l'huile essentielle de Lavandula angustifolia Mill. Ann Pharmaceutiques Francaises 47: 337–343.

Hänsel R, Keller K, Rimpler H, Schneider G (1993) Hagers Handbuch der Pharmazeutischen Praxis. Drogen E–O, 5th Edition. Springer Verlag Berlin Heidelberg, p 455.

Hänsel R, Keller K, Rimpler H, Schneider G (1994) Hagers Handbuch der Pharmazeutischen Praxis. Drogen P–Z, 5th Edition. Springer Verlag Berlin Heidelberg, pp 1067–1095.

Hänsel R, Schulz J (1982) Valerensäuren und Valerenal als Leitstoffe des offizinellen Baldrians. Dtsch Apoth Z 122: 215–219.

Hänsel R (1984) Bewertung von Baldrian-Präparaten: Differenzierung wesentlich. Dtsch Apoth Z 124: 2085.

Hänsel R, Schulz J (1985) Beitrag zur Qualitätssicherung von Baldrianextrakten. Pharm Industrie 47: 531–553.

Hänsel R, Wagener HH (1967) Versuche, sedativ-hypnotische Wirkstoffe im Hopfen nachzuweisen. Arzneim Forsch/Drug Res 17: 79–81.

Hardy M, Kirk-Smith MD, Stretch DD (1995) Replacement of drug treatment for insomnia by ambient odor. Lancet 346: 701.

Hazelhoff B (1984) Phytochemical and Pharmacological Aspects of Valeriana Compounds. Dissertation, University of Groningen.

Hendriks H, Bos R, Woerdenbag HJ, Koster AS (1985) Central nervous depressant activity of valerenic acid in the mouse. Planta Med 51: 28–31.

Hiller K-o, Zetler G (1996) Neuropharmacological studies on ethanol extracts of valeriana officinalis: behavioral and anticonvulsant properties. Phytotherapy Res 10: 145–151.

Jansen W (1977) Doppelblindstudie mit Baldrisedon. Therapiewoche 27: 2779–2786.

Kamm-Kohl AV, Jansen W, Brockmann P (1984) Moderne Baldriantherapie gegen nervöse Störungen im Senium. Med Welt 35: 1450–1454.

Koch H, Steinegger E (1980) Untersuchungen zur Alkaloid- und Flavonoidführung von Passiflora-Arten. Lecture delivered at the International Research Congress on Natural Products, Strassburg 1980. Published in Abstracts of Posters.

Krieglstein J, Grusla D (1988) Zentraldämpfende Inhaltsstoffe im Baldrian. Dtsch Apoth Z 128: 2041–2046.

Leathwood PD, Chauffard F (1983) Quantifying the effects of mild sedatives. J Psychiat Res 17: 115–122.

Leathwood PD, Chauffard F (1984) Aqueous extract of valerian reduces latency to fall asleep in man. Planta Med 50:144–148.

Maluf E, Barros HMT, Frochtengarten ML, Benti R, Leite JR (1991) Assessment of the hypnotic/sedative effects and toxicity of Passiflora edulis aqueous extract in rodents and humans. Phytother Res 5: 262–266.

Meier B (1995). Passiflorae herba – pharmazeutische Qualität. Z Phytother 16: 90–99.

Riedel E, Hänsel R, Ehrke G (1982) Hemmung des Gamma-Aminobuttersäureabbaus durch Valerensäurederivate. Planta Med 46: 219–220.

Rücker G, Tautges J, Sieek A, Wenzel H, Graf E (1978) Untersuchungen zur Isolierung und pharmakodynamischen Aktivität des Sesquiterpens Valeranon aus Nardostrachys jatamansi DC.Arzneim Forsch/Drug Res 28: 7.

Santos MS, Ferreira F, Cunha AP et al. (1994) An aqueous extract of valerian influences the transport of GABA in synaptosomes. Planta Med. 60: 278–279.

Schultze W, König WA, Hilkert A, Richter R (1995) Melissenöle. Dtsch Apoth Z 135: 557–577.

Schulz H, Stolz C, Müller J (1994) The effect of a valerian extract on sleep polygraphy in poor sleepers. A pilot study. Pharmacopsychiaty 27: 147–151.

Schulz H, Jobert M (1995) Die Darstellung sedierender/tranquilisierender Wirkungen von Phytopharmaka im quantifizierten EEG. Z Phytother Abstractband, p 10.

Speroni E, Minghetti A (1988) Neuropharmacological activity of extracts from Passiflora incarnata. Planta Med: 488–491.

Stocker HR (1967) Sedative und hypnogene Wirkung des Hopfens. Schweizer Brauerei Rundschau 78: 80–89.

Torii S, Fukuda H, Kanemoto H, Miyanchi R, Hamauzu Y, Kawasaki M (1988) Contingent negative variation (CNV) and the psychologic effects of odor. In: Van Toller St, Dodd GH (eds) Perfumery. The Psychology and Biology of Fragrance. Chapman and Hall, London New York, pp 107–146.

Tyler VE (1987) The New Honest Herbal. A sensible Guide to Herbs and Related Remedies. 2nd Edition. Stickley Co., Philadelphia, pp 125–126.

Vorbach EU, Görtelmayer R, Brüning J (1996) Therapie von Insomnien: Wirksamkeit und Verträglichkeit eines Baldrian-Präparates. Psychopharmakotherapie 3: 109–115.

Wagner H, Sprinkmeyer L (1973) Dtsch Apoth Z 113: 1159. Quoted in: Koch- Heitzmann I, Schültze W (1984) Melissa officinalis. Eine alte Arzneipflanze mit neuen therapeutischen Wirkungen. Dtsch Apoth Z 124: 2137–2145.

Wohlfart R, Wurm G, Hänsel R, Schmidt H (1983) Der Abbau der Bittersäuren zum 2-Methyl-3-buten-2-ol, einem Hopfeninhaltsstoff mit sedativ-hypnotischer Wirkung. Arch Pharmaz 315: 132–137.

Wohlfart R, Hänsel R, Schmidt H (1983) Nachweis sedativ-hypnotischer Wirkstoffe im Hopfen. 4. Mittlg. Die Pharmakologie des Hopfeninhaltsstoffes z-Methyl-3-buten-2-ol. Planta Med 48: 120–123.

3 Cardiovascular System

Phytomedicines play a significant role in the treatment of mild forms of heart failure and coronary insufficiency, in the prevention and treatment of atherosclerosis and its sequelae, and in the symptomatic treatment of chronic venous insufficiency. There are only a few herbs, however, for which safety and efficacy have been adequately proven: hawthorn (heart failure and coronary insufficiency), garlic (atherosclerosis), ginkgo extract (arterial occlusive disease), and horse chestnut extract (chronic venous insufficiency). Therefore, the bulk of this chapter is devoted to these four herbs. The closing sections deal briefly with other preparations, including herbs that contain cardioactive digitaloids and herbal remedies for angina pectoris, cardiac arrhythmias, and hypertension and hypotension.

3.1
Heart Failure and Coronary Insufficiency

The classic remedies used to treat myocardial insufficiency are the cardiac glycosides derived from purple and Grecian foxglove (Digitalis species). These compounds are colorless, bitter-tasting substances that cause local irritation. Their chemical compositions are known, and they can be synthetically produced, but for economic reasons the 14 pure glycosides or their precursors are still obtained by extraction from digitalis leaf. Because the cardiac glycosides are specific, identifiable chemical compounds that have a narrow therapeutic dose range (see Sect. 1.5.5), they are not considered phytotherapeutic agents and are outside the realm of herbal medicine. Galenic preparations made from digitalis leaves are obsolete in modern pharmacotherapy. Details on the pure glycosides and their actions can be found in textbooks of pharmacology.

3.1.1
Hawthorn

3.1.1.1
Introduction
Hawthorn (*Crataegus*, Fig. 3.1) is a proven, established remedy for heart ailments and circulatory disorders. Apparently the animal kingdom also benefits from the hawthorn, as illustrated by the following anecdote. In 1966, Klatt (quoted in Weiss, 1991) reported his observations on gypsy moths. For purposes of genetic research, Klatt had been inbreeding the moths for some time while feeding them their usual

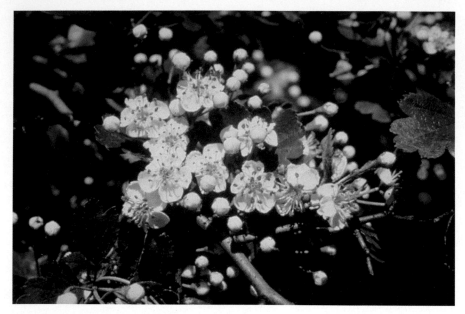

Fig. 3.1. Flowering branch of hawthorn (*Crataegus* species).

diet of alder leaves. Within a few years the insects showed retarded development, aged prematurely, and laid fewer eggs. The death of the entire colony seemed likely as a result of degeneration due to inbreeding. By chance, Klatt met a butterfly breeder who recommended feeding the insects hawthorn leaves instead of alder leaves. The colony recovered. The moths became larger and stronger and resumed normal egg-laying within a few months.

Weiss (1991), in a commentary on this study, emphasized that a positive response appeared only after the whole herb had been fed continuously for a period of several weeks. As swimming tests in rats have shown, a single dose of hawthorn does not have immediate discernible effects. A similar link between therapeutic efficacy and duration of use appears to exist in cardiac patients. The only acute effects seen after a single hawthorn dose in humans were changes in parameters having little experimental or clinical relevance (Fischer et al., 1994). A 4- to 8-week course of treatment is necessary to provide significant improvement in subjective complaints and exercise tolerance (Tauchert and Loew, 1995).

3.1.1.2
Medicinal Plant

Hawthorn is a member of the Rosaceae family, but the unpleasant aroma of its blossoms attracts only flies. The tall shrubs are distributed throughout Europe, growing at elevations up to 1600 m above sea level. They prefer hillsides and sunny slopes. The name of the plant derives from its fruits, or haws, and its sharp thorns. Only the white-blooming hawthorn is used therapeutically; the red-blooming garden variety of hawthorn has no medicinal uses.

3.1.1.3
Crude Drug and Extract

Herbs of the species Crataegus monogyna and Crataegus oxyacantha are used in the production of hawthorn-based medicines. Therapeutic efficacy has been most reliably documented for hawthorn leaves and flowers. The German Pharmacopeia *(DAB 1996)* describes the crude drug as consisting of the dried tops (about 7 cm long) of the flowering shrub. The dried herb has a faint, distinctive odor and a slightly bitter or astringent taste. A fixed combination of hawthorn flowers, leaves, and fruits has also been recognized as having therapeutic efficacy. By themselves, the dried berry-like fruits (haws) have a sweet mealy or mucilaginous taste.

The revised 1994 Commission E monograph on the hawthorn recognizes two water-and-alcohol extracts of dried hawthorn leaves and flowers (herb-to-extract ratio 5–7:1) and the fixed combination mentioned above as having therapeutic efficacy. Efficacy is deemed likely for other preparations, especially the liquid extract described in *DAB 1996* and alcoholic extracts made from leaves or flowers alone, but this has not yet been established by double-blind clinical studies.

3.1.1.4
Key Constituents, Analysis, Pharmacokinetics

The main constituents that have been isolated from hawthorn are flavonoids, procyanidins, catechins, triterpenoids, aromatic carboxylic acids, amino and purine derivatives, and various other compounds (Hänsel et al., 1992). The key constituents for testing pharmaceutical quality are the flavonoids, calculated as hyperoside according to *DAB 1996*, and the oligomeric procyanidins, calculated as epicatechin. At present there are standard analytic methods for determining the flavonoids in hawthorn but not the oligomeric procyanidins (Sticher et al., 1994). The flavonoid content of the crude drug is approximately 1 % for the leaves and flowers but only about 0.1 % for the berries. The content of oligomeric procyanidins in the leaves and flowers is believed to be about 1–3 %. The Commission E monograph recommends a daily dose of 160–900 mg hawthorn extract with a designated content of flavonoids (4–30 mg) or oligomeric procyanidins (30–160 mg).

No studies are yet available on the absorption, distribution, and metabolism of the key constituents in humans.

3.1.1.5
Pharmacology

The cardiovascular effects of hawthorn have been described in a number of original works. Most studies have dealt with aqueous and alcoholic extracts as well as various fractions and constituents. The older studies were summarized in three survey works (Ammon and Händel, 1981 a–c). Siegel and Casper (1995) summarized more recent pharmacologic studies on hawthorn.

In vitro studies of hawthorn effects on myocardial contractility have been done in isolated frog heart, isolated guinea pig heart (Langendorff preparation), and isolated atria, and in vivo studies have been done in anesthetized cats and dogs. All studies showed an increased amplitude of myocardial contractions and an increase in stroke volume. An increase in coronary blood flow was also demonstrated in isolated guinea pig heart. Studies in various anesthetized species have consistently shown a decrease in heart rate, although an increase was observed in isolated guinea pig heart.

Recent results are available from studies on models of myocardial ischemia in rats (Krzeminski and Chatterjee, 1993), isolated rat myocardial cells (Pöpping et al., 1995), human coronary arteries (Siegel et al., 1994), and isolated perfused guinea pig heart (Joseph et al., 1995).

The antiarrhythmic effects of an extract made from hawthorn leaves and flowers were tested in an ischemic model in rats (left coronary artery ischemia for 7 min, then reperfusion for 15 min). Reperfusion-induced ventricular fibrillation occurred in 88 % of the animals in the control group but in less than 20 % of the animals that had received 0.5 mg/kg or 5 mg/kg of the hawthorn extract. Significant reductions were also seen in the duration of fibrillations and the occurrence of tachycardia. The same model was used to study the effect of 100 mg/kg of the extract, administered orally for 6 days, on lethality, fibrillations, tachycardia, and CPK elevation. Reperfusion in the control group was followed by a precipitous fall in blood pressure; only 8 of the 16 animals survived, and all survivors had ventricular fibrillations. The animals treated with hawthorn had no hypotensive crises, and all survived with no episodes of ventricular fibrillation. The differences were statistically significant (Kurcok, 1992; Krzeminski and Chatterjee, 1993).

In one study, hawthorn extract increased the amplitude and duration of isolated rat myocardial cell contractions within a few minutes after exposure. The effect be-

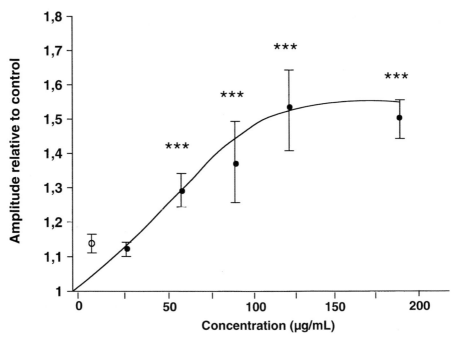

Fig. 3.2. Concentration-dependent effect of hawthorn extract on the amplitude of the contraction of isolated heart cells. The error bars indicate standard deviation from the mean (*** = p < 0.001; t-test for independent random samples) (Pöpping et al., 1995).

gan at extract concentrations of 30 μg/mL and rose steadily as the concentration was increased to about 120 μg/mL (Fig. 3.2). Calculations show that achieving this effect in an adult patient would require a daily dose of 600–900 mg, based on the assumption that the active principle is distributed in an extracellular volume of approximately 15–20 L (Pöpping et al., 1995). At concentrations of 90–180 μg/mL, the extract significantly lengthened the apparent refractory period from 144 min to 420 min (Fig. 3.3). This effect, which occurred even after prior stimulation of the cells with isoproterenol, is opposite to that of cardiac glycosides which shorten the refractory period. This difference is particularly striking when we note that agents with a positive inotropic action are generally arrhythmogenic while antiarrhythmic agents are negatively inotropic. Hawthorn extract is unique in that it is positively inotropic but appears to stabilize the heart rhythm (Pöpping et al., 1995).

The known ability of hawthorn to increase coronary blood flow was tested in isolated human coronary arteries. Wall forces and membrane potentials were measured in normal vascular segments and in atherosclerotic segments taken from heart transplants. Both parameters changed roughly in proportion to the concentration of the active principle. The degree of vascular relaxation was 14% of the resting tonus in the normal arteries and 8% in the arteries with atherosclerotic lesions (Siegel et al., 1994; Siegel and Casper, 1995).

Comparative studies were conducted in isolated perfused guinea pig hearts (Langendorff preparations) to study the effects of various inotropic agents – epinephrine

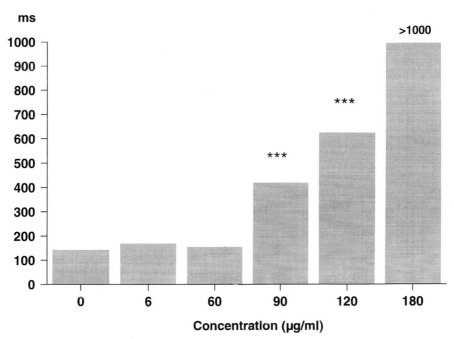

Fig. 3.3. Concentration-dependent effect of hawthorn extract (LI 132) on the apparent refractory period (*** = p < 0.001; t-test for independent random samples) (Pöpping et al., 1995).

(EPI), amrinone (AM), milrinone (MIL), digoxin (DIG), and hawthorn extract (CRA) – on selected functional parameters. Simultaneous recordings of contractile force, spontaneous heart rate, AV conduction time, coronary flow, and effective refractory period made it possible to establish cardioactive profiles for each of the agents tested. All the agents except CRA caused a concentration-dependent shortening of the effective refractory period in addition to their known inotropic effects (max. shortening: 38 % with 1×10^{-5} mol/L EPI, 26 % with 7×10^{-7} mol/L DIG, 13 % with 1×10^{-4} mol/L MIL, and 1.6 % with 5×10^{-4} mol/L AM). In terms of positive inotropism, the shortening of the refractory period was most pronounced with MIL (1.32 ms/mN), followed by AM (0.65 ms/mN), DIG (0.40 ms/mN), and EPI (0.28 ms/mN). By contrast, CRA markedly prolonged the effective refractory period, increasing it by a maximum of 10 %, i.e., by 2.54 ms/mN. Thus, CRA differs fundamentally from the reference drugs in that its inotropic action is associated with a lengthened refractory period, indicating that it may have less arrhythmogenic potential (Fig. 3.4; Joseph et al., 1995; Mül-

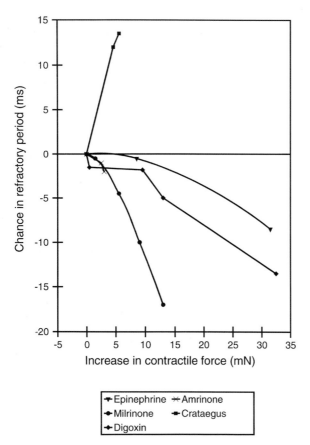

Fig. 3.4. Correlation between the change in the effective refractory period of the ventricular myocardium and the increase in the force of ventricular contraction. The graph shows the mean values of the changes relative to the initial value (Joseph et al., 1995).

ler et al., 1996). On the molecular level of action, hawthorn extract has been classified as a phytopharmacologic potassium-channel activator based on measurements in rabbit heart papillary muscle and in human coronary arteries (Siegel et al., 1996).

3.1.1.6
Toxicology

Acute toxicity studies were performed in mice and rats using a water-and-ethanol hawthorn extract (45% v/v, herb-to-extract ratio 5:1). No deaths resulted from oral or intraperitoneal doses up to 3000 mg/kg body weight. Intraperitoneal doses higher than 3000 mg/kg produced toxic symptoms consisting of sedation, dyspnea, and tremor. No toxic effects were observed after 30, 90, and 300 mg/kg/day of the same extract administered orally to rats and dogs for a period of 26 weeks. No findings have yet been published on embryonic and fetal toxicity associated with hawthorn extracts.

Several studies have been published on the mutagenicity of hawthorn preparations, but the results are inconsistent. The water-and-ethanol extract described above has been shown to be nonmutagenic in various tests. It is assumed that the mutagenic effects produced by other extracts in salmonella cultures are based on the presence of quercetin. However, the quercetin content of the herb is so low compared with the amount of quercetin normally ingested with food that it is extremely unlikely to pose an additional risk to humans (Hänsel et al., 1992; Schlegelmilch and Heywood, 1994).

3.1.1.7
Clinical Efficacy

The results of 14 clinical studies on the therapeutic efficacy of hawthorn in a total of 808 patients were published from 1981 to 1994 (Table 3.1; see also survey works by Tauchert et al., 1994; Loew, 1994; Tauchert and Loew, 1995). Alcoholic extracts of hawthorn leaves and flowers were used in 560 of these patients. Most patients were admitted to the studies with a diagnosis of stage II heart failure (NYHA classification). The parameters that proved optimal for evaluating therapeutic efficacy were exercise tolerance as measured by standard bicycle ergometry, the anaerobic threshold as measured by spiroergometry, the ejection fraction as measured by radionuclide ventriculography (Eichstädt et al., 1989), and the patients' subjective complaints, which were scored on a simple rating scale. The clinical presentation, ECG, and chest films were less useful indicators of therapeutic response. Based on ergometric performance parameters, a minimum daily dose of 300 mg extract represents the threshold of efficacy. Whether a daily dose of 900 mg extract would provide optimum efficacy remains an open question.

Almost all the studies showed improvements in clinical symptoms, even at doses less than 300 mg/day. Given the subjective nature of the complaints, however, it is reasonable to assume that significant placebo effects influenced the evaluations. As an example, Fig. 3.5 shows the frequency of symptoms and complaints in 78 patients who had been treated with either 3 × 200 mg hawthorn extract or a placebo for 8 weeks as part of a double-blind study. Despite marked placebo effects, the graph shows that significantly more patients became free of complaints while on treatment with the hawthorn extract. The semiquantitative scoring scale showed improvement

Table 3.1. Thirteen controlled clinical studies using alcoholic hawthorn extracts at doses of 160 mg–900 mg taken for periods of 21–56 days were published between 1981 and 1996. Eight of the studies used objective criteria such as exercise tolerance on the bicycle ergometer, the pressure frequence product, noninvasive measurements of the ejection fraction, or the anaerobic threshold measured by spiroergometry. These criteria indicated a clear trend toward higher doses and longer treatment times (survey in Tauchert, Siegel and Schulz, 1994, and Loew, 1994).

Year	First author	Cases	Dose (mg/day)	Days	Key parameters
1981	Iwamoto	80	180	42	B, DFP
1982	Kümmel	19	180	42	SZI
1983	Hanak	60	180	21	AT
1986	Pozenel	22	180	28	DFP
1986	O'Connolly	36	180	42	DFP
1987	O'Connolly	31	180	42	DFP
1989	Eichstädt	20	480	28	EF, AT
1992	Leuchtgens	30	160	56	B, DFP
1994	Bödigheimer	85	300	28	AT
1994	Schmidt	78	600	56	AT, B
1994	Tauchert	132	900	56	AT
1994	Förster	72	900	56	AS
1996	Weikl	126	160	56	B, DFP

B = Subjective complaints/mood; DFP = pressure-rate product; SZI = systolic interval; AT = bicycle ergometer exercise tolerance; EF = ejection fraction; AS = anaerobic threshold measured by spiroergometry.

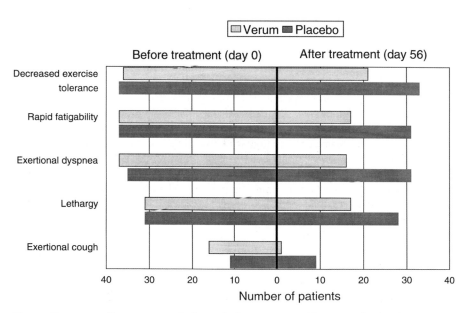

Fig. 3.5. Frequency of key symptoms before and after treatment with 600 mg/day hawthorn extract. At 56 days, patients on the drug show significantly greater symptom reductions than patients on the placebo (Schmidt et al., 1994).

from 0.90 to 0.28 in the hawthorn-treated group versus 0.92 to 0.69 in the placebo group. The difference between the groups was statistically highly significant (Schmidt et al., 1994).

Objective improvement in cardiac performance was demonstrated most clearly in three clinical double-blind studies using bicycle ergometry (Schmidt et al., 1994; Tauchert et al., 1994) or spiroergometry (Förster et al., 1994). Two of the studies tested hawthorn against a placebo, and one study with 132 patients compared the efficacy of hawthorn with that of the ACE inhibitor captopril.

The effect of hawthorn on average exercise tolerance over a 56-day treatment period is compared with a placebo in Fig. 3.6 and with captopril in Fig. 3.7. In the placebo-controlled study, the average ergometric exercise tolerance rose from 79 to 107 watts in the patients treated with hawthorn extract but rose only from 71 to 76 watts in the placebo-treated group. This indicates a highly significant superiority of the hawthorn extract over the placebo. The improvement is particularly marked at moderate levels of exertion in the range of 100–125 watts (Schmidt et al., 1994). In the study comparing hawthorn with captopril, equivalent average tolerance increases were observed in both groups: from 83 to 97 watts with hawthorn extract and from 83 to 99 watts with captopril. Thus, the hawthorn preparation offers better tolerance than the ACE inhibitor captopril while providing equal therapeutic efficacy (Tauchert et al., 1994).

Spiroergometric studies also showed statistically significant advantages of hawthorn over a placebo. One advantage was the favorable effect of hawthorn on the time of onset of the anaerobic threshold. Hawthorn therapy did not alter the resting heart rate and blood pressure, and during maximum exercise the blood pressure and

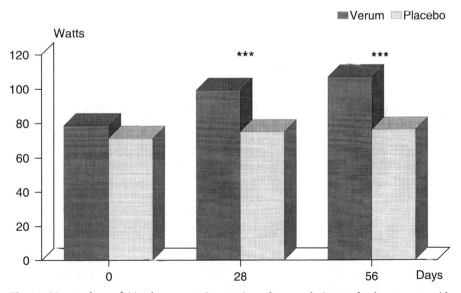

Fig. 3.6. Mean values of bicycle ergometric exercise tolerance during 56 days' treatment with 600 mg/day hawthorn extract. A statistically significant increase in exercise tolerance was noted in the hawthorn-treated group relative to the placebo (*** = p < 0.001) (Schmidt et al., 1994).

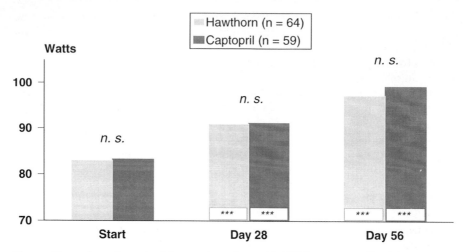

Fig. 3.7. Mean values of exercise tolerance in patients with NYHA stage II cardiac failure. Double-blind comparison of 900 mg/day hawthorn extract with 37.5 mg/day captopril. Both groups showed a highly significant increase in exercise tolerance during the course of treatment (*** = $p < 0.001$), with no statistically significant differences (Tauchert et al., 1994).

heart rate increased less with hawthorn than with the placebo, leading to significant differences in the pressure-rate product (Förster et al., 1994).

As for side effects, a review of controlled clinical studies in a total of 367 patients treated with hawthorn showed two cases each of nausea and headache and one case each of palpitations, soft stool, and migraine headache. In all cases the physicians conducting the studies questioned the relation of the complaints to the test medication. The patients and physicians consistently rated the tolerance of the medication as "good" or "excellent."

3.1.1.8
Indications, Dosages, Risks, and Contraindications
The updated 1994 Commission E monograph on hawthorn leaves and flowers states that the extract is indicated for "declining cardiac performance consistent with stage II failure according to NYHA criteria." The recommended dosage is 160–900 mg/day of the crude water-and-alcohol extract with a designated content of flavonoids (4–20 mg) or oligomeric procyanidins (30–160 mg). Hawthorn preparations should be taken orally and should be continued for at least 6 weeks. There are no known risks, contraindications, or drug-drug interactions.

3.1.1.9
Therapeutic Significance
The pharmacologic therapy of heart failure is based on three principles: increasing the efficiency of the heart muscle (cardiac glycosides), reducing the preload (diuretics), and reducing the afterload (vasodilators, ACE inhibitors). But cardiac glycosides and other positive inotropic agents (Fig. 3.4) also shorten the refractory period, thereby increasing the risk of cardiac arrhythmias. Evidence to date indicates that

Table 3.2. Comparison of the therapeutic risks of hawthorn extract and cardiac glycosides.

Therapeutic risk	Crataegus	Digitalis
Therapeutic range	Very large	Very small
Dosage errors	No danger	High risk
Arrhythmogenic potential	None	Relatively large
Renal function impairment	Not a problem	Danger of intoxication
Diuretics, laxatives	Can be safely used	Require potassium monitoring
Tolerance to oxygen deficit	Increased	Reduced

hawthorn extract is both a positive inotropic agent and a peripheral vasodilator and thus has two mutually complementary mechanisms of action. Its positive inotropic effect, unlike that of the cardiac glycosides, is associated with a lengthening of the refractory period. While a shortened refractory period predisposes to arrhythmias, the lengthening effect of hawthorn extract helps to stabilize the heart rhythm. The advantages of hawthorn extract over conventional cardioactive drugs in patients with mild forms of heart failure are summarized in Table 3.2. One disadvantage is that hawthorn extract appears to be beneficial only for NYHA stage II heart failure and is not appropriate for more advanced stages.

3.1.1.10
Drug Products
A total of 39 single-herb hawthorn preparations were listed in the *Rote Liste 1995*. Some of these products do not conform to the recommendations in the 1994 Commission E monograph, and 12 of the products are available only in liquid form. Twenty-one of the remaining hawthorn products contain leaf-and-flower extracts, and three others contain extracts of leaves, flowers, and fruits. Clinical efficacy has been demonstrated for extracts of hawthorn leaves and flowers administered in the relatively high dose range of 600–900 mg/day.

3.1.2
Herbs Containing Digitaloids

Digitaloids are cardioactive glycosides that exert a digoxin-like action but are not derived from Digitalis species. The digitaloids include, most notably, convallatoxin, cymarin, oleandrin, G- and K-strophanthin, and proscillaridin. The principal sources of digitaloids are false hellebore, lily-of-the-valley, squill bulbs, and oleander leaves. Extracts from digitaloid herbs each contain more than one cardioactive glycoside. Up to 40 structurally related glycosides may be present along with a quantitatively dominant principal glycoside. Various other compounds are extracted along with the cardiac glycosides, so digitaloid extracts can have a very complex composition. As a result, the monitoring and control of active levels is a formidable task, comparable to therapy with digitalis glycosides; this is a serious drawback given the narrow therapeutic range of cardiac glycosides.

There are no qualitative differences between the digitaloids and the classic cardiac glycosides digoxin and digitoxin in terms of their pharmacologic mechanism of action and cardiac efficacy. All these compounds are positively inotropic, negatively chronotropic, negatively dromotropic, and positively bathmotropic. Digitaloids and digitalis glycosides differ in their pharmacokinetics, however, particularly in their rates of absorption and clearance. The shorter duration of action cited by advocates as a major advantage of digitaloid preparations correlates with lower absorption rates. As a result, treatment with digitaloid herbs carries a higher overall risk than treatment with isolated cardiac glycosides. Another difficulty is that digitaloid extracts do not meet phytotherapeutic requirements for a broad therapeutic range (see Sect. 1.5.1.1 and 1.5.5). Thus, physicians who have no personal experience with these products should use them only with great caution.

3.1.2.1
False Hellabore

The crude drug is prepared by drying the aerial parts of *Adonis vernalis* gathered while the plant is in bloom. Most of the bulk herb is imported from Hungary, Bulgaria, and Russia. Standardized hellabore powder consists of pulverized crude drug whose activity in guinea pig heart corresponds to a content of 0.2% cymarin. The German Pharmacopeia *(DAB 1996)* describes the powdered drug as containing approximately 0.25% cardiac glycosides, representing a complex mixture of about 20 components. These glycosides are similar to K-strophanthin in their chemical structure and pharmacokinetic properties. The 1988 Commission E monograph states that false hellabore is indicated for "mild heart failure, especially when accompanied by nervous symptoms." The contraindications, side effects, and risks are the same as for cardiac glycosides. No single-herb products based on false hellabore are available commercially in Germany, but there are products that combine the herb with other digitaloids (e. g., Corguttin, Miroton).

3.1.2.2
Lily-of-the-Valley

The crude drug is prepared by drying the aerial parts of *Convallaria majalis* gathered during the flowering period. The standardized powdered drug has a 0.2–0.3% content of cardioactive glycosides, which number more than 30. The principal glycosides are convallatoxin and convallatoxol. Convallatoxin has an absorption rate of about 10% and a 24-h clearance rate of about 50%. The maintenance dose is 0.2–0.3 mg intravenously and 2–3 mg orally. The indications stated in the Commission E monograph of 1987 are "mild exertional failure, age-related cardiac complaints, and chronic cor pulmonale." The contraindications, side effects, and risks are the same as for cardiac glycosides. A single-herb product based on lily-of-the-valley is marketed in Germany under the brand name Convacard. Also, there are a number of combination products containing other digitaloids and other active ingredients.

3.1.2.3
Squill Powder

The crude drug is prepared by gathering the inner scales of the squill bulb *(Urginea maritima)* after the flowering season, cutting them into transverse and longitudinal strips, and drying and pulverizing them. Depending on its origin, squill powder contains 0.15–2% cardioactive glycosides. The principal glycosides are scillaren A and proscillaridin, which comprise about two-thirds of the total glycoside fraction; the other third consists of at least 25 other constituents. According to *DAB 1996*, squill powder is adjusted to an activity corresponding to 0.2 % proscillaridin.

The gastrointestinal absorption rate is about 15 % for scillaren and 20–30 % for proscillaridin. The half-life of proscillaridin is approximately 24 h. The daily dose ranges from 0.1 to 0.5 g of the standardized squill powder.

The 1985 Commission E monograph states that the indications for squill powder are "mild forms of heart failure, even in patients with impaired renal function." The contraindications, side effects, and interactions are the same as for digitalis glycosides. Single-herb products based on powdered squill are marketed in Germany under the brand names Digitalysat N Bürger and Scillamiron. There are also a number of combination products that contain other digitaloids.

3.1.2.4
Oleander Leaves

The crude drug consists of the dried leaves of *Nerium oleander*. Native to the Mediterranean, oleander derives its species name from the similarity of the shape of leaves to those of the olive tree. The cardioactive glycoside fraction of oleander leaves is dominated by oleandrin, whose aglycone is closely related to the gitoxin of the purple foxglove. Only fragmentary data are available on the pharmacokinetics of oleandrin. Commission Ein ist 1988 monograph did not recommend oleander extract as a medicinal agent, but in 1993 the Commission did ascribe therapeutic value to a fixed combination of false hellebore liquid extract, lily-of-the-valley powdered extract, squill powdered extract, and oleander-leaf powdered extract based on clinical studies of the commercial product (Miroton). The indication was described as "mild forms of heart failure with circulatory lability." The following contraindications were noted: NYHA stage III or IV heart failure, treatment with digitalis glycosides, digitalis intoxication, hypercalcemia, potassium deficiency states, bradycardia, and ventricular tachycardia.

3.1.3
Other Cardioactive Plant Drugs

Extracts from *Ammi visnaga* fruits and the compounds isolated from them, khellin and visnagin, improve myocardial perfusion by increasing blood flow through the coronary vessels. These actions form the basis for the use of visnaga extract in relieving angina due to coronary heart disease. Reports of adverse effects (isolated cases of pseudoallergic reactions, reversible cholestatic jaundice, elevated hepatic transaminase levels) prompted Commission E in 1993 to withdraw its 1986 claim that ammi visnaga extract was appropriate for the treatment of "mild angina pectoris."

Antiarrhythmic agents of plant origin include the drugs ajmaline (alkaloid obtained from the root of *Rauwolfia* species), quinidine (alkaloid obtained from the bark of *Cinchona* species), and sparteine (alkaloid obtained from the broom shrub). The treatment risks associated with these compounds are similar to those of synthetic antiarrhythmic drugs. Hence it is better to use the substances in pure, isolated form rather than in the form of herbal extract-based preparations. Further information on the medicinal uses of ajmaline, quinidine, and sparteine as isolated compounds can be found in textbooks of pharmacology.

Extracts from the perennial herb motherwort *(Leonurus cardiaca)* are recommended for the treatment of nervous heart conditions. The 1986 Commission E monograph recommends an average daily dose of 4.5 g of the crude drug. The cut and dried aerial parts of motherwort occur as ingredients in "cardiovascular teas" (from Kneipp and other manufacturers), and motherwort extract is an ingredient of several combination products (e.g., Crataezyma, Oxacant).

Mixtures of herbal cardiotonics and volatile oils containing 3–12 ingredients are available for local external application. There is some rationale for products that contain ingredients with local irritating properties. Products such as Cor-Selekt ointment or Kneipp Heart Ointment are rubbed into the dermatome that is associated with the heart (an area on the left side of the chest extending down to the costal arch, and an area on the left side of the back extending roughly from the base of the neck to the inferior angle of the scapula).

References

Ammon HPT, Händel M (1981) Crataegus, Toxikologie und Pharmakologie. Part 1: Toxizität. Planta Med 43: 105–120.
Eichstädt H, Bäder M, Danne O, Kaiser W, Stein U, Felix R (1989) Crataegus-Extrakt hilft dem Patienten mit NYHA II-Herzinsuffizienz. Therapiewoche 39: 3288–3296.
Fischer K, Jung F, Koscielny J, Kiesewetter H (1994) Crataegus-Extrakt vs. Methyldigoxin. Einfluß auf Rheologie und Mikrozirkulation bei 12 gesunden Probanden. Münch Med Wschr 136 (Suppl 1): 35–38.
Förster A, Förster K, Bühring M, Wolfstädter HD (1994) Crataegus bei mäßig reduzierter linksventrikulärer Auswurffraktion. Ergospirometrische Verlaufsuntersuchung bei 72 Patienten in doppelblindem Vergleich mit Plazebo. Münch Med Wschr 136 (Suppl 1): 21–26.
Hänsel R, Keller K, Rimpler H, Schneider G (eds) (1992) Hagers Handbuch der Pharmazeutischen Praxis. Vol. 4, Drogen A–D. 5th Ed. Springer Verlag, Berlin Heidelberg, pp 1040–1056.
Joseph G, Zhao Y, Klaus W (1995) Pharmakologisches Wirkprofil von Crataegus-Extrakt im Vergleich zu Epinephrin, Amrinon, Milrinon und Digoxin am isoliert perfundierten Meerschweinchenherzen. Arzneim Forsch/Drug Res 45: 1261–1265.
Krzeminski T, Chatterjee SS (1993) Ischemia and early reperfusion-induced arrhythmias: beneficial effects of an extract of Crataegus oxyacantha L. Pharm Pharmacol Lett 3: 45–48.
Kurcok A (1992) Ischemia- and reperfusion-induced cardiac injury, effects of two flavonoid-containing plant extracts possessing radical scavenging properties. Naunyn-Schmiedebergs's Arch Pharmacol 345 (Suppl RB 81) Abstr 322.
Loew D (1994) Crataegus-Spezialextrakte bei Herzinsutfizienz. Kassenarzt 15: 43–52.
Müller A, Linke W. Zhao Y, Klaus W (1996) Crataegus extract prolongs action potential duration in guinea pig papillary muscle. Phytomedicine 3: 257–261.
Pöpping S, Rose H, Ionescu I, Fischer Y, Kammermeier H (1995) Effect of a hawthorn extract on contraction and energy turnover of iolated rat cardiomyocytes. Arzneim Forsch/ Drug Res 45: 1157–1161.
Schlegelmilch R, Heywood R (1994) Toxicity of crataegus (hawthorn) extract (WS 1442). J Am Coll Toxicol 13: 103–111.
Schmidt U, Kuhn U, Ploch M, Hübner WD (1994) Wirksamkeit des Extraktes Ll 132 (600 mg/Tag) bei 8 wöchiger Therapie. Plazebokontrollierte Doppelblindstudie mit Weißdorn an 78 herzinsuffizienten Patienten im Stadium 11 nach NYHA. Münch Med Wschr 136 (Suppl 1):13–20.
Siegel G, Casper U, Schnalke F, Hetzer R (1996) Molecular physiological effector mechanisms of hawthorn extract in cardiac papillary muscle and coronary vascular smooth muscle. Phytother Res 10: 195–198.
Siegel G, Casper U (1995) Crataegi folium cum flore. In: Loew D, Rietbrock N (eds) Phytopharmaka in Forschung und klinischer Anwendung. Steinkopff Verlag, Darmstadt, pp 1–14.

Siegel G, Casper U, Walter H, Hetzer R (1994) Weißdorn-Extrakt LI 132. Dosis-Wirkungs-Studie zum Membranpotential und Tonus menschlicher Koronararterien und des Hundepapillarmuskels. Münch med Wschr 136 (Suppl 1): 47–56.

Sticher O, Rehwald A, Meier B (1994) Kriterien der pharmazeutischen Qualität von Crataegus-Extrakten. Münch Med Wschr 136 (Suppl 1): 69–73.

Tauchert M, Ploch M, Hübner WD (1994) Wirksamkeit des Weißdorn-Extraktes Ll 132 im Vergleich mit Captopril. Multizentrische Doppelblindstudie bei 132 Patienten mit Herzinsuffizienz im Stadium II nach NYHA. Münch Med Wschr 136 (Suppl 1): 27–34.

Tauchert M, Loew D (1995) Crataegi folium cum flore bei Herzinsuffizienz. In: Loew D, Rietbrock N (eds) Phytopharmaka in Forschung und klinischer Anwendung. Steinkopff Verlag, Darmstadt, pp 137–144.

Tauchert M, Siegel G, Schulz V (1994) Weißdorn Extrakt als pflanzliches Cardiacum (Vorwort). Neubewertung der therapeutischen Wirksamkeit. Münch Med Wschr 136 (Suppl 1): 3–5.

Weikl A, Assmus KD, Neukum-Schmidt A, Schmitz J, Zapfe G, Noh HS, Siegrist J (1996) Crataegus-Spezialextrakt WS 1442. Objektivierter Wirksamkeitsnachweis bei Patienten mit Herzinsuffizienz (NYHA II). Fortschr Med 114: 291–296.

Weiss RF (ed) (1991) Lehrbuch der Phytotherapie. 7th Ed., Hippokrates Verlag Stuttgart, p 223.

3.2
Hypotension and Hypertension

Hypotension and hypertension are not considered primary indications for phytotherapy. Nevertheless, some herbal medications are suitable for short-term use in the symptomatic treatment of orthostatic complaints associated with low blood pressure and for longer-term use as a supportive therapy in patients with high blood pressure.

3.2.1
Phytotherapy of Hypotension

Hypotension ordinarily refers to blood pressures less than 100 mm Hg systolic and 60 mm Hg diastolic. Low blood pressure has no pathologic significance in itself and is even beneficial in inhibiting atherosclerotic disease. Hypotension requires treatment only if it is associated with orthostatic symptoms such as dizziness, grogginess, headache, and fatigue. Physical therapy (e.g., physical training, Kneipp regimens) and dietary measures (increased fluid and salt intake) are the mainstays of treatment, and medications are used only temporarily in a supportive role. Dihydroergotamine, a hydrogenation product of the alkaloid ergotamine, is believed to increase the tonus of capacitance vessels by the stimulation of α-adrenergic receptors, resulting in increased venous return and a rise in blood pressure. However, dihydroergotamine is a modified pure plant constituent and, as such, is not considered a phytotherapeutic agent. Pharmacology textbooks may be consulted for more details on this compound.

On the other hand, preparations made from caffeine-containing herbs and certain aromatic herbs containing volatile oils are correctly classified as herbal antihypotensives.

Extracts from the broom shrub (Scotch broom; *Cytisus*) can no longer be recommended for antihypotensive therapy. Commission E approved this herb for "functional cardiovascular complaints" in its 1991 monograph, but the main alkaloid constituent of broom, sparteine, has shown a narrow range of therapeutic utility. Also, sparteine is poorly metabolized in a significant percentage of the population who have a congenital enzyme defect, delaying the excretion of this compound by a factor of 1000 so that even low doses can pose a significant health risk. A final problem with broom extract is that its therapeutic efficacy has not been adequately documented (Eichelbaum, 1986).

3.2.1.1
Caffeine-Containing Herbs and Beverages

Caffeine and caffeine-containing beverages are agents with unpredictable antihypotensive effects. It is a common experience, however, for people with low blood pressure to feel better after drinking their morning coffee or tea. Caffeine and other methylxanthines act directly on the pressor centers of the circulatory system; they also exert mild positive inotropic and chronotropic effects on the heart. Their duration of action is approximately 1–3 h.

A morning coffee infusion is prepared with 5–8 g of roasted coffee per cup (150 mL). Roasted coffee has a caffeine content of about 1–2%, so a total of about 100 mg of caffeine is ingested in one cup of coffee.

Dried tea leaves contain 2–5% caffeine. But given the smaller amount of herb that is used, and the method of extraction (infusion) one cup of black tea contains only about 30–50 mg of caffeine. Other caffeine-containing herbs are guarana seeds, cola seeds, maté leaves, and cocoa beans. The amounts of methylxanthines contained in these herbs are shown in Table 3.3. Extracts from guarana and cola seeds are sold over the counter in the form of chewable tablets or drink mixtures. Due to the unpredictable risks, especially to children and adolescents (lethal caffeine dose between 3 and 10 g!), efforts are being made to restrict the over-the-counter availability of guarana products.

Caffeine is lipid-soluble, so it is readily absorbed from the gastrointestinal tract. The monographs state that caffeine and caffeine-containing herbs are useful for the short-term relief of symptoms due to mental or physical fatigue. None of the monographs address the treatment of hypotension or orthostatic complaints, but we know from experience that many hypotensive patients respond positively to caffeine and caffeine-containing herbs. The possible side effects of caffeine-containing herbs include stomach upset, nervousness, and sleeplessness.

Table 3.3. Percentage content of methylxanthines in dried herbs. n. d. = not detectable (Ploss, 1994).

Herbal drug	Caffeine	Theobromine	Theophylline
Coffee	0.9–2.6	0.002	0.0005
Cola nut	2.00	0.05	n.d.
Tea leaf	2.5–5.5	0.07–0.17	0.002–0.013
Cocoa bean	0.2	1.2	n.d.
Maté	0.5–1.5	n.d.	n.d.
Guarana	2.95–5.8	0.03–0.17	0.02–0.06

3.2.1.2
Essential Oils

Analeptic is an older term denoting a restorative remedy for states of weakness that are frequently accompanied by dizziness and fainting (Aschner, 1986). Traditional formulas for analeptics contained aromatic substances that stimulated the olfactory nerve and the sensory trigeminal nerve endings, causing a reflex stimulation of respiration and circulation. Among these substances were essential oils derived from aromatic herbs (plants containing volatile oils). The Commission E monographs recommend rosemary leaves (indicated for circulatory problems) and lavender leaves (indicated for functional circulatory disorders) as aromatic herbs for external use in balneology. Rosemary leaves contain at least 1.2 % volatile oil. A hot infusion is prepared from about 50 g of the crude drug and is added to the bath. Lavender leaves also contain at least 1.5 % volatile oil. About 100 g of lavender leaves are used to prepare a hot infusion for adding to bathwater. The Commission E monograph on camphor cites hypotensive regulatory disorders as one of its indications. Camphor is obtained from the wood of the camphor tree *(Cinnamomum camphora)* by steam distillation and consists of at least 96 % 2-bornanone.

It is likely that these aromatic herbs are effective only when the molecules of their volatile oils come in contact with the nasal mucosa through inhalation. The classic prototype is smelling salts, a preparation that is no longer manufactured today. But a homemade version can be prepared by placing 1–4 drops of essential oil on a sugar cube that is then slowly dissolved in the mouth. Rubbing the oil into the temples can also be beneficial. Essential oils should not be used in infants and small children due to the danger of reflex respiratory arrest.

3.2.2
Phytotherapy of Hypertension

According to the WHO definition, hypertension is present when the blood pressure exceeds 160 mm Hg systolic and 95 mm Hg diastolic. Blood pressures in the range of 140–160 systolic and 90–95 diastolic are classified as borderline hypertension, which is usually managed by nonpharmacologic means (weight loss, low-salt diet, exercise). An herbal remedy that has been used in the treatment of mild to moderate hypertension is the whole extract made from the dried roots of Indian snakeroot (Rauwolfia serpentina), an evergreen shrub native to tropical Asia. The extract contains more than 50 different alkaloids, including the sympatholytic agent reserpine. Reserpine is not only one of the oldest antihypertensive agents, it is still one of the most economical. Because of its association with objectionable side effects, particularly at doses higher than 0.2 mg/day (depression, fatigue, impotence, nasal stuffiness), the use of reserpine has declined in industrialized countries, but it is still included as a standard antihypertensive agent in the WHO list of essential drugs. Because reserpine is an isolated compound with a known chemical composition, it is not considered a phytotherapeutic agent.

The whole extract derived from Indian snakeroot has the same actions and side effects as reserpine when properly standardized and administered in the proper dose. Because of its narrow therapeutic range, however, rauwolfia extract does not meet the safety criteria of an acceptable phytomedicine (see Sect. 1.5.1.1, 1.5.4, and 1.5.5). Besides two combination products that cannot be recommended, the *Rote Liste 1994* cites only one standardized rauwolfia-extract-based product (Arte Rautin forte M drops) that is still marketed in Germany. The product is standardized to 7% total alkaloids. It has no apparent advantage over reserpine therapy which is easier to control.

Several older antihypertensives that have de facto approval in Germany contain preparations made from European mistletoe, olive leaves, and rhododendron leaves as their active ingredients. The parenteral use of mistletoe preparations may cause a transient fall in blood pressure, but this is due to an allergic response based on the release of biogenic amines and may not signify real therapeutic benefit for hypertension. The antihypertensive effect of orally administered mistletoe preparations has not been adequately documented. Palliative use of parenteral mistletoe preparations in cancer patients is discussed in Chap. 9.

The dried leaves of the olive tree are used in Italian folk medicine as a remedy for high blood pressure (Poletti et al., 1982), but clinical studies have not furnished definite proof of their therapeutic efficacy in hypertension.

Rhododendron leaves contain grayanotoxins, which lower blood pressure. But these compounds are highly toxic, causing nausea, vomiting, diarrhea and, at higher doses, muscular and respiratory paralysis. Consequently, rhododendron leaf extract is not considered an acceptable herbal antihypertensive.

It has been shown that spontaneously hypertensive rats can be made normotensive by adding garlic powder to their feed (Jacob et al., 1991). In a meta-analysis of eight clinical studies with coated garlic powder tablets, three of which specifically included hypertensive patients, four of the studies showed a significant reduction in diastolic blood pressures while three showed a significant reduction in systolic pressures (Silagy and Neil, 1994). In an observational study of some 2000 patients taking 300 mg of garlic powder three times daily, 1.3% of the patients developed new orthostatic symptoms while on that therapy (Beck and Grünwald, 1993). In summary, it may be concluded that garlic powder preparations taken in an adequate dose (600–1200 mg/day of active ingredient) have mild antihypertensive effects that are significant both therapeutically and with regard to possible side effects and drug-drug interactions (additive effects with other antihypertensives). Based on information currently available, garlic powder preparations are the only phytomedicines that can be recommended as adjuncts in the treatment of hypertensive patients. The vasoactive properties of garlic are discussed more fully in Sect. 3.3 below.

References

Aschner B (1986) Lehrbuch der Konstitutionstherapie. Hippokrates Stuttgart, p 311.

Beck E, Grünwald J (1993) Allium sativum in der Stufentherapie der Hyperlipidämie. Med Welt 44: 516–520.

Eichelbaum M (1986) Pharmakogenetische Aspekte der Arzneimitteltherapie. In: Dölle W, Müller-Oerlinghausen B, Schwabe U (eds) Grundlagen der Arzneimitteltherapie. Wissenschaftsverlag Bl, Mannheim Vienna Zürich, pp 438–448.

Jacob R, Ehrsam M, Ohkubo T, Rupp H (1991) Antihypertensive und kardioprotektive Effekte von Knoblauchpulver (Allium sativum). Med Welt (Suppl 7a): 39–41.

Ploss E (1994) Guarana semen – Guaranasamen. Wissenschaftliche Bewertung (unpublished).

Silagy C, Neil A (1994) A meta-analysis of the effect of garlic on blood pressure. J Hypertension 12: 463–468.

3.3
Atherosclerosis and Arterial Occlusive Disease

Some phytomedicines are useful in the prevention or symptomatic treatment of atherosclerosis and its sequelae. Particular value is ascribed to certain *Allium* species (garlic, onion, ramson) in the prevention of atherosclerosis, and the effects of garlic have been extensively documented by pharmacologic and clinical research. The antiatherosclerotic effects of garlic are based mainly on its vasodilating, rheologic, and lipid-reducing actions. It has been discovered that garlic lowers blood lipids by inhibiting cholesterol synthesis. Other lipid-reducing plant constituents for the secondary prophylaxis of atherosclerosis are phospholipids derived from soybeans, oat bran, and guar gum.

Special extracts from *Ginkgo biloba* leaves have value in the symptomatic treatment of peripheral arterial occlusive disease. Another major application of these ginkgo extracts is in the symptomatic treatment of cognitive deficits secondary to organic brain disease (see Sect. 2.1).

3.3.1
Garlic

3.3.1.1
Historical Background

Garlic is a traditional herb. Some of the earliest references to this medicinal and culinary plant are found on Sumerian clay tablets dating from 2600–2100 BC. Garlic was an important medicine to the ancient Egyptians, appearing in 22 of the more than 800 remedies listed in the famous Ebers papyrus (ca. 1550 BC). The Greek historian Herodotus, who traveled through Egypt in about 450 BC, reported that the workers who built the pyramids were given large rations of onions, radishes, and garlic. A sum of 1600 silver talents (equivalent to about $ 10 million) was spent over a 20-year period to supply some 360,000 workers with these provisions. Herodotus went on to explain that large amounts of garlic were necessary to protect the pyramid builders from febrile illnesses.

The Israelites learned about garlic from the Egyptians. After the Hebrew slaves had been led out of Egypt, they bemoaned the loss of this valuable medicine and spice with these words:

> "We remember the fish we ate in Egypt for nothing, the cucumbers, the melons, the leeks, the onions, and the garlic; but now our strength is dried up, and there is nothing at all . . ."   (Numbers 11: 5–6)

Garlic has been known in Europe as a healing herb since the Middle Ages. It owed much of its popularity to the Benedictine monks who grew garlic in their monastery gardens. Garlic was thought to be a valuable remedy for communicable diseases, and many references are found to its use in plagues. When Basel was struck by the plague, the Jewish population who consumed garlic regularly, reportedly fared much better than other citizens. In 1721 the plague was rampant in Marseilles. During this time a band of thieves looted the city, robbing the sick and dead alike, without contracting the disease themselves. When one of the thieves was caught, he explained that his band had regularly consumed garlic soaked in wine and vinegar.

Besides its antimicrobial properties, garlic was prized by the peoples of Europe and the Orient for its effects on the heart and circulation. For example, garlic was commonly recommended as a remedy for "dropsy" (cardiac insufficiency). The lipid-reducing and antiatherosclerotic effects of garlic – a focal point of current interest – were unknown in ancient and medieval medicine because atherosclerosis did not become an important disease entity until the Industrial Age. Koch and Hahn (1988) published a detailed account of the history of the medicinal uses of garlic.

3.3.1.2
Botanical Description

A member of the lily family, garlic (*Allium sativum*, Fig. 3.8) traces its origins to Central Asia. Today it is known only in its cultivated form. The subterranean garlic bulb is not laminar like an onion but is a composite structure consisting of 4–20 cloves, each enclosed within a dry, white leaf skin. The weight of one clove is highly variable, averaging about 1 g. Rising from the cloves are unbranched, quill-like stalks about 30–90 cm high topped by flowers arranged in a loose, globular cluster. This flower head is surrounded by a cylindrical, sharply tapered leaf, or spathe, resembling a pointed cap. The cluster is an umbel composed of about 5–7 pale flowers that bloom from June to August. Among the flowers are about 20–30 bulbils or "brood bulbs" up to 1 cm in size. Because the flowers are almost always sterile, the bulbils perform an important reproductive function.

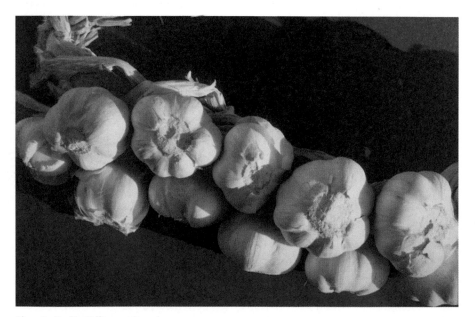

Fig. 3.8. Garlic *(Allium sativum).*

3.3.1.3
Crude Drug

Only the garlic bulb has culinary and medicinal applications. Today it is entirely a product of commercial cultivation (Fig. 3.9). World production is approximately 2 million tons annually, with about 60% grown in Asia (mostly China), 20% in Europe, and 10% each in North America and Africa (Fenwick and Hanley, 1985).

Most garlic is processed into a powdered form immediately after harvesting. Garlic powder is produced by peeling the cloves, cutting them into slices, and drying them for 3–4 days at a maximum temperature of 50 °C to a residual moisture content of less than 5%. During this process the garlic loses about two-thirds of its fresh weight (Heikal et al., 1972). Drying destroys very little of the sulfur-containing constituents or the enzyme alliinase that causes their breakdown (see Sect. 3.3.1.4); but the residual moisture in the garlic powder leads to a gradual but constant enzymatic decomposition and subsequent volatilization of the sulfur-containing compounds that contribute to garlic's medicinal effects. This process limits the shelf life of fresh garlic and of garlic-based medications.

Besides the powdered herb, there are other preparations that are used in medicinal garlic products. In terms of practical significance, the most important are garlic oil macerations (cold oil infusions) using fatty oils. In this process the garlic cloves are ground, covered with a vegetable oil such as corn oil or wheat germ oil, and allowed to stand so that lipophilic compounds can dissolve into the oil. A press is then used to separate the oil from the solid residues. These preparations do not contain the water-soluble constituents of garlic.

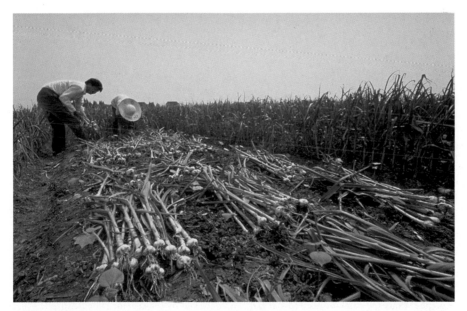

Fig. 3.9. All garlic for commercial use is cultivated.

Another process uses steam distillation to obtain essential garlic oil from freshly ground garlic. Garlic bulbs have about a 0.1–0.5% content of water-soluble compounds. Analogous to cold oil infusions, the compounds present in essential garlic oil no longer correspond to the original plant constituents as enzymatic and thermal breakdown transform alliin and other thiosulfinates (see Sect. 3.3.1.4) into sulfur-containing products. While garlic-oil preparations are known to have certain therapeutic effects, they are not nearly as effective as garlic powder and other medicinal garlic preparations.

Garlic fermentation products (aged garlics) have been available on the pharmaceutical market for several years now. These odor-free products are fermented for several months in the presence of moisture and atmospheric oxygen, resulting in the conversion of all reactive garlic constituents into more or less inert degradation products. One would not expect these fermented products to have significant medicinal actions, nor have such actions been demonstrated in pharmacologic or clinical studies.

3.3.1.4
Key Constituents, Analysis, Pharmacokinetics

The constituents of garlic are ordinarily divided into two groups: sulfur-containing compounds and non-sulfur-containing compounds. Most of the medicinal effects of garlic are referable to the sulfur compounds and the alliin-splitting enzyme alliinase. Thus, commercial garlic preparations are often adjusted or standardized to sulfur-containing ingredients, particularly to the amino acid alliin contained in garlic powder.

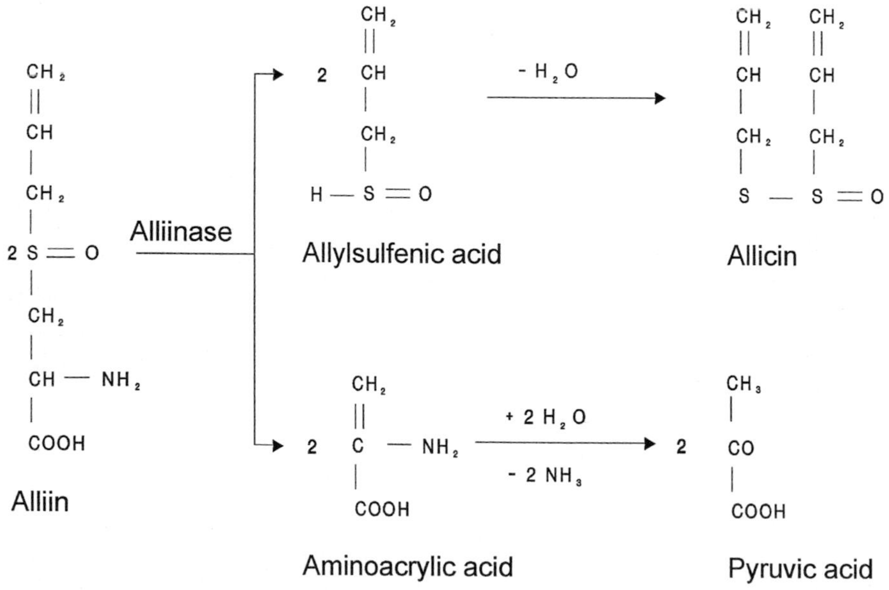

Fig. 3.10. Alliin, the natural constituent of garlic, is converted by the enzyme alliinase to allicin and pyruvic acid.

Garlic cloves typically contain about 0.35% total sulfur (about 1% of dry weight) and about 1% total nitrogen. The organic sulfur compounds in garlic are derived from the amino acid cysteine or its derivatives and can be subdivided into S-allylcysteine sulfoxide and γ-glutamyl-S-allylcysteines. Apparently the cysteine sulfoxides are stored in the form of γ-glutamylcysteines, which undergo a gradual hydrolytic cleavage during germination of the garlic bulb and in products that are stored. Thus, freshly harvested garlic differs markedly from stored garlic, especially in its content of γ-glutamylcysteines.

Fresh garlic contains about 0.5–1% cysteine sulfoxides, mostly alliin, and an equal amount of γ-glutamylcysteines. Garlic powder that has been carefully dried may contain up to twice the concentrations of these constituents. Garlic powder products are usually standardized to a specified content of alliin or of the allicin that is released from alliin by the action of the enzyme alliinase (Fig. 3.10). Alliin is separated from alliinase while it is still in the cells of an intact garlic bulb. But when the bulb is chopped or crushed, damage to the cells allows the alliin to come into contact with alliinase, and within minutes the enzyme converts the alliin into the volatile compound allicin. Allicin has an aromatic odor but is unstable in aqueous and oily solution, and within a few hours it degrades into vinyldithiins and ajoene. Cold oil infusions and distilled garlic oils contain only the products of alliin degradation.

The amount of sulfur-containing constituents in fresh garlic is highly variable (Fig. 3.11); hence it is important to standardize garlic-powder preparations to a specified concentration range of alliin. This standardization may well account for the positive, reproducible results that have been obtained in recent years with garlic-powder tablets in controlled clinical studies (see Sect. 3.3.7).

The non-sulfur-containing constituents of garlic include alliinase and other enzymes. These enzymes appear to have significant bearing on the bioavailability of

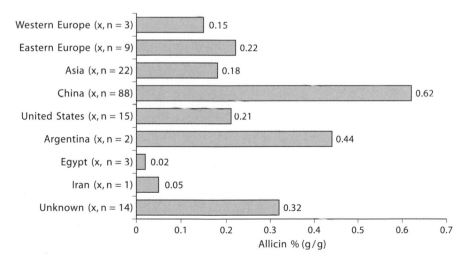

Fig. 3.11. Quantity of allicin released from garlic samples obtained from various regions of the world. The tests were performed between 1984 and 1990. Quantitative allicin release varied by up to a factor of 31 among different samples (Chinese vs. Egyptian garlic) (Pfaff, 1991).

garlic principles, and the garlic should be dried in a manner that preserves the enzymes (e. g., avoiding air temperatures in excess of 50 °C). Other non-sulfur-containing garlic constituents are various amino acids, proteins, lipids, steroids, vitamins, and 12 trace elements (Block 1992; Reuter and Sendl, 1994).

Pharmacokinetic studies were performed in rats using ^{35}S-labeled alliin, allicin, and vinyldithiin. Each compound was administered in a dose of 8 mg/kg, and the activity levels were determined in terms of ^{35}S-alliin. Blood levels were measured over a 72-h period along with excretion levels in the urine, feces, and expired air. Whole-animal autoradiographs were also obtained to assess organ distribution. It was found that the rates of absorption and elimination for ^{35}S-alliin were markedly higher than for the other garlic constituents. Maximum blood levels were reached within 10 min after oral administration (by stomach tube). The measured urinary levels indicated a minimum absorption rate of 65 % for allicin and 73 % for the vinyldithiins. Approximately 20 % was found in the stool, and traces were detectable in the expired air (Lachmann et al., 1994).

3.3.1.5
Experimental Pharmacology

To date, some 100 original papers have been published on the experimental pharmacology of garlic and its preparations, so it is not possible to provide here a complete listing of bibliographic references. (Surveys may be found in Reuter et al., 1994, 1995.)

Most pharmacologic studies in the past 20 years have been done in animal models and have dealt mostly with the antiatherogenic, lipid-reducing, and antihypertensive effects of garlic; its inhibitory effects on cholesterol synthesis; its properties as a vasodilator and antioxidant; and its capacity to activate fibrinolysis and inhibit platelet aggregation. Older studies tended to focus on the antimicrobial properties of garlic.

3.3.1.5.1
Effects on Atherogenesis and Lipid Metabolism

Five groups of authors (Jain, 1975, 1977; Bordia et al., 1977; Chang et al., 1980; Kamanna et al., 1984; Mand et al., 1985) studied the effects of the long-term (2–9 months) feeding of garlic and garlic preparations to rabbits with experimental atherosclerosis induced by a high-cholesterol diet. Most of the authors found that dietary garlic supplementation caused a statistically significant reduction of atheromatous lesions, particularly in the aorta, that averaged about 50 %. The duration of use was a highly significant factor, and a period of months was necessary to inhibit atherogenesis. Comparative studies with various garlic preparations showed that the antiatheromatous effects were due mainly to the lipophilic fractions in the garlic, with hydrophilic fractions playing a lesser role. Other authors who studied specific garlic constituents (Fujiwara et al., 1972; Itokawa et al., 1973; Zhao et al., 1983) showed that the sulfur-containing compounds have special significance in inhibiting atherogenesis. Heinle and Betz (1994) documented antiatheromatous effects in live rats, and Orekhov et al. (1995) observed similar effects on atherosclerotic plaque in human aortas. Jacob et al. (1993) demonstrated cardioprotective effects in rats with experimental myocardial infarction that had been fed garlic powder for 10 weeks.

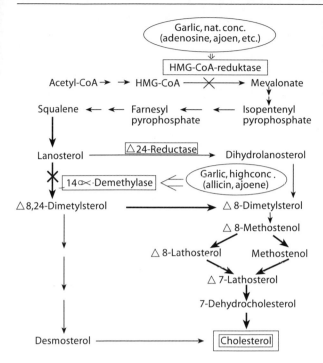

Fig. 3.12.
Metabolic pathways of cholesterol biosynthesis. Garlic constituents inhibit cholesterol synthesis in an early phase (HMG-CoA-reductase) and in a late phase (14α-demethylase) (Gabhardt, 1993).

The inhibitory effects of garlic on cholesterol biosynthesis were first documented by Quereshi et al. (1983) in chicken hepatocytes and monkey livers. These authors also conducted comparative studies with three extract fractions. At equivalent doses, both the whole herb and its lipophilic and hydrophilic fractions caused a 50–75 % inhibition of two key enzymes in cholesterol biosynthesis. In experiments with rat hepatocytes, Gebhardt et al. (1993, 1994) identified the steps in cholesterol biosynthesis that are influenced by garlic and its sulfur-containing constituents (Fig. 3.12). The studies of Quereshi and Gebhardt are particularly noteworthy. Their results show that the inhibition of endogenous cholesterol biosynthesis occurs as a physiologic response to the ingestion of certain plant constituents.

3.3.1.5.2
Effects on Vascular Resistance, Fibrinolysis, and Platelet Aggregation
Chandorkar and Jain (1973) and Malik et al. (1981) demonstrated the ability of garlic preparations to lower blood pressure in experimental dogs.

Jacob et al. (1991) tested the effects of garlic powder added to the feed of spontaneously hypertensive rats for periods of 2 weeks to 11 months. The results of this study (Fig. 3.13) provide very impressive evidence of the antihypertensive effect of garlic, which was accompanied by a reduction in secondary myocardial injury.

Besides the inhibition of plaque formation, the antihypertensive properties of garlic appear to be based partly on a direct vasodilating action of garlic constituents. Siegel et al. (1991, 1992) investigated these effects in isolated strips from canine carotid arteries and in isolated vascular muscle cells. They found that aqueous garlic extracts and some sulfur-containing compounds produced a strong membrane-po-

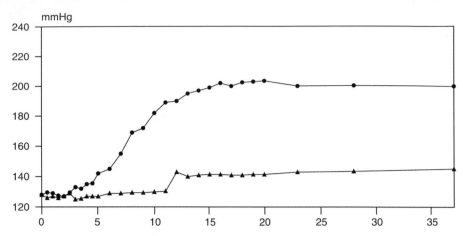

Fig. 3.13. Progression of blood pressure readings in spontaneously hypertensive rats. Time 0 corresponds to delivery of the experimental animals (at about 3 weeks of age). The animals were observed for approximately 9 months. The upper curve represents the control animals; the lower curve represents animals given an average dose of 1 g/kg b.w. garlic powder daily added to their standard feed (Jacob et al., 1991).

larizing effect, suggesting that certain garlic constituents may act as potassium channel openers. A recent study showed that garlic is a potent activator of endogenous nitric oxide synthesis (Das et al., 1995). Nitric oxide is known as a powerful vasodilator whose functions include physiologic vasodilatation in response to muscular exercise (Bode-Böger et al., 1994).

The activating effect of garlic on fibrinolysis and its inhibitory effect on platelet aggregation have been demonstrated in a total of 16 experimental studies, some done in live animals and some performed in vitro. These studies and their results are reviewed in Reuter et al. (1994, 1995, 1996). Most of these studies showed that various garlic preparations as well as certain sulfur-containing metablic products of alliin act to stimulate endogenous fibrinolysis and inhibit platelet aggregation. A therapeutic trial in patients with increased platelet aggregation showed an absence of acute effects; treatment had to be continued for 2–4 weeks to achieve a significant response (Kiesewetter et al., 1993). Das et al. (1995) identified the activation of calcium-dependent nitric oxide synthetase as the mechanism by which garlic inhibits platelet aggregation.

3.3.1.5.3
Antimicrobial Properties

A number of predominantly older studies showed that garlic and its aqueous preparations had marked antibacterial and antifungal properties, with a few studies even showing evidence of antiviral activity. These studies are reviewed in Reuter et al. (1994, 1995). The antimicrobial properties of garlic are mainly of historical interest (see Sect. 3.3.1) and have no practical significance for treatment of infectious diseases today, at least in industrialized countries. However, garlic could also prevent arteriosclerosis by acting against chlamydia pneumoniae.

3.3.1.5.4
Other Actions

Various experimental models in rabbits, rats, and guinea pigs have demonstrated the antihypertensive properties of garlic (Mathew et al., 1973; Jain, 1977; Zacharias et al., 1980; Chang et al., 1980). The groups of Mathew and Chang concluded from their findings that garlic stimulates insulin production, but therapeutic studies (see Sect. 3.3.7) have shown no evidence that garlic has antidiabetic properties in human patients.

Five studies have described antitoxic effects of garlic in cases of carbon tetrachloride, isoproterenol, and heavy metal poisoning. Garlic has exhibited tumor-inhibiting properties in 12 other studies, showing the greatest effects in sarcomas, bladder tumors, liver cell carcinomas, and isolated colon carcinoma cells. Two relatively recent studies report on the antioxidant effects of garlic preparations (Popov and Lewin, 1994; Török et al., 1994).

Because the therapeutic implications of the antitoxic, antitumor, and antioxidant properties of garlic are still unclear, we shall not present further details of these studies; the interested reader may consult the survey in Reuter and Sendl (1994).

3.3.1.6
Toxicology

Tests of the acute toxicity of allicin in mice indicated LD_{50} values of 60 mg/kg by intravenous injection and 120 mg/kg by subcutaneous injection (Cavallito and Bailey, 1944). A more recent study on the acute toxicity of a garlic extract in rats and mice showed lethal effects following the oral, intraperitoneal, and subcutaneous administration of doses higher than 30 mL/kg (Nakagawa et al., 1984).

In another study, rats fed up to 2000 mg/kg of a garlic extract for 6 months showed no weight loss but did show a slightly reduced food intake relative to controls. There were no changes in renal function, hematologic parameters, or selected serologic parameters, and there was no evidence of any pathologic changes in organs or tissues (Sumiyoshi et al., 1984).

A study testing for genotoxicity in mouse bone marrow cells after the oral administration of garlic showed no significant changes in comparison with untreated controls (Abraham and Kesavan, 1984).

A review of other studies on the toxicology of garlic may be found in Koch (1988, 1996).

In summary, available toxicologic findings raise no significant concerns about the therapeutic use of garlic in humans.

3.3.1.7
Clinical Studies

Twenty-eight controlled clinical studies on garlic preparations were published from 1985 to 1995. Two of these studies were done with garlic oil or an oil maceration; the rest used coated garlic powder tablets adjusted to an alliin content of 1.0–1.4 % (Table 3.4). Further discussions in this chapter pertain exclusively to studies that used standardized garlic powder tablets. The results of these studies cannot be validly applied to other garlic preparations due to differences in pharmaceutical quality. Recently, several surveys and meta-analyses have been published that provide de-

Table 3.4. Review of 18 clinical studies in a total of 2920 patients taking standardized garlic powder pills (coated tablets). Sixteen of these studies were completed after release of the Commission E monograph on garlic. The standardized garlic powder was administered in a daily dose of 300–1200 mg for a period of 2–24 weeks. The references can be found in Koch et al. (1995) and Reuter (1995, 1996).

First author, year	Number of patients		mg/day	Weeks	Key parameters
	Total	Taking garlic			
Ernst, 1986	20	10	600	4	CH, TG
König, 1986	53	53	600	4	CH, TG, PVD, RR
Kandziora, 1988a	40	20	600	12	CH, TG, RR
Kandziora, 1988b	40	20	600	12	CH, TG, RR
Harenberg, 1988	20	20	600	4	CH, TG, FL, RR
Schwartzkopff, 1988	40	20	900	12	Lipid fractions, RR
Auer, 1989	47	24	600	12	CH, TG, RR
Brosche, 1989	40	40	600	12	Lipid fractions
Vorberg, 1990	40	20	900	16	CH, TG, RR, B
Zimmermann, 1990	23	23	900	3	CH, TG
Kiesewetter, 1990	64	32	800	12	PVD, TAH, PV, CH, RR
Mader, 1991	221	111	800	16	CH, TG, RR
Kiesewetter, 1992	60	30	800	5	TAH, EF, PV, RR
Holzgartner, 1992	94	47	900	12	CH, TG, HDL, LDL, RR
Rotzsch, 1992a	24	12	900	6	TG (postprandial)
Rotzsch, 1992b	1931	1061	600	6	CH (vs. diet)
Schmidt, 1992b	111	111	300–1200	2	Garlic odor
Almeida-Santos, 1992	52	25	900	24	CH, TG, LDL, HDL, RR, B

Abbreviations: CH = cholesterol reduction; TG = triglyceride reduction; B = improvement in mood; PVD = improvement in peripheral arterial occlusive disease symptoms; RR = blood pressure reduction; FL = activation of fibrinolysis; TAH = inhibition of platelet aggregation; PV = reduction of plasma viscosity; EF = increase in erythrocyte flow rate.

tailed, tabulated information on the various studies (Reuter and Sendl, 1994; Reuter et al., 1995; Silagy and Neil, 1994; Warshafsky et al., 1993).

The antiatherosclerotic effects of garlic can be directly demonstrated only in animal models, not by clinical studies in patients. Because atherosclerosis develops gradually over a period of many years or decades, the direct demonstration of anti-atherosclerotic effects in humans poses serious methodologic problems. Such research would have to be conducted in large numbers of patients over a prolonged period of time to allow for the large methodologic variations that are inherent in the few diagnostic procedures that are available (e.g., ultrasound measurement of plaque volumes in the carotid artery).

Thus, the criteria used in the clinical studies on garlic preparations consisted entirely of indirect, surrogate parameters of atherosclerosis such as hyperlipidemia, hypertension, decreased fibrinolysis, or increased platelet aggregation. One study used increased walking distance in patients with peripheral arterial occlusive disease as its key parameter (Kiesewetter et al., 1993).

3.3.1.7.1
Effects on Blood Lipids
Table 3.4 lists 18 therapeutic studies that were performed with coated garlic powder tablets of standard quality. A total of 2920 patients participated in these studies. Four studies did not use control groups, two compared coated garlic tablets with a

reference therapy, and 12 were double-blind and placebo-controlled. The usual daily dose was in the range of 600–900 mg garlic powder, and the duration of treatment in most studies was 4–12 weeks.

Table 3.5 lists 11 studies that showed a reduction in cholesterol during the course of treatment. In nine of the studies the reduction was statistically significant. Eight of the 11 studies allowed a statistical comparison with control groups. Again, all these studies showed a reduction in cholesterol, with 5 studies showing a statistically significant reduction, 1 study showing a tendency toward reduction, and 2 studies showing an insignificant decrease. It is noteworthy that the significant results were all achieved after 1989, presumably owing to the use of higher doses or larger case numbers than in earlier studies (Table 3.4).

Table 3.6 shows analogous results for triglyceride levels. These results showed greater variation than the cholesterol findings, but most of the studies (8 of 11) indicated marked reductions in plasma triglycerides. Due to the greater variation in the progression and interindividual scatter of triglyceride levels, only 5 of the 8 controlled studies showed statistically significant differences, especially in relation to the control groups. Again, the post-1989 studies are of greater value in demonstrating efficacy.

The most comprehensive placebo-controlled study, involving 261 patients, is that of Mader et al. (1990). These authors found significant reductions in total cholesterol compared with placebo-treated controls over a 16-week course of treatment. The most pronounced effects were seen in patients whose initial cholesterol levels were between 250 and 300 mg/dL.

Holzgartner et al. (1992) conducted a 3-month double-blind study comparing the efficacy of 3 × 200 mg bezafibrate with that of 3 × 300 mg garlic powder in 94 pa-

Table 3.5. Efficacy of standardized garlic powder pills (coated tablets) in patients with hyperlipidemia. Review of the principal results on cholesterol reduction in 11 studies that were completed or published after release of the Commission E monograph on garlic. The garlic powder was administered in a daily dose of 600–900 mg. The references can be found in Koch et al. (1995) and Reuter (1995, 1996).

Author, year, design c)	Cholesterol a) before:after (mg/dL)	Difference b)	
		During course of treatment (%)	Relative to controls (%)
Harenberg, 1988	278:258	−7*	
Kandziora, 1988, K	314:294	−6 f	−5 ns
Schwartzkopff, 1988, R	278:274	−1 ns	−3 ns
Auer, 1989, R	268:230	−14*	−6 +
Brosche, 1989	260:240	−8***	
Vorberg, 1990, R	259:233	−21***	−17***
Kiesewetter, 1990, R	267:234	−12***	−8*
Mader, 1990, R	266:235	−12***	−9***
Holzgartner, 1992, K	282:210	−25***	
Rotzsch, 1992b, K	261:253	−3***	−2***
Almeida-Santos, 1992, R	267:243	−5*	−6*

a) Mean values at beginning and end of treatment with garlic powder.
b) Significance levels of p values: +: <0.1; *: <0.05; **: <0.01; ***: <0.001; ns: not significant; f: significance not indicated.
c) R: double-blind study using placebo; K: drug vs. control group.

Table 3.6. Same as Table 3.5, but here reviewing the study data on triglyceride reduction. All but two of the studies showed reductions in plasma triglyceride levels during the course of treatment or relative to controls. However, due to the strong variations in triglyceride levels both diurnally and among different individuals, the reductions were statistically significant in only 7 of the 11 studies, including 5 studies comparing treatment groups. References can be found in Koch et al. (1995) and Reuter (1995, 1996).

Author, year, design c)	Triglycerides a) before:after (mg/dL)	Difference b) During course of treatment (%)	Relative to controls (%)
Harenberg, 1988	231:240	+4 ns	
Kandziora, 1988, K	213:197	−8 f	−7*
Schwartzkopff, 1988, R	140:160	+14 ns	+22 ns
Auer, 1989, R	171:140	−18*	−12*
Brosche, 1989	207:174	−16***	
Vorberg, 1990, R	206:156	−24 f	−19***
Kiesewetter, 1990, R	184:177	−4 ns	−4 ns
Mader, 1990, R	226:188	−17***	−15***
Holzgartner, 1992, K	218:144	−34***	
Rotzsch, 1992 a, R	134:104	−22 ns	−40*
Almeida-Santos, 1992, R	130:134	+4 ns	−34 ns

a) Mean values at start and end of treatment with garlic powder.
b) Significance levels of p values: +: <0.1; *: <0.05; **: <0.01; ***: <0.001; ns: not significant; f: significance not indicated.
c) R: double-blind study using placebo; K: drug vs. control group.

tients with hyperlipidemia. No significant difference was found between the two therapies in terms of total cholesterol reduction or in reducing the LDL cholesterol fraction and increasing the HDL fraction.

Two recently published meta-analyses of the studies in hyperlipidemic patients both concluded that garlic is effective in reducing blood lipid levels in humans. Allowing for placebo effects, it was concluded that garlic produced an average reduction of 9% (Warshafsky and Russel, 1993) or 12% (Silagy and Neil, 1994) in total serum cholesterol. The average reduction in triglycerides versus a placebo was 13% (Silagy and Neil, 1994). This applies to doses of 600–900 mg garlic powder taken daily for at least 4 weeks.

3.3.1.7.2
Blood Pressure Reduction
Blood pressure changes were investigated as an associated parameter in a total of 12 studies. Table 3.7 reviews the average blood pressures measured in garlic-treated subjects at the start and conclusion of the treatment periods. The percentage differences in blood pressures measured before and after treatment are indicated. The last column in Table 3.7 shows the statistical significance relative to a placebo or controls. The table indicates that, except for one study, all the researchers noted blood pressure reductions in the subjects who took coated garlic tablets. The reductions ranged from 2% to 17% of the initial values.

A meta-analysis of eight studies, including three that specifically included hypertensive patients, showed a significant reduction of diastolic blood pressure in four

Table 3.7. Mean blood pressure readings before and after treatment with garlic powder pills (coated tablets). The data pertain to patients on garlic therapy whose blood pressure had been measured as an accompanying parameter. In 11 of these 12 studies, a mean statistical reduction in blood pressure was measured in the patients on garlic therapy. A statistical group comparison was possible in 8 studies, and in 7 it showed significant reductions compared with control or placebo-treated groups. References can be found in Koch et al. (1995) and Reuter (1995, 1996).

Author, year, design	Mean BP Patients on garlic therapy			Significance Garlic vs. placebo
	Before	After	Diff.%	
König, 1986	167/107	156/97	−6/−5	−
Harenberg, 1988	137/86	126/81	−8/−9	−
Kandziora, 1988 a	174/99	158/83	−9/−16	−
Kandziora, 1988 b, K	178/100	167/85	·6/−15	−
Schwartzkopff, 1988, R	128/82	130/84	+2/+2	n.s.
Auer, 1989, R	171/101	151/90	−12/−11	*
Vorberg, 1990, R	144/90	138/87	−4/−3	*
Kiesewetter, 1990 b, R	152/85	150/82	−2/−3	*
Kiesewetter, 1991, R	116/73	108/67	−7/−9	*
Mader, 1991, R	151/92	143/85	−5/−8	*
Holzgartner, 1992, K	143/83	135/79	−6/ 5	*
Almeida-Santos, 1992, K	145/90	120/80	−17/−11	*

Abbreviations: BP = blood pressure, K = garlic vs. control group, R = randomized double-blind study using placebo, * = statistically significant (p < 0.001–0.05).

studies and a significant reduction of systolic blood pressure in three studies (Silagy and Neil, 1994). These authors concluded from the studies that garlic can slightly lower blood pressure when taken in doses equivalent to 600–900 mg of powder daily but that this effect is not adequate for specific antihypertensive therapy in patients with high blood pressure.

3.3.1.7.3
Antiatherosclerotic Effects in Humans

Drugs that reduce lipid levels, lower blood pressure, and inhibit platelet aggregation are useful mainly for the prevention of atherosclerosis and its sequelae. The pathogenic significance of reducing these risk factors is difficult to quantify in any given case, however. Thus, testing the efficacy of an antiatherosclerotic agent should not be limited to the measurement of surrogate parameters as stated above but should be supplemented by a direct follow-up of the progression of atherosclerotic disease. This type of evidence requires long-term observations conducted over a period of several years using suitable noninvasive techniques. One such technique is the measurement of pulse-wave velocity, which increases in proportion to the degree of sclerosis of the aorta and the loss of its *"windkessel"* function (Breithaupt et al., 1992).

The efficacy of a daily dose of at least 300 mg of a standardized garlic powder (brand name Kwai) was tested in a crossover study in two age- and gender-matched populations, one of which was treated with the garlic product. Each group of 101 adults 50–80 years of age consisted of matched pairs that were randomly assigned to either the treatment group or the control group. Pulse-wave velocities were determined in a standard protocol based on measurements taken in the carotid and fe-

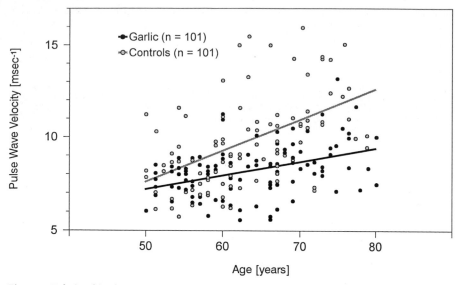

Fig. 3.14. Relationships between age and pulse wave velocity (PWV) in the garlic users (•) and control subjects (○). The slope of the lines relating age and PWV was different between the two groups (p < 0.0001). The linear regression line was less steep in the garlic group than in the control group; garlic group: PWV = 0.08 (SD, 0.017) age +3.03 (SD, 1.081); control group: PWV = 0.18 (SD, 0.029) age − 1.25 (SD, 1.822) (Breithaupt-Grögler et al., 1997).

moral arteries. Statistical analysis of the data showed that the average pulse-wave velocity was significantly lower in the garlic-treated group than in the control group (at rest: 8.3 ± 1.46 m/s vs. 9.8 ± 2.45 m/s, p < 0.0001). Pulse-wave velocities in both groups showed a significant positive correlation with age (garlic r = 0.44, control r = 0.52) and systolic blood pressure (garlic r = 0.48, control r = 0.54). The pulse-wave velocities for both treatment groups, correlated with blood pressure, are shown in Fig. 3.14 (Breithaupt-Grögler et al., 1997).

3.3.1.7.4
Further Clinical Studies

A placebo-controlled study was performed in a total of 80 patients with Fontaine stage II peripheral arterial occlusive disease. For 12 weeks the patients took either a daily dose equivalent to 800 mg of garlic powder or a placebo. All the patients received gait training as a basic therapy in addition to the garlic or placebo. The pain-free walking distance in the patients taking garlic increased by 46 m (from 161 ± 65 m to 207 ± 80 m); this was a significantly better outcome than in the placebo-treated patients, whose walking distance increased by 41 m (from 162 ± 61 m to 203 ± 73 m) (Kiesewetter et al., 1993).

Another study was performed in 60 subjects who had an increased propensity for spontaneous platelet aggregation. These subjects took a daily dose equivalent to 800 mg of garlic powder or a placebo for 4 weeks in a double-blind, placebo-controlled protocol. The differences between the two treatment groups at the end of 4 weeks were statistically significant (Kiesewetter et al., 1993).

A total of seven clinical pharmacologic studies in healthy subjects have dealt with the effects of garlic on endogenous fibrinolysis, plasma viscosity, arteriolar caliber, and blood flow velocity as determined by direct light microscopy at the nail fold. These techniques were used to test the dose-dependence of the response to a single dose of 100–2700 mg. It was found that 300 mg of the garlic powder preparation constituted the threshold dose for significant pharmacodynamic effects. Increasing the dose to 1200 mg led to proportionate increases in the demonstrable effects (Kiesewetter et al., 1993; survey in Reuter et al., 1994).

3.3.1.8
Side Effects and Garlic Odor

An observational study in 1993 investigated the side effects of a regimen of 3 × 300 mg/day garlic powder, taken in the form of coated tablets, in a total of 1997 patients. The participants were questioned at the start of the study and after 8 and 16 weeks of treatment. The difference between the reports on admission and the maximal reports at 8 or 12 weeks was interpreted as a specific effect of garlic use (Table 3.8). Gastrointestinal discomfort was the most frequent complaint, followed by orthostatic complaints, and allergic reactions. Other reported side effects included bloating, headache, dizziness, and outbreaks of sweating (Beck and Grünwald, 1993).

A double-blind study using a 5-fold crossover design was conducted in 123 patients to determine the incidence of garlic odor as a function of the ingested dose. The study period was divided into 2-week segments during which the participants took daily doses of 0 mg, 300 mg, 600 mg, 900 mg, and 1200 mg of garlic powder in tablet form. All the participants kept an odor log. Figure 3.15 shows the dose-dependent percentage of subjects who had an offensive garlic smell. As the graph indicates, daily doses of 900–1200 mg were associated with about a 50% incidence of garlic odor – a side effect that is known to prompt many patients to reduce their daily intake below the prescribed dose (Schmidt et al., 1992).

Table 3.8. During the course of an observational study, the side effects occurring in a total of 1997 patients on treatment with the commercial product Sapec (300 mg garlic powder per coated tablet) were systematically recorded. The recommended dosage was 1 tablet taken three times daily. The patients were questioned on admission to the study, at 8 weeks, and at 16 weeks. The differences between statements made on admission and at 8 and 12 weeks were interpreted as possible therapy-related side effects. Gastrointestinal complaints (6% reported nausea) and allergic reactions (1.1%) were confirmed as known adverse effects of garlic therapy. Surprisingly, there were relatively frequent reports of orthostatic circulatory problems (1.3% incidence of hypotension), underscoring the need to caution users about possible hypotensive effects in the prescribing literature and in package inserts for garlic medications. In the "other" category, bloating, headaches, dizziness, and outbreaks of sweating were reported somewhat more frequently during treatment than on admission (Beck and Grünwald, 1993).

Adverse side effects	Number of cases (% of 2010)		
	Admission (A)	Maximum (M)	Difference (M-A)
Nausea	149 (7%)	262 (13%)	113 (6%)
Hypotension	28 (1.4%)	54 (2.7%)	26 (1.3%)
Allergy	12 (0.6%)	35 (1.7%)	23 (1.1%)
Other	11 (0.5%)	27 (1.3%)	16 (0.8%)

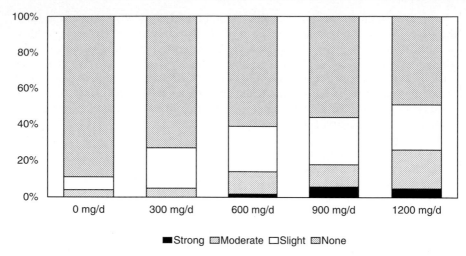

■Strong ▨Moderate ☐Slight ▨None

Fig. 3.15. Randomized double-blind study in 123 subjects using a 5-part crossover design; 111 of the protocols could be statistically evaluated. The subjects took 0 mg, 300 mg, 600 mg, 900 mg, and 1200 mg/day garlic pills for 14 days, and each participant kept an odor diary. The graph shows the percentage of subjects in the various dosage groups who perceived a garlic odor. The frequency of this complaint rises in proportion to the dosage, with about 50 % of subjects reporting garlic odor at a dosage of 1200 mg/day (Schmidt et al., 1992).

Unauthorized dose reductions may well have occurred in the therapeutic studies as well, suggesting that the efficacy demonstrated in those studies may have been based on daily doses lower than those stated in the published protocols.

3.3.1.9
Indications, Dosages, Risks, and Contraindications

The monograph on the garlic bulb published by Commission E in 1988 states that garlic preparations are indicated "as an adjunct to dietary measures in patients with elevated blood lipids and for the prevention of age-related vascular changes." In the years since this monograph was published, the results of 28 controlled clinical studies have become available. Most of these studies involved patients with hyperlipidemia, and two recently published meta-analyses have evaluated and summarized the results (Warshafsky and Russell, 1993; Silagy and Neil, 1994). Their findings: treatment with the garlic preparations led to an average reduction of 9–12 % in total cholesterol levels and a 13 % reduction in triglyceride levels relative to a placebo. Thus, both meta-analyses substantiate the first indication stated in the Commission E monograph.

Most of the clinical studies used coated garlic powder tablets taken in doses of 600–900 mg daily. This dose range is equivalent to eating about 2400–2700 mg of fresh garlic. The test preparations were standardized garlic powder tablets that had been adjusted to an alliin content of 1.0–1.4 %. Thus, the average daily dose recommended in the monograph of July 6, 1988, equivalent to 4 g of fresh garlic bulb, should be interpreted as a range of doses rather than a fixed mean value; Commission E states, in fact, that a dose of 2700 mg of fresh garlic, equivalent to 900 mg of garlic powder, is within the proper range of dosages when a high-quality preparation is used.

Meanwhile, studies in humans documenting the ability of garlic preparations to lower blood pressure, inhibit platelet aggregation, promote fibrinolysis, reduce lipid levels, and provide vasodilating and antioxidant effects are consistent with the anti-atherosclerotic effects of garlic that have been directly demonstrated in experiments with animals. This supports the second indication stated in the 1988 Commission E monograph: "... the prevention of age-related vascular changes." Of course, the phrase "age-related vascular changes" does not conform to standard medical terminology and should be replaced by the term atherosclerosis.

The 1988 monograph characterizes the side effects of garlic preparations as "infrequent gastrointestinal complaints, allergic reactions, and a garlic odor of the breath and skin." This list is confirmed in its nature and sequence by the results of an observational study (Table 3.8), except that hypotensive circulatory reactions, which have an incidence of more than 1%, should be added to the list after allergic reactions. Although Commission E claimed that there were no known drug-drug interactions, there is a possibility that garlic may potentiate the effect of antihypertensive and anticoagulant medications.

3.3.1.10
Therapeutic Significance
In the prescribing of medications by office practitioners, only high-dose coated garlic tablets (200-mg or preferably 300-mg coated tablets, daily dose equivalent to 900 mg garlic powder) have true significance as herbal lipid-reducing agents. They provide an alternative to synthetic lipid-reducing prescription drugs in patients with milder forms of hyperlipidemia. This particularly applies to patients who have an aversion to synthetic drugs. Garlic odor may be a problem for younger patients and patients who are employed (Fig. 3.15), but many older patients do not find it objectionable. Thus, the pros and cons of this therapy for the individual patient should always be weighed in consultation with the physician. Treatment with garlic preparations is a relatively low-cost option compared with other lipid-reducing drugs.

The great majority of garlic preparations are purchased and used without a prescription, mostly by older individuals. Since it is very likely that garlic has a prophylactic effect against atherosclerosis, this preventive therapy should be recommended to patients as a form of doctor-assisted self-medication.

3.3.1.11
Drug Products
Eight single-herb commercial garlic products are mentioned in the *Rote Liste 1995*, five of them based on garlic powder and three based on garlic oil or an oil maceration. Suitably designed clinical studies have been performed using standard garlic-powder products taken in doses of 600–900 mg/day, and their results are particularly useful for evaluating the lipid-reducing properties of garlic.

References

Abraham SK, Kesavan PC (1984) Genotoxicity of garlic, turmeric and asafoetida in mice. Mutat Res 136: 85–88.
Beck E, Grünwald J (1993) Allium sativum in der Stufentherapie der Hyperlipidämie. Med Welt 44: 516–520.
Block E (1992) The organosulfur chemistry of the genus Allium – implications for the organic chemistry of sulfur. Angew Chem Int Ed Engl 31: 1135–1178.
Bode-Böger SM, Böger RH, Schröder EP, Frölich JC (1994) Exercise increases systemic nitric oxide production in man. J Cardio Risk 1:173–178.
Bordia AK, Verma SK, Vyas AK, Khabya BL, Rathore AS, Bhu N, Bedi HK (1977) Effect of essential oil of onion and garlic on experimental atherosclerosis in rabbits. Atherosclerosis 26: 379–386.
Breithaupt K, Belz SG, Sinn W (1992) Noninvasive assessments of compliance of the aortic windkessel in man derived from pulse pressure/storage volume ratio and from pulse-wave velocity. Clin Physiol Biochem 9: 18–25.
Breithaupt-Grögler K, Ling M, Boudoulas H, Belz GG (1997) Protective effect of chronic garlic intake on the elastic properties of the aorta in the elderly. Circulation 96, No 7, in press.
Brosche T, Platt D (1990) Knoblauch als pflanzlicher Lipidsenker: Neuere Untersuchungen mit winem standardisierten Knoblauchtrockenpulver-Präparat. Fortschr Med 108: 703–706.
Cavallito CJ, Bailey JH (1944) Allicin, the antibacterial principle of Allium sativum. 1. Isolation, physical properties and antibacterial action. J Am Chem Soc 66:1950–1954.
Chandorkar AG, Jain PK (1973) Analysis of hypotensive action of Allium sativum (garlic). Indian J Physiol Pharmacol 17: 132–133.
Chang MLW, Johnson MA (1980) Effect of garlic on carbohydrate metabolism and lipid synthesis in rats. J Nutr 110: 931–936.
Das I, Khan NS, Sooranna SR (1995) Potent activation of nitric oxide synthase by garlic: a basis for its therapeutic applications. Curr Med Res Opin 13: 257–263.
Fenwick GR, Hanley AB (1985) The Genus Allium – Part 1. Crit Rev Food Sci Nutri 22 (3): 199–235.
Fujiwara M, Itokawa Y, Uchino H, Inoue K (1972) Anti-hypercholesterolemic effect of a sulfur-containing amino acid, S-methyl-L-cysteine sulfoxide, isolated from cabbage. Experientia 28: 254–255.
Gebhardt R. (1993) Multiple inhibitory effects of garlic extracts on cholesterol biosynthesis in hepatocytes. Lipids 28 (6): 613–619.
Gebhardt R, Beck H, Wagner KG (1994) Inhibition of cholesterol biosynthesis by allicin and ajoene in rat hepatocytes and HepG2 cells. Biochem Biophys Acta 1213: 57–62.
Heikal HA, Kamel Sl, Awaad KE, Khalil NF (1972) A study on the dehydration of garlic slices. Agri Res Rev 50: 243–253.
Heinle H, Betz E (1994) Effects of dietary garlic supplementation in a rat model of atherosclerosis. Arzneimittelforschung/Drug Res 44 (1): 614–617.
Holzgartner H, Schmidt U, Kuhn U (1992) Wirksamkeit und Verträglichkeit eines Knoblauchpulver-Präparates im Vergleich mit Bezafibrat. Arzneimittelforschung/Drug Res 42: 1473–1477.
Itokawa Y, Inoue K, Sasagawa S, Fujiwara M (1973) Effect of S-methylcysteine sulfoxide, S-allylcysteine sulfoxide and related sulfur-containing amino acids on lipid metabolism of experimental hypercholesterolemic rats. J Nutr 103: 88–92.
Jacob R Ehrsam M, Ohkubo T, Rupp H (1991) Antihypertensive und kardioprotektive Effekte von Knobiauchpulver (Allium sativum). Med Welt (Suppl 7a): 39–41.
Jacob R, Isensee H, Rietz B, Makdessi S, Sweidan H (1993) Cardioprotection by dietary interventions in animal experiments: Effect of garlic and various dietary oils under the conditions of experimental infarction. Pharm Pharmacol Lett 3: 131–134.
Jain RC (1975) Onion and garlic in experimental cholesterol atherosclerosis in rabbits 1. Effect on serum lipids and development of atherosclerosis. Artery 1: 115–125.
Jain RC (1977) Effect of garlic on serum lipids, coagulability and fibrinolytic activity of blood. Am J Clin Nutr 30: 1380–1381.
Kamanna VS, Chandrasekhara N (1984) Hypocholesteremic activity of different fractions of garlic. Indian J Med Res 79: 580–583.
Kiesewetter H, Jung EM, Mrowietz C, Koscielny J, Wenzel E (1993) Effect of garlic on platelet aggregation in patients with increased risk of juvenile ischemic attack. Eur J Clin Pharmacol 45: 333–336.
Kiesewetter H, Jung F, Jung EM, Blume J, Mrowietz C, Birk A, Koscielny J, Wenzel E (1993) Effects of garlic coated tablets in peripheral arterial occlusive disease. Clin Invest 71: 383–386.
Kiesewetter H, Jung F, Mrowietz C, Wenzel E (1993) Wirkung von Knoblauch (Allium sativum L.), insbesondere rheologische und hämostaseologische Effekte. Hämostaseologie 13: 3–12.

Koch HP, Hahn G (1988) Knoblauch – Grundlagen der therapeutischen Anwendung von Allium sativum L. Urban & Schwarzenberg Verlag Munich, Vienna, Baltimore.

Koch HP, Lawson DL (1996) Garlic – The Science and Therapeutic Application of Allium sativum L. and Related Species. 2nd Edition. Williams & Wilkins Baltimore.

Lachmann G, Lorenz D, Radeck W, Steiper M (1994) Untersuchungen zur Pharmakokinetik der mit ^{35}S markierten Knoblauchinhaltsstoffe Alliin, Allicin und Vinyldithiine. Arzneimittelforschung/Drug Res 44: 734–743.

Lewin G, Popov I (1994) Antioxidant effects of aqueous garlic extract, 2nd communication: inhibition of the Cu^{2+}-initiated oxidation of low-density lipoproteins. Arzneimittel-Forschung/Drug Research 44 (1): 604–607.

Mader FH, Auer W, Becker W, Böhm W, Brüchert E, Deutsch S (1990) Hyperlipidämie-Behandlung mit Knoblauch-Dragees. Der Allgemeinarzt 12: 435–440.

Malik ZA, Siddiqui S (1981) Hypotensive effect of freeze-dried garlic (Allium sativum) SAP in dog. JPMA 31: 12–13.

Mand JK, Gupta PP, Soni GL, Singh R (1985) Effect of garlic on experimental atherosclerosis in rabbits. Indian Heart J 37: 183–188.

Mathew PT, Augusti KT (1973) Studies on the effect of allicin (diallyl disulphide-oxide) on alloxan diabetes: Part I – Hypoglycemic action & enhancement of serum insulin effect & glycogen synthesis. Indian J Biochem Biophys 10: 209–212.

Nakagawa S, Masamoto K, Sumiyoshi H, Harada H (1984) Acute toxicity test of garlic extract. J Toxicol Sci 9: 57–60.

Orekhov AN, Tertov VV, Sobenin IA, Pivovarova EM (1995) Direct antiatherosclerosis-related effects of garlic. Ann Med 27: 63–65.

Pfaff K (1991) Allicin-Freisetzung und Lagerungsstabilität: Bestimmung anhand von frischem Knoblauch und Knoblauchpulver mit einer spezifischen HPLC-Methode. Dtsch Apoth Z (Suppl 24): 12–15.

Popov I, Blumstein A, Lewin G (1994) Antioxidant effects of aqueous garlic extract, 1st communication: direct detection using photochemiluminescence. Arzneimittel-Forschung/Drug Research 44 (1): 602–604.

Quereshi AA, Abiurmeileh N, Din ZZ, Elson CE, Burger WC (1983) Inhibition of cholesterol and fatty acid biosynthesis in liver enzymes and chicken hepatocytes by polar fractions of garlic. Lipids 18: 343–348.

Reuter HD, Sendl A (1994) Allium sativum and Allium ursinum: chemistry, pharmacology and medical applications. Econo Med Plant Res 6: 56–108.

Reuter HD (1995) Allium sativum und Allium ursinum: Part 2. Pharmacology and medicinal application. Phytomedicine 2: 73–91.

Reuter HD (1996) Therapeutic effects and applications of garlic and its preparations. In: Koch HP, Lawson DL (eds) Garlic – The Science and Therapeutic Application of Allium sativum L. and Related Species. 2nd Edition. Williams & Wilkins Baltimore, pp 135–212.

Schmidt U, Schenk N (1992) Geruchsbildung bei repetierter Einnahme von standardisierten Knoblauchpulver-Dragees Kwai (LI 111) in Abhängigkeit von der Tagesdosis. Scientific Report, Lichtwer Pharmaceuticals, Berlin.

Siegel G, Emden J, Schnalke F, Walter A, Rückborn K, Wagner KG (1991) Wirkungen von Knoblauch auf die Gefäßregulation. Med Welt (Suppl 7 a): 32–34.

Siegel G, Emden J, Wenzel K, Mironneau J, Stock G (1992) Potassium channel activation in vascular smooth muscle. In: Frank GB (ed) Excitation-Contraction Coupling in Skeletal, Cardiac and Smooth Muscle. Plenum Press, New York, pp 53–72.

Silagy C, Neil A (1994) A meta-analysis of the effect of garlic on blood pressure. J Hypertension 12: 463–468.

Silagy C, Neil A (1994) Garlic as a lipid-lowering agent – a meta-analysis. J R Coll Physicians 28 (1): 2–8.

Sumiyoshi H, Kanezawa A, Masamoto K, Harada H, Nakagami S, Yokota A (1984) Chronic toxicity test of garlic extracts in rats. J Toxicol Sci 9: 61–75.

Török B, Belagyi J, Rietz B, Jakob R (1994) Effectiveness of garlic on radical activity in radical generating systems. Arzneimittelforschung/Drug Research 44 (I): 608–611.

Warshafsky S, Kamer RS, Sivak L (1993) Effect of garlic on total serum cholesterol. Ann Inter Med 119: 599–605.

Zacharias NT, Sebastian KL, Philip B, Augusti KT (1980) Hypoglycemic and hypolipidaemic effects of garlic in sucrose fed rabbits. Ind J Physiol Pharmac 24: 151–154.

Zhao F, Chen H, Shen Y, Liu Z, Chen Y, Sun X, Cheng G, Lang L (1983) Study of synthetic allicin in the prevention and treatment of atherosclerosis. Chem Abst 98: 209–844.

3.3.2
Ginkgo Special Extract for Peripheral Arterial Occlusive Disease

The Commission E monograph of 1994 lists only two special extracts made from *Ginkgo biloba* leaves (acetone-and-water extracts with an average herb-to-extract ratio of 50:1) that are recommended for therapeutic use. The extracts are designated in the technical literature as EGb 761 (produced by Dr. Willmar Schwabe GmbH) and LI 1370 (produced by Lichtwer Pharma GmbH). Details on the history, pharmacy, pharmacology, and clinical aspects of these ginkgo extracts are presented in Sect. 2.1. Their use for the symptomatic treatment of peripheral arterial occlusive disease (PAOD) is considered here.

The 1994 Commission E monograph states that ginkgo special extracts are indicated in the treatment of PAOD "to improve pain-free walking distance in patients with Fontaine stage II peripheral arterial occlusive disease (intermittent claudication) as an adjunct to physical therapy, particularly gait training."

Generally, patients with stage II PAOD have a pain-free walking distance in the range of 30–300 m. When this limit is reached, the oxygen deficit in the leg muscles causes the onset of pain and intermittent claudication. In cases that are not amenable to surgical correction (reopening or bypassing the stenosed segments in larger vessels), physical therapy with an emphasis on gait training is the most effective therapeutic measure. The training benefits peripheral arterial disease mainly by enlarging the caliber of the collateral arteries and increasing metabolic activities, i. e., promoting capillarization and increasing intracellular mitochondrial density to improve oxygen utilization.

Pharmacologic agents that promote blood flow act mainly by improving the rheologic properties of the blood. Ginkgo extracts are known to produce such an effect (see Sect. 2.1.6). The pharmacologic action profile of ginkgo extracts implies that ginkgo should be of benefit in the symptomatic treatment of PAOD.

The increase in walking distance seen in placebo-controlled double-blind studies following the administration of vasoactive agents is clinically relevant for the majority of patients, as the gain in walking distance provided by pharmacotherapy is roughly equal to that achieved with an equal period of gait training in comparable clinical populations.

To date, 13 therapeutic studies have been completed dealing with the therapeutic efficacy of ginkgo special extracts in patients with Fontaine stage II peripheral arterial disease. Most of these studies had a randomized, placebo-controlled, double-blind design. The studies began with a 2- to 6-week run-in phase followed by a 3- to 6-month course of treatment with ginkgo extracts taken in daily doses of 120–160 mg. By July of 1994, most of these studies had been evaluated by Commission E and its consultants for preparation of the Commission monograph. It was concluded that, in four of the placebo-controlled studies, the increase in pain-free walking distance achieved with ginkgo therapy was both statistically significant and clinically relevant (e. g., Blume et al., 1996). Published meta-analyses indicate gains in walking distance of 34–109 m (Letzel and Schoop, 1992) and 24–161 m (Schneider, 1992) in comparison to treatment with a placebo.

In some cases, ginkgo extracts have shown somewhat less efficacy in PAOD than synthetic drugs, and in others their effects have been comparable. The basic advantage of ginkgo lies in the fact that its preparations are significantly better tolerated than synthetic drugs (see Table 2.3).

References

Blume J, Kieser M, Holscher U (1996) Placebokontrollierte Doppelblindstudie zur Wirksamkeit von Ginkgo-biloba-Spezialextrakt EGb 761 bei austrainierten Patienten mit Claudicatio intermittens. VASA 25: 265–274.
Letzel H, Schoop E (1992) Ginkgo-biloba-Extrakt EGb 761 und Pentoxifyllin bei Claudicatio intermittens. VASA 21: 403–410.
Schneider B (1992) Ginkgo-biloba-Extrakt bei peripheren arteriellen Verschlußkrankheiten. Arzneim Forsch/Drug Res 42: 428–436.

3.3.3
Other Herbs with Antiatherosclerotic Properties

The 1986 Commission E monograph states that onion (Allium cepa), like garlic, is useful "for the prevention of age-related vascular changes" (i.e., atherosclerosis). It must be taken in significantly higher doses than garlic, however, the Commission recommending an average daily dose of 50 g fresh onion bulb or 20 g dried herb. Onion is described as having antibacterial, lipid-reducing, antihypertensive, and platelet-aggregation-inhibiting properties.

The chemistry of the onion bulb resembles that of garlic. Instead of alliin, onion contains methyl and propyl compounds of cysteine sulfoxide. These chemicals are transformed by fermentation into the familiar eye-irritating compounds that induce lacrimation (cepaenes). In one study, the decrease in fibrinolytic activity caused by a fatty meal could be reversed by feeding the subjects onions (Menon et al., 1968). The ingestion of onion was also shown to inhibit platelet aggregation (Baghurst et al., 1977). More recent placebo-controlled studies comparable to those with garlic have not yet been conducted on the effects of onion.

Phospholipids derived from soybeans consist of an enriched extract containing 73–79 % phosphatidylcholine. The 1994 Commission E monograph states that this phospholipid extract is useful for the treatment of mild forms of hypercholesterolemia in cases that are not adequately managed by diet and other nonpharmacologic measures (e.g., exercise and weight loss) alone. In addition, soybean phospholipids have shown hepatoprotective properties in numerous experimental models of acute toxic liver damage (e.g., caused by ethanol, carbon tetrachloride, or galactosamine). The pharmacokinetics of orally administered phospholipids have been investigated with radiolabeled agents in experimental animals. It has been shown that phospholipid is degraded to lyso-phosphatidylcholine while still in the intestine and is mainly absorbed in that form. Most phosphatidylcholine circulating in the plasma is bound to albumin. It is likely that most of the metabolites of administered soybean phospholipids are integrated into endogenous phospholipids within a few hours. Thirty-two clinical studies were evaluated in preparation for the monograph; nine were placebo-controlled studies in patients with hyperlipoproteinemia. Four of the nine placebo-controlled studies demonstrated efficacy, consisting of a reduction in total cholesterol (7–19 % of initial levels). Three studies showed significant reductions in LDL cholesterol. Triglycerides and HDL cholesterol were unaffected. The studies employed doses of 1–3 g of phospholipids per day. Lipostabil 300 forte is one example of a suitable commercial product.

Oat bran (from *Avena sativa*) was found to reduce total cholesterol by 13 % when taken in a daily dose of about 100 g for 3 weeks (Gold and Davidson, 1988). A similar study using the same daily dose administered for 14 weeks showed a 16 % total cholesterol reduction accompanied by a 21 % reduction in LDL (Fischer et al., 1991). The cholesterol-lowering effect of oat bran is apparently based on its content of gel-forming dietary fiber; wheat bran does not produce this effect.

Guar gum, a reserve polysaccharide derived from the Indian guar plant *(Cyamopsis tetragonolobus)*, lowered cholesterol levels by 6–8 % and triglyceride levels by 13–17 % when taken in a dose of 15 g/day. As in the case of oat bran, this effect apparently results from the binding of primarily liver-excreted cholesterol to nonabsorbable bulk materials. Owing to their lipid-reducing effects, both of these sources of dietary fiber may be beneficial in the secondary prophylaxis of atherosclerosis (Fischer et al., 1991).

References

Baghurst Kl, Raj MI, Truswell AS (1977) Onions and platelet aggregation. Lancet 101: 1051.
Fischer S, Berg A, Keul J, Leitzmann C (1991) Einfluß einer ballaststoffangereicherten Kost auf die Ernährungsgewohnheiten und die Blutfettwerte bei Hypercholesterinämikern. Aktuelle Ernährungsmedizin 16: 303–308.
Gold KK, Davidson DM (1988) Oat bran as a cholesterol-reducing dietary adjunct in a young, healthy population. West J Med 148: 299–302.
Menon IS, Kendal RY, Dewar HA, Newell DI (1968) Effects of onion on blood fibronolytic activity. Brit Med J 3: 351.

3.4
Chronic Venous Insufficiency

Chronic venous insufficiency is the term applied to a syndrome resulting from the obstruction or persistent incompetence of deep veins or perforating veins in the lower extremities. The symptoms range from edema, cyanosis or dermatosclerosis to atrophic skin changes and crural ulceration, depending on the severity and duration of the impaired venous return and associated impairment of metabolic exchange. Chronic venous insufficiency is divided into three stages based on its degree of severity (Marshall and Loew, 1994).

Causal therapy in the form of vascular surgery is possible only in a small percentage of patients. Conservative treatment options consist of elastic compression (support stockings) and symptomatic pharmacotherapy with so-called venous remedies.

Most pharmacologic and clinical studies on herbs used in the treatment of venous disorders have dealt with horse chestnut extracts and their constituent aescins. These agents act less on the veins and venules than at the capillary level, where they exert antiexudative and antiedematous effects. Commercial products vary widely in quality, however, and only some contain active levels of antiexudative constituents. This variable quality of herbal venous remedies is a major reason why their clinical efficacy remains a controversial matter.

Proof of safety and efficacy by controlled clinical studies requires a differentiated approach to patient evaluation and follow-up. Instrumental diagnostic techniques may consist of more general procedures such as Doppler and duplex scanning, phlebodynamometry, and venous occlusion plethysmography or of more specialized procedures, such as volumetry, that can detect pharmacologic actions. Since pharmacologic therapy can influence functional vascular changes but cannot reverse pathoanatomic changes, proof of clinical efficacy must rely on techniques for determining capillary permeability, such as venous occlusion plethysmographic volumetry. Emphasis should also be placed on the follow-up of subjective complaints. Tired, heavy legs, a tense or bursting sensation, and calf pain are not mood disorders but symptoms that have major pathologic significance. If instrumental diagnostic techniques as well as clinical follow-up indicate a positive response to herbal therapy, it is reasonable to conclude that these preparations can be important in the treatment of lower-extremity venous disorders (Marshall and Loew, 1994).

3.4.1
Horse Chestnut Seed Extract

3.4.1.1
Introduction
The horse chestnut, Aesculus hippocastanum (family Hippocastanaceae), was introduced into northern Europe from the Near East in the sixteenth century. Extracts from horse chestnut seeds were already used therapeutically in France in the early 1800's. Several French works published between 1896 and 1909 reported successful outcomes in the treatment of hemorrhoidal ailments. Even then it was assumed that the active components belonged to the saponin class of glycosides (Hitzenberger, 1989).

3.4.1.2
Crude Drug and Extract
The German Pharmacopeia *(DAB 1996)* describes the crude drug as consisting of the dried seeds of the horse chestnut tree (Fig. 3.16). Preparations made from other parts of the tree (leaves, bark) have also been used medicinally, but their efficacy has not been adequately proven. For simplicity, the term horse chestnut extract will hereafter refer to the extract derived from horse chestnut seeds.

The fully ripe seeds are predried by spreading them out in a thin layer in a well-ventilated area. Then they are split open and dried rapidly at a temperature of 60 °C to obtain a powdered crude drug containing 3–5 % saponins. Water-and-alcohol mixtures are used to prepare powdered extracts, which are adjusted as needed by the addition of dextrins. to a triterpene glycoside content of 16–20 % (m/m), calculated as aescin.

3.4.1.3
Chemistry and Pharmacokinetics of Aescin
Aescin is considered the main active constituent of horse chestnut extract, and isolated aescin has shown clinical efficacy on administration (Fink Serralde et al., 1975). The triterpene saponins in horse chestnut seeds form a complex mixture of

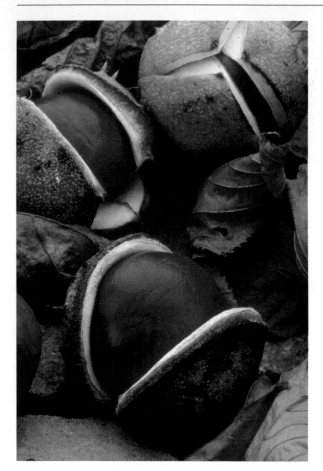

Fig. 3.16.
Horse chestnut *(Aesculus hippocastanum),* opening fruits with seeds.

saponins. The part of the mixture that tends to crystallize, called β-aescin, is itself a mixture of several glycosides. These glycosides contained in β-aescin are derived from two aglycones. Aescin is fairly soluble in water but is poorly soluble in lipid solvents. Glycoside determinations employ a method developed in 1966 and slightly modified for pharmaceutical purposes; it is based on a color reaction of triterpene glycosides with ferric chloride.

Orally administered aescin is either sparingly absorbed or undergoes a substantial first-pass effect. Its relative bioavailability compared with i.v. administration is less than 1%. It has an absorption half-life of about 1 h and an elimination half-life of about 20 h. In subjects who took 50 mg of aescin in capsule form (brand name Venostasin retard), maximum plasma levels of approximately 20–30 ng/mL were measured 2–3 h after ingestion of the capsule (Hänsel et al., 1992).

3.4.1.4
Pharmacology

Studies in an animal model (rat paw edema) showed that whole horse chestnut extract was 100 times more active than the same extract with the aescin removed (Lorenz and Marek, 1960). Since then, it has been repeatedly confirmed that aescin is responsible for the antiexudative properties of horse chestnut extract, even in inflammatory and stasis-related edema (Hitzenberger, 1989).

Several authors showed that horse chestnut extract increased the tonicity of isolated veins (Annoni et al., 1979; Locks, 1974; Longiave et al., 1978). This effect was not blocked by phentolamine, proving that it is not mediated by α-adrenergic receptors. There is no evidence to date, however, that horse chestnut can significantly affect venous capacity in patients with venous insufficiency (Rudofsky et al., 1986; Bisler et al., 1986).

3.4.1.5
Toxicology

Horse chestnut extract and aescin have been tested for acute toxicity in several animal species (mouse, rat, guinea pig, rabbit, dog). The "no effect" dose is approximately 8 times higher than the dose recommended for therapeutic use in patients. Tests for chronic toxicity (34 weeks in rats and dogs) showed no cumulative toxic effects or any evidence of embryotoxic or teratogenic effects. The results of animal studies are corroborated by decades of use in patients with no reports of harmful effects due to overdosing. No studies have been published on mutagenicity or carcinogenicity (Hänsel et al., 1992).

3.4.1.6
Actions and Efficacy in Subjects and Patients

3.4.1.6.1
Studies in Healthy Subjects

Pauschinger (1987) investigated the effects of a standardized horse chestnut extract (single dose of 600 mg) on capillary filtration in a double-blind, placebo-controlled study of 12 healthy subjects. The parameters of interest were vascular capacity and the filtration coefficient as measured by venous occlusion plethysmography. While both parameters remained unchanged in the placebo-treated group, the subjects taking the extract showed a decrease in vascular capacity and filtration coefficient.

Among the clinical pharmacologic studies in healthy subjects is that of Marshall et al. (1987), who conducted a double-blind study on the development of foot and ankle edema in 19 subjects following a long-distance flight. They found that edema was significantly reduced in subjects who had taken a prophylactic dose of 600 mg horse chestnut extract prior to the flight.

3.4.1.6.2
Therapeutic Studies in Patients

Seven placebo-controlled double-blind studies were carried out with a standardized horse chestnut extract to assess its therapeutic efficacy in patients with chronic venous insufficiency. These studies, listed in Table 3.9, included a total of 558 evaluable

Table 3.9. Placebo-controlled double-blind studies using a standardized horse chestnut extract (brand name Venostasin retard). The dose in all studies was 100 mg aescin per day. Except for Lohr et al., all the authors used a crossover design for their studies. $* = p < 0.05$; $** = p < 0.01$; $*** = p < 0.001$; ns. = not significant.

First author, year	Number of patients	Duration (days)	Key parameters and statistical results of drug vs. placebo
Alter, 1973	96	2 × 20	Palpable findings, skin color, venous prominence, edema, dermatoses, pain, feeling of heaviness, and itching significantly improved in most patients.
Neiss, 1978	212	2 × 20	Complaint scale (0–3): Edema** Calf spasms ns. Pain** Itching ns. Feeling of heaviness*
Friedrich, 1978	95	2 × 20	Complaint scale (0–3): Edema* Calf spasms** Pain** Itching ns. Feeling of heaviness*
Steiner, 1986	20	2 × 14	Leg volume[1] ** Subjective complaints**
Lohr, 1986	74	56	Leg volume[1] ** Subjective complaints**
Bisler, 1986	22	2 × 1	Filtration coefficient[2] *** (−22%) Venous capacity[2] ns. (−5%)
Rudofsky, 1986	39	28	Extravascular volume[1] [3] *** Venous capacity[2] ns. Subjective complaints*
Diehm, 1996	240	84	Leg volume[1] **

[1] Water plethysmography, [2] venous occlusion plethysmography, [3] measured on the foot and distal lower leg.

patient treatment cycles. All the studies used daily doses of approximately 600 mg of horse chestnut extract, equivalent to 100 mg/day aescin. Most of them used a crossover design in which each patient received both the extract and the placebo in separate treatment cycles.

The study by Alter (1973) is of limited value, despite its double-blind design, due to significant methodologic and statistical deficiencies. Subsequent studies by Neiss et al. (1976) and Friedrich et al. (1978) are of considerably greater interest. Both studies had a similar design, and both used a 0–3 point scale to rate the severity of symptoms typically associated with chronic venous insufficiency. A 4-field test was used for statistical significance. The majority of symptoms showed significantly greater improvement in the patients taking the horse chestnut extract than in patients taking a placebo.

Four additional studies were published in 1986. Steiner and Hillemanns (1986) treated 13 women diagnosed with pregnancy-related varicose veins and 7 women diagnosed with chronic venous insufficiency. Leg volumes were determined by water plethysmography, and leg circumferences were measured at three levels. The leg volumes did not change in placebo-treated patients, but treatment with horse chestnut extract led to a significant average reduction of 114 mL and 126 mL in the two patient groups. The subjective complaints and overall physician-rated efficacy were also significantly better in patients treated with the extract than in patients given a placebo.

Lohr et al. (1986) conducted a study in 74 patients with chronic venous insufficiency and proneness to lower extremity edema. Leg volumes were determined by water plethysmography and leg circumferences were directly measured before and after the provocation of edema. The provocative increase in leg volume fell from 32 mL to 27 mL in the group treated with horse chestnut but rose from 27 mL to 31 mL in the placebo-treated group. Subjective symptoms were also significantly improved.

Bisler et al. (1986) and Rudofsky et al. (1986) studied the effects of horse chestnut on the intravascular volume of the lower extremity veins and on interstitial filtration (measured indirectly by venous-occlusion or water plethysmography) in patients with chronic venous insufficiency.

Bisler et al. (1986) tested the effects of a single dose of 600 mg horse chestnut extract versus a placebo. In patients taking the placebo, transcapillary filtration rose from 8.2 to 8.3 scale units over a 3-h period, but it fell from 9.4 to 7.4 units in the patients treated with horse chestnut extract. This indicated a significant 22 % reduction in the transcapillary filtration coefficient. The decrease in intravascular volume (−5 %) was not significant. This led the authors to conclude that the vein-toning action of horse chestnut extract is of far less importance than its ability to reduce capillary permeability.

Rudofsky et al. (1986) documented similar effects of horse chestnut extract over a 28-day treatment period. Whereas venous capacity before and after the therapy showed no significant differences between the extract- and placebo-treated groups, the extravascular volume changes measured in the foot and ankle at 14–28 days showed highly significant intergroup differences (Fig. 3.17). Four weeks' treatment with the horse chestnut extract also led to significant improvement in most subjective symptoms (feeling of tension, pain, leg fatigue, itching) and in the finding of leg edemas. The symptom of calf muscle spasms did not improve.

Diehm et al. (1996) carried out a study to compare the efficacy (oedema reduction) and safety of compression stockings class II and dried horse chestnut seed extract (HCSE, 50 mg aescin, twice daily). Equivalence of both therapies was examined in a novel hierarchical statistical design in 240 patients with chronic venous insufficiency. Patients were treated over a period of 12 weeks in a randomized, partially blinded, placebo-controlled, parallel study design. Lower leg volume of the more severely affected limb decreased on average by 43.8 mL (n = 95) with HCSE and 46.7 mL (n = 99) with compression therapy, while it increased by 9.8 mL with placebo (n = 46) after 12 weeks therapy for the intention-to-treat group (Fig. 3.18). Significant edema reductions were achieved by HCSE (p = 0.005) and compression (p = 0.002) compared to placebo, and the two therapies were shown to be equivalent (p = 0.001); in this design, however, compression could not be proven as standard with regard to edema reduction in the statistical test procedure. Both HCSE and compression therapy were well tolerated and no serious treatment-related events

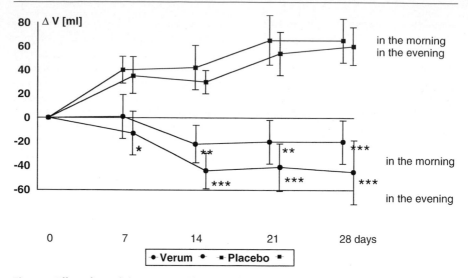

Fig. 3.17. Effect of 4 weeks' treatment with 600 mg horse chestnut extract, corresponding to 100 mg/day aescin, on volume changes in the foot and distal lower leg with a fixed, reduced blood volume (change in extravascular volume). Mean values ± SEM for n = 19 patients (horse chestnut extract) and n = 20 patients (placebo). * = p < 0.05, ** = p < 0.01, *** = p < 0.001 (significance comparing extract vs. placebo) (after Rudofsky et al., 1986).

were reported. These results indicate that compression stocking therapy and HCSE therapy are alternative therapies for the effective treatment of patients with edema resulting from chronic venous insufficiency.

3.4.1.7
Indications, Dosages, Risks, and Contraindications

There appears to be sufficient evidence to prove the therapeutic efficacy of horse chestnut extract in reducing leg edema and improving the typical subjective complaints associated with chronic venous insufficiency. Thus, the Commission E monograph on horse chestnut seeds published in the April 15, 1994, issue of *Bundesanzeiger* states that a standardized powdered extract of horse chestnut seeds *(DAB 1996)* adjusted to a triterpene glycoside content of 16–20% (calculated as anhydrous aescin) is appropriate for the "treatment of complaints relating to diseases of the lower extremity veins (chronic venous insufficiency) such as pain and a feeling of heaviness in the legs, nocturnal calf muscle spasms, itching, and swelling of the legs."

The monograph further states that other noninvasive physician-prescribed measures such as elastic compression or cold water treatments should definitely be continued.

There are no known contraindications to the use of horse chestnut extract. Isolated instances of itching, nausea, and stomach discomfort have been reported as side effects.

With regard to tolerance, it should be emphasized that high tolerance has been demonstrated only for the controlled-release dosage form. The saponins contained

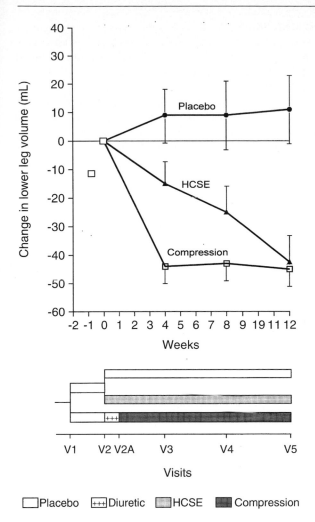

Fig.3.18.
Study design (lower) and differences (mean SEM) in lower leg volume versus baseline (upper) of the study of Diehm et al. (1996) with 240 patients. Significant reductions of lower leg volume were achieved by horse chestnut seed extract (HCSE, p = 0.005) and compression (p = 0.002) compared to placebo. The two therapies were shown to be equivalent (p = 0.001).

in non-controlled-release preparations of horse chestnut extract tend to cause stomach upset when the extract is taken at therapeutic doses of 250–313 mg twice daily, equivalent to 100 mg of aescin.

3.4.1.8
Therapeutic Significance

Horse chestnut extract is the most widely prescribed oral antiedema venous remedy in Germany. Semisynthetic derivatives of plant constituents such as hydroxyethylrutin, calcium dobesilate, troxerutin, and trimethylhesperidin chalcone are also used individually or in combinations; but single-herb products, especially those based on horse chestnut seed extract, are the most commonly prescribed (Fricke, 1995).

The therapeutic efficacy of orally administered venous remedies is still controversial. Attitudes of caution or outright rejection alternate with frank enthusiasm. This applies particularly to standardized horse chestnut extract, which controlled clinical studies have shown to be effective, especially in the amelioration of subjective complaints (Hitzenberger, 1989). The Commission E monograph of April, 1994, pertains only to preparations that supply a daily dose of 100 mg aescin, corresponding to about 300 mg of extract in a controlled-release dosage form. Other preparations made from horse chestnut leaves, bark, and flowers have been negatively appraised and should no longer be prescribed. Extracts from other herbs (butcher's broom rhizome, sweet clover, buckwheat, grape leaves) are traditional remedies that have not been proven by up-to-date clinical studies. Caution is advised in prescribing these herbs as well as any combination products that are offered for the treatment of venous disorders.

As for chemically modified isolated plant constituents, which by definition are not phytotherapeutic agents in the strict sense (Sect. 1.2 and 1.3), the compound hydroxyethylrutin has shown at least short-term efficacy in ameliorating the subjective complaints of chronic venous insufficiency. Thus it can be recommended as an alternative to horse chestnut seed extract, although there have been isolated reports of hair loss in patients using hydroxyethylrutin. One case of agranulocytosis was reported following the use of calcium dobesilate. The side effects of horse chestnut seed extract (gastrointestinal complaints, allergic skin reactions) are relatively harmless by comparison.

In contrast to herbal and semisynthetic antiedema agents, the use of diuretics is only occasionally indicated to clear venogenic edema in patients with chronic venous insufficiency. Also, a number of contraindications exist to diuretic therapy. Given the potential for hemoconcentration with impairment of venous drainage and the risk of stasis predisposing to thrombosis, diuretics are inappropriate for the long-term treatment of edema due to venous insufficiency.

3.4.2
Topical Venous Remedies

The most commonly prescribed topical venous remedies are products containing heparin. Combination products containing herbal extracts or plant constituents from the group of saponins (e. g., aescin) or flavonoids (e. g., rutin) are also used. The topical application of these agents does not produce systemic therapeutic levels of the active principle. Their therapeutic effects may be based largely on the ointment base and the tissue massage that occurs when the ointment is applied. Patients frequently experience subjective improvement in their complaints, but the benefits are not referable to specific plant constituents because all but one of the commercial preparations (Venostasin N ointment, active ingredient: horse chestnut extract) are combination products.

It is unclear whether extracts from arnica flowers are topically active and, if so, how they exert their effects. They are used as additives in the form of ethanol extracts (e. g., Arnica Kneipp Gel, Vasotonin Gel). Arnica extracts contain a volatile oil with bicyclic sesquiterpenes of the helenalin type as characteristic constituents.

Helenalins cause local irritation of the skin and mucous membranes, yet they are considered to have an anti-inflammatory action. Arnica flowers induce hyperemia when applied topically to the skin in the form of a tincture or infusion.

Assessment of the efficacy of topical venous remedies is still based primarily on experience with practical use. To date there has been insufficient proof of efficacy, especially with regard to the prevention of thrombosis and the improvement of its sequelae. While local therapeutic agents are of unquestioned benefit in the treatment of chronic venous disorders, they are also associated with risks in the form of allergic sensitization and contact eczema.

3.4.3
Drug Products

Twenty-two single-herb venous remedies for internal use were included in the *Rote Liste 1995*. Five products based on horse chestnut conform to the recommendations of the Commission E monograph on horse chestnut seeds. Other products do not conform to Commission recommendations, especially with regard to dosage. Five other single-herb products contain preparations of sweet clover, butcher's broom, or buckwheat as active ingredients. There are also three combination products that rank among the most commonly prescribed herbal medications (see Appendix).

References

Alter H (1973) Zur medikamentösen Therapie der Varikosis. Z Allg Med 49 (17): 1301–1304.
Annoni F, Mauri A, Marincola 17, Resele LF (1979) Venotonic activity of aescin on the human saphenous vein. Arzneim Forsch/Drug Res 29: 672.
Bisler H, Pfeifer R, Klüken N, Pauschinger P (1986) Wirkung von Roßkastaniensamenextrakt auf die transkapilläre Filtration bei chronischer venöser Insuffizienz. Dtsch Med Wschr 111: 1321–1328.
Diehm C, Trampisch HJ, Lange S, Schmidt C (1996) Comparison of leg compression stocking and oral horse-chestnut seed extract therapy in patients with chronic venous insufficiency. Lancet 347: 292–294.
Fink Serralde C, Dreyfus Cortes GO, Colo Hernandez, Marquez Zacarias LA (1975) Valoracion de la escina pura en el tratamiento del sindrome des estasis venosa cronica. Münch Med Wschr (Spanish edition) 117(1): 41–46.
Fricke U (1995) Venenmittel. In: Schwabe U, Paffrath D (eds) Arzneiverordnungs-Report '95. Gustav Fischer Verlag, Stuttgart Jena, pp 421–430.
Friederich HC, Vogelsberg H, Neiss A (1978) Ein Beitrag zur Bewertung von intern wirksamen Venenpharmaka. Z Hautkrankheiten 53 (11): 369–374.
Hänsel R, Keller K, Rimpler H, Schneider G (1992) Hagers Handbuch der Pharmazeutischen Praxis. 5th Ed., Drogen A-D. Springer Verlag, Berlin Heidelberg New York, pp 108–122.
Hitzenberger G (1989) Die therapeutische Wirksamkeit des Roßkastaniensamenextraktes. Wien Med Wschr 139 (17): 385–389.
Locks H, Baumgartner H, Konzett H (1974) Zur Beeinflussung des Venentonus durch Roßkastanienextrakte. Arzneim Forsch 24: 1347.
Lohr E, Garanin G, Jesau P, Fischer H (1986) Ödemprotektive Therapie bei chronischer Veneninsuffizienz mit Ödemneigung. Münch Med Wschr 128: 579–581.
Longiave D, Omini C, Nicosia S, Berti F (1978) The Mode of Action of aescin on isolated veins: Relationship with $PGF_{2\alpha}$. Pharmacol Res 10: 145.
Lorenz D, Marek ML (1960) Das therapeutisch wirksame Prinzip der Roßkastanie (Aesculus hippocastanum). Arzneim Forsch 10: 263–272.
Marshall M, Loew D (1994) Diagnostische Maßnahmen zum Nachweis der Wirksamkeit von Venentherapeutika. Phlebol 23: 85–91.

Marshall M, Dormandy JA (1987) Oedema of long distant flights. Phlebol 2: 123–124.

Neiss A, Böhm C (1976) Zum Wirksamkeitsnachweis von Roßkastaniensamenextrakt beim varikösen Symptomenkomplex. Münch Med Wschr 7: 213–216.

Pauschinger P (1987) Klinisch experimentelle Untersuchungen zur Wirkung von Roßkastaniensamenextrakt auf die transkapilläre Filtration und das intravasale Volumen an Patienten mit chronisch venöser Insuffizienz. Phlebol Proktol 16: 57–61.

Rudofsky G, Neiß A, Otto K, Seibel K (1986) Ödemprotektive Wirkung und klinische Wirksamkeit von Roßkastaniensamenextrakt im Doppelblindversuch. Phlebol Proktol 15: 47–54.

Steiner M, Hillemanns HG (1986) Untersuchung zur ödemprotektiven Wirkung eines Venentherapeutikums. Münch Med Wschr 31: 551–552.

4 Respiratory System

4.1
Cold Syndrome (Flulike Infection)

A cold (common cold, upper respiratory infection, flulike infection) is a benign catarrhal inflammation of the upper and middle respiratory tract caused by a viral infection. It may present as rhinitis, pharyngitis, laryngitis, laryngotracheobronchitis, or less commonly as sinusitis or tracheobronchitis.

4.1.1
Risk Factors

It is widely believed that people are more likely to contract a cold after being exposed to low temperatures – hence the popular term for the disease. Yet experiments under controlled conditions have failed to prove that lowering the body temperature induces colds or even increases susceptibility to a rhinoviral infection. Nevertheless, there is ample evidence to support a link between exposure to cold and a decreased resistance to infection. In one study, for example, the incidence of colds among crew members on modern, air-conditioned cargo ships was almost twice that seen in workers on non-air-conditioned ships of the same line traveling the same route (Schwaar, 1976). The most likely explanation is that workers on the air-conditioned vessels were exposed to greater and more frequent ambient temperature changes, especially in tropical regions.

Experiments have shown that cooling of the feet is associated with a transient, reflex fall in the temperature of the oral, pharyngeal, and tracheal mucosae (Demling et al., 1956; Pollmann, 1987; Schmidt and Kairies, 1932). The partial restriction of blood flow, leading to cooling of the mucous membranes and a local decrease in mucosal resistance, could promote invasion by pathogenic organisms already adherent to the mucosal surfaces (see Sect. 4.1.2).

Whether the infection will incite a symptomatic illness or will be successfully combated with no overt symptomatology depends on preexisting nonspecific host defense mechanisms as well as the condition of the mucosa, the mucosal blood flow, the thickness and condition of the epithelium, the thickness and composition of the mucous layer, the local concentration of antibodies and interferon, the commensal flora colonizing the mucosae, the replication factors in the host cells, and the virulence of the pathogenic microorganisms. Every viral infection impairs the mucociliary clearance mechanism of the upper respiratory tract, paving the way for the bacterial invasion of areas normally free of bacteria, such as the paranasal sinuses, middle ear, and tracheobronchial tree (Germer, 1985).

4.1.2
Viruses and Host Defenses

All told, there are about a dozen different groups of viruses with more than 150 serotypes that have a demonstrable association with upper respiratory infections. The viruses that show a predilection for the respiratory mucosa include rhinoviruses, coronaviruses, respiratory syncytial (RS) viruses, adenoviruses, and parainfluenza viruses.

The confinement of rhinoviruses to the surfaces of the upper airways is due in part to the very limited temperature range that is optimum for their growth (Mims, 1976): they proliferate well at 33°C, the temperature of the nasal epithelium, and less well at the normal body temperature of 37°C. In theory, inhaling hot steam (which may contain essential oils, Sect. 4.2.2.2) could alter the temperature milieu of the nasal mucosa and make it less hospitable to viruses. There is still no experimental proof of this hypothesis, however.

In evaluating the efficacy of immunostimulants (Chap. 9), it is helpful to review the strategy that has emerged in the conflict between cold viruses and specific host immune responses during the course of their joint evolution. There are two mechanisms by which cold viruses attempt to evade host defenses:

- By very rapid proliferation combined with a very short incubation period of 1–2 days. The host organism needs 5–7 days to produce specific antibodies, and usually the infection has already run its course by the time the host has mounted a specific response (Fig. 4.1).
- By antigenic variations that constantly generate new viral types, delaying and weakening the primary response of the immune system.

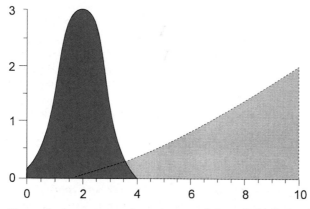

Fig. 4.1. Immune response to an upper respiratory viral infection. Through rapid proliferation, the infecting viruses evade much of the immune response. Dark area: proliferation of viruses; light area: host immune response (antibody formation).

It is likely that interferon plays a major role in the active host defenses against cold viruses. It has been shown that interferon can protect the organism within a few hours after the onset of an infection (Jork, 1979). When a cell is invaded by viruses, it responds by releasing interferon for several hours prior to its own destruction. The interferon from the doomed cell travels to healthy neighboring cells by diffusion, and its interaction with the cells confers absolute protection from viruses for about a 24-h period. It has not yet been proven that this interferon induction mechanism actually checks the cold viruses. There are no known cases in which a congenital defect of interferon production would allow observation of the progress of a cold in a human body unprotected by interferon. Nor are there any suitable animal models in which the effects of interferon could be selectively eliminated for experimental purposes. The mechanism of action of interferon suggests that its antiviral activity is protective and not curative. Clinical studies with human leukocyte interferon support this view, showing that intranasally applied interferon protects against respiratory viral infection (Merigan et al., 1973). There have been no reports of curative effects.

4.2
General Phytotherapeutic Measures

Herbal remedies can make a significant contribution to the relief of cold symptoms. Remedies should be selected that do not further compromise the mucociliary clearance mechanism of the upper respiratory tract. Disruption of this mechanism by the viral infection can promote the bacterial invasion of normally germ-free areas (paranasal sinuses, inner ear, tracheal mucosa). If bacterial complications arise, herbal medications can be administered as an adjunct to antibiotic therapy.

4.2.1
Teas for Cold Relief

A proven and recommended home remedy for the initial stages of a cold (scratchy throat, malaise) consists of hot teas and gradient foot baths (starting at about 33 °C and increasing the water temperature over a 20-min period according to tolerance) followed by warm bed rest to promote diaphoresis. Teas made from elder flowers, linden flowers, and meadowsweet flowers are particularly recommended for colds. Willow bark is also a component in many tea formulas (see Sect. 4.2.1.5).

4.2.1.1
Elder Flowers

Elder flowers are derived from *Sambucus nigra* (Fig. 4.2), a deciduous shrub that is widely distributed in Europe and central Asia. The flowering tops, which are flat compound cymes, are gathered, dried, and separated by sifting into individual flowers and peduncles and pedicels. These latter are then discarded. A crude drug of low-

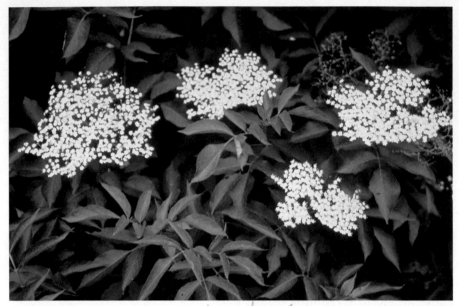

Fig. 4.2. Cymes of *Sambucus nigra.* *potvrdené*

er quality is made by drying and cutting the flowering tops, without separating the flowers from the peduncles and pedicels. Elder flowers have a faint, distinctive odor, an initially sweet taste, and an acrid aftertaste. It has not been proven that elder flowers contain diaphoretic principles. Elder flower tea is prepared as follows according to the German Standard Registration: pour boiling water (150 mL) over about 2 teaspoons (3 g) of dried elder flowers, steep for 5 min, and strain; drink 1–2 cups very hot.

4.2.1.2
Linden Flowers
Linden flowers are derived from two species of linden tree that are native to Europe and are often planted ornamentally along city streets: the early blooming summer linden (*Tilia platyphyllos,* Fig. 4.3) and the winter linden (Tilia cordata), which blooms about 2 weeks later. The crude drug from both species is made by gathering and drying the fully developed, whole flowering tops including the bracts.

Dried linden flowers have a pleasant, distinctive odor different from that of the fresh blossoms. They have a pleasant, faintly sweet, mucilaginous taste.

The pleasant taste is based on the interaction of astringent tannins (about 2 %) with mucilage and aromatics. However, the flowers have not been shown to have constituents with a specific diaphoretic action. The diaphoretic effect of linden flower tea (like that of elder flower tea) is based at least partly on the heat of the liquid itself combined with warm bed rest. It should be noted that the response to thermal

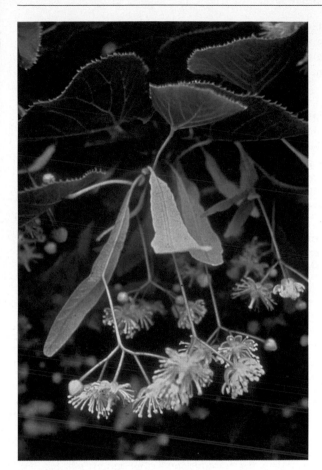

Fig. 4.3.
Drooping cymes of the linden
(*Tilia platyphyllos*).

stimuli follows a marked diurnal pattern. Hildebrandt et al. (1954) found that heat applied in the morning had little or no effect, while heat applied in the afternoon and evening induced profuse sweating.

4.2.1.3
Meadowsweet Flowers

The crude drug consists of the dried flowers of *Filipendula ulmaria* (formerly *Spiraea ulmaria*), an herbaceous perennial of the Rosaceae family native to northern Europe. The dried herb consists mostly of brownish yellow petals accompanied by numerous unopened buds. Commercial herb of good quality has a faint odor of methylsalicylate and a bitter, astringent taste. Meadowsweet flowers contain 0.5% flavonol glycosides, mostly quercetin-4'-glucoside (spiraeoside). The astringent taste is due to the presence of tannins. Hexahydroxydiphenic acid esters of glucose have been identified as components of the tannin fraction. The aromatic fraction consists of salicylaldehyde, phenylethyl alcohol, anisaldehyde, and methylsalicylate (methyl ester of salicylic acid).

Meadowsweet flowers are used in the form of a tea infusion, either alone or mixed with other tea herbs, in the supportive therapy of colds. Infusions contain only trace amounts of salicylates, so meadowsweet tea is considered an aromatic remedy rather than a salicylate medication.

4.2.1.4
Willow Bark and Salicylates

The treatment of inflammatory disorders with salicin-containing plant extracts was known to the physicians of ancient Greece. Dioscorides (ca. 50 AD), in his book *De Materia Medica* recommended willow bark preparations as a remedy for gout and other inflammatory joint diseases, suggesting that it be taken "with some pepper and wine." Extracts from parts of the willow tree (*Salix* species) were also used in medieval folk medicine for their pain-relieving and fever-reducing properties. In 1829, the French pharmacist Leroux isolated the glycoside salicin as the active principle in these extracts. Six years later the German chemist Löwig was the first to synthesize salicylic acid. Because he had extracted the parent compound, salicylaldehyde, from plants of the genus *Spiraea*, he named the product spiric acid. This name later became the root for aspirin (*a*-acetyl, *-spir-* spiric acid, *-in* suffix), first marketed in 1896. Acetylsalicylic acid is better tolerated than salicylic acid and has made salicin-containing plant drugs obsolete.

The following calculation illustrates the problems posed by the continued use of willow bark preparations: A single aspirin dose of at least 500 mg is necessary for effective analgesia. Allowing for differences in molecular weights, 500 mg of aspirin is equivalent to 794 mg of salicin – an amount contained in no less than 88 g of willow bark. Moreover, when the powdered herb is used, salicin is not released quantitatively. As far as orthodox scientific medicine is concerned, willow bark is purely of historical interest today.

Willow bark is indicated in phytotherapy for "febrile diseases, rheumatic complaints, and headache" according to the Commission E monograph of 1992. Accordingly, the herb is a common ingredient in diaphoretic and antirheumatic teas. The source plant, identified simply as willow bark, has not been specifically defined. Various *Salix* species and varieties with a high salicin content are used, most notably *Salix alba* (white willow), *Salix fragilis* (brittle willow), and *Salix purpurea* (purple willow). In addition to salicin, willow bark contains 8–20% tannins. Presumably, the bitter taste and known irritant effect of tannins on the gastric mucosa would limit the use of higher doses in the form of powdered herb or infusions.

4.2.1.5
Tea Formulas

Indications: Febrile upper respiratory infections in which diaphoresis is desired.
Preparation and dosing guidelines: Pour boiling water (about 150 mL) over 1 tablespoon or 1–2 teaspoons of the dried herb, cover and steep for about 10 min, and strain. Drink one fresh cup several times daily.
Directions to patient: Take 1–2 teaspoonsful per cup (about 150 mL) as an infusion several times daily.

Diaphoretic tea according to DRF (German Prescription Formula Index)

Rx	Elder flowers	
	Linden flowers	aa 25.0
	Mix to make tea	
	Directions (see above)	

Diaphoretic tea according to Meyer Camberg

Rx	Linden flowers	
	Elder flowers	aa 30.0
	Chamomile flowers	40.0
	Mix to make tea	
	Directions (see above)	

Diaphoretic tea in Swiss Pharmacopeia 6

Rx	Linden flowers	40.0
	Elder flowers	30.0
	Peppermint leaves	20.0
	Pilocarpus leaves	10.0
	Mix to make tea	
	Directions (see above)	

Cold-relief tea I according to German Standard Registration

Rx	Linden flowers	30.0
	Elder flowers	30.0
	Meadowsweet flowers	20.0
	Rose hips	20.0
	Mix to make tea	
	Directions (see above)	

Cold-relief tea IV according to German Standard Registration

Rx	Willow bark	35.0
	Elder flowers	30.0
	Thyme	20.0
	Rose hips	5.0
	Licorice root	5.0
	Mallow flowers	5.0
	Mix to make tea	
	Directions (see above)	

Diaphoretic tea according to Suppl. Vol. 6 (German Pharmacopeia)

Rx	Willow bark	20.0
	Birch leaves	20.0
	Elder flowers	20.0
	Linden flowers	20.0
	Meadowsweet flowers	10.0
	Chamomile flowers	0.5
	Pilocarpus leaves	0.5
	Mix to make tea	
	Directions (see above)	

4.2.2
Essential Oils

There is much empirical evidence to show that essential plant oils such as peppermint oil and eucalyptus oil are beneficial for subjective complaints involving the nasopharynx, particularly nasal airway obstruction. Surprisingly, rhinomanometric measurements after menthol inhalation showed no objective change in nasal airflow, which seems to contradict general experience. But when a patient with a stuffy nose has the sensation of being able to breathe more easily after inhaling peppermint oil and is able to sleep better after this therapy, the response must be characterized as something more than a placebo effect (Eccles et al., 1988).

Essential oils for topical application are available in various forms: nasal ointments, nosedrops, aerosol inhalants, steam inhalants, or as an ingredient of lozenges, troches, or gargles.

4.2.2.1
Nasal Ointments and Nosedrops

Menthol, camphor, and essential oils are lipophilic substances that, when processed into medicines, can be incorporated only into lipophilic bases. White petroleum jelly or lanolin alcohols are used for nasal ointments, and fatty plant oils are used for nosedrops. As a rule, rhinologic medications should not disrupt the normal protective functions of the nasal mucosa. Hydrophilic preparations are preferable in this regard as they do not disrupt the normal function of the ciliary apparatus. Fatty preparations have two serious disadvantages: they do not mix with the nasal mucous so they do not make adequate contact with the mucosa, and the high viscosity of hydrophobic bases can significantly retard ciliary motion.

The effect of menthol on the nasal mucosa appears to depend on the concentration. Higher concentrations ($> 5\%$), which generally are not used, cause local irritation. According to Nöller (1967), the application of menthol to the nasal mucosa elicits a two-phase response: an initial phase lasting about 30 min in which the nasal air passage becomes constricted or even obstructed, followed by a period of improved nasal airflow. Despite the initial, objective increase in mucosal swelling, test subjects consistently report a pleasant, cooling sensation and a feeling of being able to breath more easily. This purely subjective improvement in rhinitis-associated complaints by menthol application may relate partly to the action of menthol on temperature and pain receptors (Bromm, 1995; Göbel, 1995). Cold, fresh air has a similar effect on nasal stuffiness, most noticeable on walking outdoors from a heated room (Fox, 1977).

The effects of camphor and eucalyptus oil are similar to those of menthol. Detailed investigations (Burrow et al., 1983; Eccles and Jones, 1982; Eccles et al., 1987, 1988) showed that all three substances stimulate the cold receptors in the nasal mucosa and lead to subjective improvement of complaints, despite the fact that there is no measurable decongestant effect. The absence of this effect is advantageous, however, when one considers that the inflammatory response is a natural process and that suppressing it could delay or prolong recovery.

Interestingly, Bromm et al. (1995) and Göbel et al. (1995) found significant differences between the effects of peppermint oil (main component: menthol) and eucalyptus oil (main component: cineol) on temperature and pain receptors when applied topically to the scalp.

In summary, the local application of peppermint oil and eucalyptus oil can significantly improve subjective nasal stuffiness without compromising natural host defenses. So far, no comparable studies have been done on other essential oils contained in cold remedies. The anhydrous bases used in many formulations (fatty oils, petroleum jellies, paraffins) are incompatible with normal functioning of the ciliary apparatus. Ciliary motion is not hampered by dosage forms that deliver the active ingredient to the mucosa through inhalation (chest rubs, cold balsams, inhalant solutions, nasal sprays) (see Sect. 4.2.2.2).

Camphor, menthol, and other medications that contain highly aromatic substances or their essential oils should not be applied to the face and especially the nasal region of infants and children under 2 years of age due to the risk of glottic spasm and respiratory arrest.

4.2.2.2
Inhalation Therapy

Essential oils reach the nasal mucosa in much lower concentration when administered by inhalation than when applied topically. Unfortunately, no studies have yet been published on the effects of inhaled essential oils on the nasal mucosa. It is conceivable, for example, that small amounts of essential oils reaching the mucosa could actually stimulate ciliary motion rather than suppress it. In one clinical study, the inhalation of cineol led to significant improvement in ciliary clearance in patients with chronic obstructive bronchitis (Dorow, 1989). Extrapolating observations on the expectorant effects of inhaled alcohol (Boyd and Sheppard, 1970) on the nasal mucosa suggests that essential oils could stimulate the flow of secretions. The fact that secretions inhibit drying of the nasal mucosa is important because mucosal dryness can seriously disable the ciliary apparatus. For this reason, keeping the mucosae moist is perhaps the most important supportive measure in the management of colds.

Two basic methods are available for administering essential oils by inhalation: steam inhalation and dry inhalation. Steam inhalation is a simple, effective method when applied by any of three techniques:

- simmering chamomile, peppermint leaves, or anise in a pot and inhaling the rising vapors while the head is covered with a towel (head steam bath);
- adding 1 teaspoon of lemon balm spirit to a steam vaporizer; chamomile extracts and other products containing essential oils can also be used;
- taking a hot bath to which a bath salt containing essential oils has been added.

Inhalation devices can be purchased and used for dry inhalation, but a simpler method is to place several drops of peppermint oil on a handkerchief or on the pillow near the head at bedtime and inhale the vapors through the nose. Several breaths should be enough to produce a sensation of easier breathing. As menthol stimulates the cold receptors in the nasal mucosa, it intensifies the patient's sensation and awareness of air streaming through the nose. This is a subjective response that need not be accompanied by an objective change in the nasal air passage (Burrow et al., 1983; Eccles et al., 1987, 1988). Meanwhile, it is a physiological fact that thermoregulation is linked to vasoregulation, i.e., cold stimuli tend to induce vasoconstriction. Therefore, it may be hypothesized that essential oils, by activating cold receptors in the nose, can induce reflex vasoconstriction and thus exert a decongestive effect (Leiber, 1967). Hamann and Bonkowsky (1987) supported this hypothesis by demonstrating objective improvement in the nasal airway.

Risks and contraindications to the topical use of essential oils should be noted. In particular, various mint oils, including peppermint oil, should not be used in the facial region of infants and small children, especially near the nose, due to the risk of inducing reflex respiratory arrest. Spruce needle oil, pine needle oil, and turpentine oil may exacerbate bronchial spasms in asthmatics and in patients with whooping cough.

4.2.2.3
Lozenges, Troches, and Gargles

Lozenges, troches, and gargles are used to soothe local inflammation in the mouth and throat and inhibit the urge to cough.

The cough accompanying a common cold may develop as a result of nasal airway obstruction. As the pharyngeal mucosa dries out, the cough receptors in the throat become more irritable. Even in the absence of objective clinical studies, it is reasonable to assume that lozenges, by promoting the flow of saliva, can keep the mucosa moist and indirectly quiet the cough.

A major ingredient of throat lozenges is sugar, which may be in the form of sucrose, corn syrup, glucose, maltose, fructose, or the substitutes sorbitol and xylitol.

Troches differ from ordinary tablets in their significantly longer dissolving time, achieved by omitting the disintegrants and forming the troches under much higher pressure. Another difference is that the troche masks the taste of the drug substance itself (e. g., plant mucilage). Besides the sugars, essential oils also serve as flavor correctives and thus perform a dual function.

Gum lozenges derive their name from their content of the raw material gum arabic. The base consists of sugar, gum arabic, and possibly other hydrocolloids. The liquid mass is mixed with solid drug substances, plant extracts, and essential oils and formed by pouring into molds. Essential oils may be the only medicinal substances that are incorporated into cough drops and gum lozenges. The most important essential oils are anise oil, eucalyptus oil, fennel oil, menthol, peppermint oil, thyme oil, and tolu balsam (Table 4.1).

Cough drops and gum lozenges are held in the mouth for 20–30 min while they dissolve. One function of the essential oils in them is to impart a pleasant flavor that stimulates salivation. The increased salivation promotes more frequent reflex swallowing, although voluntary swallowing is also useful for suppressing an imminent urge to cough.

Gargling involves taking a fluid into the mouth without swallowing it and holding it suspended in the throat by forcing air through it while exhaling. Gargling exerts a massaging action that is mostly confined to the pharyngeal ring and largely spares the tonsils. Thus, gargles are indicated for inflammatory diseases of the oropharynx and have two essential functions: to cleanse the mouth and pharynx while exerting an anti-inflammatory action on inflamed mucous membranes. The most common ingredients in gargles are essential oils and aromatic herbs that contain volatile oils. Herbs with anti-inflammatory properties are also used, most notably chamo-

Table 4.1. Essential oils commonly used in cough remedies.

Essential oil (Latin name)	Source	Main constituents	Sensory qualities
Anise oil (Anisi aetheroleum)	Ripe seeds of *Pimpinella anisum* (aniseseed)	90% *trans*-anethole	Spicy odor of anise; sweet taste.
Eucalyptus oil (Eucalypti aetheroleum)	Fresh leaves of *Eucalyptus* species that contain cineol	70% Cineole (= eucalyptol)	Camphor-like odor; taste is initially acrid, then cooling.
Fennel oil (Foeniculi aetheroleum)	Ripe fruits of sweet fennel, *Foeniculum vulgare var. vulgare*	50–70% *trans*-anethole, 10–23% fenchone	Odor similar to anise; taste is initially sweet, then becomes bitter and camphor-like.
Peppermint oil (Menthae piperitae aetheroleum)	Flowering tops of *Mentha piperita* (peppermint)	40–55% Menthol, 10% esters of menthol, 10–35% menthone	Pale yellowish liquid with the pleasant, refreshing odor of the peppermint plant; taste is initially acrid, then cooling.
Thyme oil (Thymi aetheroleum)	Fresh flowering tops of *Thymus vulgaris* (thyme)	30–70% Thymol, 3–15% carvacrol	Colorless liquid that gradually turns red; has a phenolic (medicinal) smell and acrid taste.
Tolu balsam (Balsamum tolutanum)	Balsamic resin seeps from the damaged bark of *Myroxylon balsamum*	Esters of benzoic and cinnamic acid (not well analyzed)	Doughy, reddish-brown mass with an odor reminiscent of vanilla; has a somewhat bitter, acrid taste.

mile and tannin-containing herbs. Oral antisepsis is no longer considered a therapeutic goal, for it is known that only transient antiseptic effects are obtained even when highly active concentrations are used.

The gargle may be used in the form of a warm tea infusion or a liquid commercial product. The phytotherapeutic components of commercial gargles include essential oils as well as extracts from chamomile (anti-inflammatory), sage (essential oils, bitters, and tannins), or tormentil rhizome (tannins). Partially evaporated aqueous extracts from Iceland moss are also used.

4.3
Herbal Cough Remedies

Three basic methods are available for the purely symptomatic treatment of cough:

- reduction of local throat irritation,
- peripheral suppression of the cough reflex,
- central suppression of the cough reflex.

Cough as a response to local throat irritation can be treated by physical and pharmacologic measures or a combination of both. Physical measures include humidification of the air, steam inhalation, oral fluid intake, and baths. Pharmacologic measures include adding herbs or essential oils to baths or inhalants and the use of mucilaginous herbs in antitussive teas.

Inhibition of the cough reflex by pharmacologic cough suppression is appropriate for a persistent, dry, nonproductive cough. It should be noted that the cough reflex is part of the normal defense mechanism for cleansing the tracheobronchial tree. Caution is advised in suppressing a productive cough as this may cause an undesired and potentially hazardous retention of airway secretions.

Some herbal remedies act as peripheral cough suppressants, the primary example being ephedra (Hosoya, 1985; Aviado, 1972).

There are no true examples of medicinal herbal extracts among the central-acting cough suppressants – a group that includes the opium-derived alkaloids codeine and noscapine, their transformation products (ethylmorphine, hydrocodone, dihydrocodeine), and purely synthetic drugs such as levopropoxyphene and normethadone.

4.3.1
Mucilaginous Herbs in Antitussive Teas

Coughing as a reflex act is triggered by mechanical irritation of the respiratory mucosa. The pharynx, larynx, and trachea contain receptors that are highly sensitive to mechanical stimuli (Gysling, 1976; Hahn, 1987). The mucilages in plants can inhibit cough by forming a protective coating that shields the mucosal surface from irritants (Kurz, 1989). This effect is limited to the pharynx, however, since plant mucilages probably are not absorbed as macromolecules and thus cannot reach the tracheobronchial mucosa following oral administration. Mucilaginous herbs have no known adverse effects, although coltsfoot leaves may be contraindicated due to their content of pyrrolizidines (hence the omission of this herb from Table 4.2). While it is true that the content of potentially carcinogenic pyrrolizidine alkaloids is very low, implying a very small risk, it is always possible that products may contain varieties of coltsfoot leaves that have a higher alkaloid content or are mixed with butterbur leaves *(Petasites hybridus)*, which contain pyrrolizidine alkaloids. Thus it is best to avoid the use of coltsfoot altogether, especially since mallow leaves and english plantain leaves make acceptable substitutes. Other suitable mucilaginous herbs are listed in Table 4.2.

Besides containing mucilaginous herbs to reduce local irritation, most cough-soothing tea mixtures also contain herbs that serve as odor and flavor correctives. Thus, antitussive teas have basically the same composition as bronchial teas, and both are often referred to collectively as cough and bronchial teas. Formulas for these teas are listed in Sect. 4.4.5.

4.3.2
Essential Oils in Cough Remedies

Throat lozenges and other intraoral cough remedies may contain essential plant oils singly or in combination with other medicinal agents. Anise oil, eucalyptus oil, fennel oil, menthol, peppermint oil, thyme oil, and tolu balsam are commonly used (Ta-

Table 4.2. Mucilaginous herbs used in teas or lozenges to soothe coughs and sore throat.

Herb (Latin name)	Source plant (family)	Constituents	Preparation
Marshmallow root (Althaeae radix)	*Althaea officinalis* (Malvaceae)	5–10% Mucilage	2–5% Infusion or cold-water maceration (1–2 teaspoons/150 mL)
Iceland moss (Lichen islandicus)	*Cetraria ericetorum* and *C. islandica* (Parmeliaceae)	About 50% mucilage of glucan type, including lichenin as the main component	1–2% Infusion (1–2 teaspoons/150 mL)
Mullein flowers (Verbasci flos)	*Verbascum densiflorum* and *V. phlomoides* (Scrophulariaceae)	3% Mucilage of unknown structural type	1–2% Infusion (3–4 teaspoons/150 mL)
Mallow leaf (Malvae folium)	*Malva sylvestris* and *M. neglecta* (Malvaceae)	About 8% mucilage of unknown tertiary structure; arabinose, glusoe, galactose, and galacturonic acid also occur as basic components	2–3% Infusion (3–4 teaspoons/150 mL)
Mallow flowers (Malvae flos)	*Malva sylvestris* ssp. *mauritaniana* (Malvaceae)	About 10% mucilage as in mallow leaves	2% Infusion (2 teaspoons/150 mL)
Plantain (Plantaginis lanceolatae herba)	*Plantago lanceolata* (Plantaginaceae)	About 6% mucilage, including a rhamnogalacturonan, an arabinogalactan, and a glucomannan; iridoid glycosides including 1–2% aucubin	2% Infusion (3–4 teaspoons/150 mL)

ble 4.1). The function of the essential oils is to produce a pleasing taste sensation that stimulates the production and secretion of saliva, which in turn activates the swallowing reflex. Voluntary swallowing can also suppress an impending cough. Lozenges and cough drops can aid patients in their efforts at voluntarily controlling the urge to cough (Walther, 1979).

4.3.3
Ephedra

The crude drug consists of the dried, young stems of *Ephedra sinica* and other Ephedra species that contain ephedrine, such as *E. equisetina* and *E. intermedia*. Ephedra species are herbaceous perennials (family Ephedraceae) that grow to a height of 1 m and resemble horsetail. Ephedra tops contain up to 2% alkaloids with (-) ephedrine as the principal alkaloid.

Preparations made from ephedra stems exert the peripheral vasoconstricting, bronchodilating, and central stimulatory actions of ephedrine. Whole herb extracts reportedly have a less pronounced hypertensive action than pure (-)-ephedrine (*Brit Herb Pharmacopoeia* 1983, p 83).

Coughing induced by stimulation of the tracheal or bronchial mucosa in anesthetized animals is suppressed by ephedra extracts (Hosoya, 1985) much as it is suppressed by ephedrine itself (0.01 mg/kg b.w.). This suppression of the cough reflex results from the bronchodilating action of ephedrine, although a pronounced antitussive effect is obtained even in nonasthmatic subjects (Aviado, 1972). One disadvantage is that ephedrine lacks an expectorant action and has even been shown to reduce airway secretions in laboratory animals.

The indications for ephedra preparations are mild forms of airway disease, especially those resulting from spastic disorders. A single dose of ephedra extract should deliver 15–30 mg of alkaloids, calculated as ephedrine. The maximum daily dose for adults is 300 mg total alkaloids calculated as ephedrine. The maximum daily dose for children is 2 mg/kg body weight. Today ephedrine is usually administered in pure form rather than as one component of a whole plant extract. Potential adverse effects are palpitations, blood pressure elevation, sleeplessness, anorexia, and urinary difficulties.

Conditions that would contraindicate ephedra preparations or limit their use are hypertension, thyrotoxicosis, pheochromocytoma, narrow-angle glaucoma, and prostatic adenoma with urinary retention.

In the United States, the central-nervous-system stimulation effects of ephedra are often potentiated by the addition of caffeine-containing botanicals. Such combination products have frequently been used on a chronic basis to promote weight loss or to enhance athletic performance. Very high doses of these products have also been employed as euphoriants or intoxicants, so-called legal highs. As of 1996, the Food and Drug Administration had recorded some 800 adverse reactions, including 22 deaths, which it attributed to such misuse of ephedra products (Dickinson, 1996).

Following two meetings of special advisory groups, the Agency indicated it would act on ephedra's continued marketability prior to 1997. However, no action was taken before the self-imposed deadline. In the meantime, several states have passed legislation restricting the availability of ephedra.

There is also concern in the U.S. that clandestine chemists may use ephedra as a starting material for the synthesis of illegal designer drugs, such as methamphetamine. Although possible, it is not likely because of the difficulty in separating the product from accompanying plant material. A much more likely starting material is pseudoephedrine which is readily available in pure form. Large-scale sales of that alkaloid are now monitored by the Drug Enforcement Agency.

4.4
Herbal Expectorants

4.4.1
Mechanisms of Action

Often in practical use a strict distinction cannot be drawn between antitussives (Sect. 4.3) and expectorants. Mucus in the bronchi stimulates coughing, so expectorants produce an indirect antitussive effect. Conversely, vigorous coughing intensifies the secretion of mucus, so antitussives can reduce excess mucus production

(Kurz, 1989). According to their pharmacologic definition, expectorants are agents that can influence the consistency, formation, and transport of bronchial secretions.

Herbal expectorants have been used on an empirical basis for centuries. They are believed to act by three mechanisms: a reduction of mucus viscosity (owing partly to the water content of tea preparations), a gastropulmonary reflex mechanism, and the liquefaction of secretions, which is accomplished mainly by direct effects of the essential oils on the bronchial glands (Ziment, 1985).

4.4.1.1
Reduction of Mucus Viscosity by Water

The ability of expectorants to reduce mucus viscosity is due at least partly to the fluid that is ingested with certain preparations. This particularly applies to many bronchial teas, 3 or more liters of which may be consumed daily in a palatable form without causing undesired pharmacologic effects (like those of caffeine in caffeinated beverages).

The quantity of water administered by inhalation is very small by comparison. With a standard regimen of 20 min of inhalation 3 or 4 times daily, water aerosols should have no impact on mucociliary clearance. Thus, inhaled water would appear ineffectual for hydrating airway secretions or altering their rheologic properties (Medici, 1980).

Although animal experiments have failed to confirm the efficacy of increased water intake in liquefying airway secretions (Irwin et al., 1977), this is widely acknowledged to be one of the most important benefits of expectorant medications (Nolte, 1980; Dorow, 1984; Endres and Ferlinz, 1988).

4.4.1.2
Neural Mechanism Based on the Gastropulmonary Reflex

It is known that irritation of the upper digestive tract induces vomiting as afferent impulses are relayed to the vomiting center from visceral sensory fibers in the gastric mucosa. Vomiting starts with increased salivation and a feeling of nausea. Reflex expectorants are administered in a dose sufficient to induce a preliminary stage in which a thin, watery secretion is produced in the goblet cells and in the bronchial glands.

All substances that induce vomiting when taken in large amounts can act as expectorants when taken in a smaller dose (1/10 of the emetic dose). The prototype for this drug action is emetine, an alkaloid obtained from ipecac root. The saponin-containing herbs may have a comparable mechanism of action (see Sect. 4.4.2). Reflex expectorants include acrid-tasting spices that irritate the gastric mucosa and induce nausea when taken in large doses. Spices such as long pepper, cubeb, ginger, and curcuma are common ingredients of cough remedies in traditional Indian and Chinese medicine. Onions and garlic, cooked in milk, are used in European folk medicine as mucolytic agents to help clear congested airways.

4.4.1.3
Liquefaction of Secretions by Direct Action on the Bronchial Glands

Bronchomucotropic agents (Ziment, 1985) directly stimulate the bronchial glands and increase their activity. These agents may be inhaled externally or administered orally for subsequent excretion (and action) via the bronchial tree. Essential oils and aromatic herbs have bronchomucotropic properties.

A study of the direct actions of the terpene preparation Ozothin (see Sect. 4.4.3) on the bronchial glands showed that this agent selectively stimulates the serous glands but depresses the function of the mucous glands. The net result of these actions is a liquefaction of bronchial secretions (Lorenz and Ferlinz, 1985).

Ethyl alcohol is an effective expectorant when inhaled in low concentrations (Boyd and Sheppard, 1969) and is classified as a mucotropic agent. Like the essential oils, alcohol acts as a local irritant, but its overall action is probably based partly on its surfactant properties, i.e., its ability to alter surface tension.

A solution of essential oils in ethanol, rather than essential oils alone, can be added to a steam vaporizer in order to utilize the expectorant effects of both substances (e.g., a tablespoon of citronella spirit or the compound spirit described in German Pharmacopeia 6). The ethanol dose in these spirits, at about 4 g, is too small to produce central alcohol effects in adults.

4.4.2
Saponin-Containing Herbs

Saponins are glycosidic plant constituents with a terpenoid agylcone component. They are like detergents in their tendency to form a durable foam when shaken with water. Saponins have an acrid and/or bitter taste and are irritating to mucous membranes. In finely powdered form, saponins cause sneezing, eye inflammation, and lacrimation. In addition to their surfactant properties, saponins alter the permeability of all biologic membranes. Higher concentrations entering the blood or tissues have a generally toxic effect on cells. Due to their polar nature, saponins are only sparingly absorbed from the gastrointestinal tract so they usually produce no systemic effects when administered orally. Their expectorant action is thought to be mediated by the gastric mucosa, which reflexly stimulates mucous glands in the bronchi via parasympathetic sensory pathways. Higher doses of saponin-containing expectorants cause stomach upset, nausea, and vomiting. Even ordinary doses may cause adverse side effects in patients with a sensitive stomach.

The saponin-containing herbs that are most commonly used as expectorants are listed in Table 4.3. The list does not include licorice root. The glycyrrhizin contained in licorice root is often classified as a saponin, and its chemical composition would support this. But licorice does not have all the biologic and pharmacologic properties that are characteristic of saponins. As a result, licorice root and its preparations are not included in the class of reflex expectorants. The mechanism by which glycyrrhizin exerts its expectorant action requires further study. In any case, licorice and licorice extracts are useful as flavor correctives in teas and cough syrups.

Some combination products contain preparations from *Gypsophila* species as their saponin component. These plants are perennial herbs or subshrubs that prefer a dry climate (e.g., tall gypsophyll). Gypsophila-derived saponin is a complex chemical mixture. It is the standard saponin used to determine the hemolytic index as described in pharmacy texts.

Small amounts of saponins are also contained in grindelia, a tincture of which is a component of several combination products. The aerial parts of *Grindelia* species, native to the southwestern U.S., are gathered during the flowering season and dried to

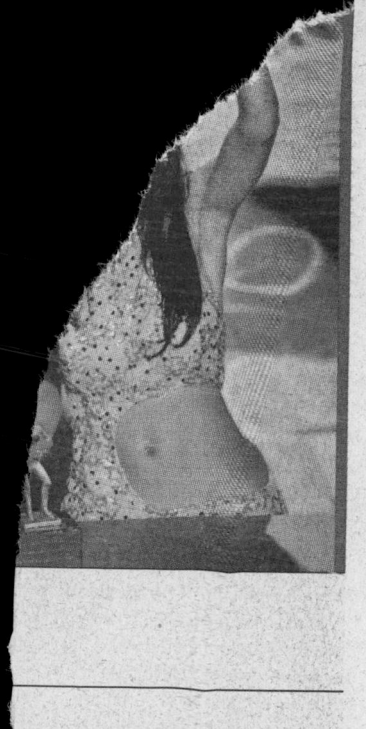

ge**ther**

Table 4.3. Saponin-containing herbs that are used as expectorants.

Herb (Latin name)	Source plant (family)	Type of saponin	Remarks
Ivy leaf (Hederae folium)	*Hedera helix* (Araliaceae)	Neutral bis-desmosides, termed hederacosides, with oleanolic and 28-hydroxyoleanolic acid as aglycone; also hederin type of monodesmosides; total saponin content 3–6 %	Not used as an infusion. Extracts used in drug products, with daily dose equal to 0.3 g of crude drug. Fresh leaves can cause skin irritation; the contact allergen is falcarinol, an aliphatic C_{17} alcohol with acetylene bonds
Primula root (Primulae radix)	*Primula veris* and/or *P. elatior* (Primulaceae)	Monodesmosidic triterpene saponins (5–10 %), including the principal saponin primulic acid A	Used as an infusion or tincture, with daily dose equal to 1 g of crude drug.
Soap bark (Quillajae cortex)	*Quillaja saponaria* (Rosaceae)	Triterpene saponins (10 %)	Single dose of 0.2 g of crude drug corresponds to 10 g of decoction (2 %) or 1.0 g of tincture
Senega snake-root (Polygalae radix)	*Polygala senega* (Polygalaceae)	6–10 % Bisdesmosidic triterpene saponins	Single dose of 1 g of crude drug corresponds to 20 g of decoction (5 %) or 2.5 g of tincture (1:5)

make the crude drug, which also contains 0.3 % volatile oil. Grindelia is believed to act as an expectorant, although relevant pharmacologic studies have not been performed.

4.4.3
Essential Oils as Expectorants

The principal essential oils that are used as expectorants are reviewed in Table 4.4. These oils cannot be strictly differentiated from essential oils that are used as antitussives (Table 4.1). The essential oils are well absorbed after oral administration and are partially excreted via the lungs. As the exhaled molecules pass through the bronchial tree, they can act on the bronchial mucosa to stimulate the serous glandular cells and ciliated epithelium.

Irritation of the mucous membranes is a property shared by all essential oils. Even trace amounts that have little or no detectable odor can exert demonstrable local effects on mucosal surfaces (Boyd and Sheppard, 1970 a). The specificity of the effects of essential oils is demonstrated by studies with Ozothin, a turpentine oil that has been purified with oxidants. Chemically, Ozothin represents a mixture of monoterpene alcohols, aldehydes, and ketones, most notably verbenol, verbenone, myrtenol, myrtenal, and pinocarveol. Its actions can be summarized as follows:

- stimulates serous bronchial gland function and suppresses mucous glandular cell activity following i.v. administration (Bauer, 1973);
- reduces surface tension (surfactant effect) (Zänker and Blümel, 1983);

Table 4.4. Essential oils that are used as expectorants in inhalants, cold ointments, or capsules. See also Table 4.1.

Essential oil (Latin name)	Source plant (family)	Main constituents	Remarks
Spruce-needle oil (Piceae aetheroleum)	*Pinus excelsa, Abies species* (Pinaceae)	20–40 % Bornyl acetate along with α- and β-pinene and β-phellandrene	
Cajuput oil (Cajuputi aetheroleum rectificatum)	Leaves of *Melaleuca* species (Myrtaceae)	65 % Cineole (= eucalyptol)	Reminiscent of eucalyptus oil (see Table 4.1)
Pine-needle oil (Pini aetheroleum)	*Pinus silvestris* (Pinaceae)	80 % Monoterpene hydrocarbons, including α-pinene and 3-carene	
Myrtol	Exact botanical origin unknown	Mainly cineole (= eucalyptol), α-pinene and limonene	
Niaouli oil	*Melaleuca viridiflora* (Myrtaceae)	Like cajuput oil; principal constituent cineole (= eucalyptol)	
Rectified turpentine oil (Terebinthinae aetheroleum rectificatum)	*Pinus palustris* and other P. species (Pinaceae)	90 % Monoterpene hydrocarbons: α- and β-pinene	Starting material is the tree trunk gum turpentine.
Citronella oil (Citronellae aetheroleum)	*Cymbopogon winterianus* and *C. nardus* (Poaceae)	Monoterpene alcohols such as geraniol, nerol, and corresponding aldehydes such as citral and citronellal	Often sold under the name of lemon grass oil or Indian grass oil.

- improves mucociliary activity and tracheobronchial clearance in concentrations of 10^{-7} g/mL or higher (Iravani, 1972).

Controlled clinical studies have been done to test the efficacy of certain medicinal products containing essential oils. A placebo-controlled double-blind study was done in patients with chronic obstructive bronchitis who were being managed with theophylline and a beta-adrenergic drug. This regimen was supplemented by treatment with an ointment containing menthol, camphor, eucalyptus oil, and conifer oil as its active ingredients. Statistical analysis showed that this regimen was significantly better than a placebo-supplemented regimen in terms of objective parameters (pulmonary function, quantity of sputum) as well as subjective parameters (cough, breathing difficulties, lung sounds) (Linsenmann and Swoboda, 1986). Placebo-controlled double-blind studies in patients with acute tracheobronchitis showed improved mucolysis following the administration of essential oils in capsule form (containing anethole, cineole, and dwarf pine needle oil) compared with a placebo (Stafunsky et al., 1989; Linsemann et al., 1989). Another study in patients with chronic obstructive airway disease showed that an orally administered combination of pine oil, lemon oil, and cineole was effective as ambroxol in increasing mucociliary clearance (Dorow et al., 1987).

When stimulus-response relationships are present, ordinary dose-response relationships hold only within a limited range. The expectorant action of essential oils is subject to a marked reversal effect in which very low doses are mucotropic (stimulate bronchial gland activity) while higher doses are inhibitory. This was first shown experimentally for citral and geraniol (Boyd and Sheppard, 1970).

Adverse effects and allergic reactions (type IV) are known to occur with essential oils. Inhalation can provoke bronchospasms, particularly in children and asthmatics. This danger can be reduced by placing the vaporizer farther from the patient and gradually increasing the inhaled concentration by moving the device progressively closer (Kurz, 1989).

Besides the familiar essential oil preparations listed in Tables 4.1 and 4.4, saxifrage root (Pimpinella saxifraga) is also considered an aromatic herb, and its preparations are found in several combination products. It contains 0.4–0.6 % volatile oil with isoeugenol esters as a characteristic component.

4.4.3.1
Dosage Forms

Bronchial teas. There is no strict dividing line between antitussive teas and bronchial teas (see Sect. 4.3.1). Also, the efficacy of antitussive and bronchial teas is based only in part on specific pharmacodynamic actions. An essential part of any expectorant therapy is increased fluid intake; this measure, plus humidification of the air, helps keep bronchial secretions in a relatively nonviscid state and prevents drying of the mucous membranes. About 2–3 L of water should be consumed daily, except in cases where fluid intake is restricted due to heart failure or impaired renal function.

Oral dosage forms. Coated tablets, capsules, and drops allow for accurate dosing. They also permit the use of extracts that contain nonvolatile components.

Inhalations. These agents are administered by steam inhalation. The simplest method is to place about 1 L of water in a pan, bring it to a boil, let it cool slightly, and add the prescribed amount of agent to the hot water. The patient bends over the vessel and inhales the rising vapors as deeply as possible. A towel should be draped over the head and vessel to ensure that the essential oils in the inhalation do not evaporate too quickly. Since the water temperature falls rapidly, an adequate amount of steam is obtained only initially. Commercial steam vaporizers will keep the inhalation solution at a high temperature for a longer period.

Physically, the steam consists of water-saturated air mixed with essential oil vapors and possibly alcohol vapors, depending on the temperature of the medium. The gradient between the temperature in the water vessel and the temperature of the body will cause part of the rising steam to condense. The concentrations of water vapor and volatile medicinal agents (essential oils, ethyl alcohol) that reach the airways depend on the local partial vapor pressure at body temperature, with lower concentrations occurring in the lower respiratory tract. This is probably not a disadvantage with essential oils, however, since low concentrations exert a stronger mucotropic action than higher ones (the "reversal effect"). Boyd and Sheppard (1970) note that the rising vapors should have a barely perceptible odor.

Percutaneous application. Most medications classified as chest rubs or cold balsams are ointments; some are oil- or paraffin-base solutions that incorporate essential

oils. The designated amount is applied to the skin of the chest and back. As lipophilic compounds, portions of the oils penetrate the skin, enter the circulation, and
reach the bronchial mucosa. An unknown percentage evaporates on the warm skin
and is inhaled.

Bath salts and oils. Essential oils are available in several forms for adding to bathwater: bath salts, bath oils, and essences (i. e., essential oils without other additives).
The very large surface area of exposed skin allows for more extensive absorption
and distribution than chest rubs. Portions of the absorbed essential oil components
are excreted via the lungs, producing an expectorant action in the bronchial tree.
The percutaneously absorbed and exhaled doses are further supplemented by the inhalation of essential oils from the air over the bathwater.

Observations in aromatherapy (Jackson, 1989) are consistent with the dose-response relationship found in experimental animals (Boyd and Sheppard, 1970) and
support the value of moderate dosing. Just 7–9 drops of essential oil, equivalent to
about 150–200 mg, is recommended for a whole bath consisting of about 30 L water.

Favorite essential bath oils for respiratory tract diseases are eucalyptus oil, pine
needle oil, spruce needle oil, thyme oil, and cypress oil.

4.4.3.2
Cineole (Eucalyptol)

Approximately 70 % of eucalyptus oil is cineole (Table 4.1). Cineole is an ambiguous
term, referring either to the pure chemical substance that is isolated from cineole-con-
taining eucalyptus oils by fractional crystallization or distillation, or to the commercial medication known as cineol. The pharmaceutical product has a cineole content
of only 80–90 % and is produced simply by treating eucalyptus oils with lye. This
yields a clear, colorless liquid with a camphor-like odor and a pungent, cooling taste.

Cineole has antispasmodic, secretagogic, secretolytic, rubefacient (antimicrobial),
and fungicidal properties. Experiments with cineole inhalation in rabbits showed that
it exerts a surfactant-like action by reducing surface tension (Zänker et al., 1984).

Römmelt et al. (1988) investigated the pharmacokinetics of 1,8-cineole following
10 min exposure to a terpene-containing ointment (9.17 % cineole) administered by
steam inhalation. The C_{max} in the venous blood following alveolar absorption was
200 ng/mL; the half-life was 35.8 min. Concentrations as low as 10 ng/mL were associated with an increase in ciliary frequency.

As for adverse effects, rare instances of stomach upset have been reported following the internal use of cineole, and external use occasionally causes hypersensitivity
reactions of the skin. The LD_{50} in rats is 3480 mg/kg b.w. Cineole has a wide therapeutic range, and there have been almost no reports of cineole toxicity. Patel and
Wiggins (1980) reported one case of medicinal poisoning with eucalyptus oil.

The usual therapeutic dose for adult patients is 0.3–0.6 g cineole daily.

4.4.3.3
Myrtol

Myrtol, an essential oil with a pleasant odor reminiscent of turpentine oil and eucalyptus oil, is a component of a drug product that has the following manufacturer-
listed ingredients: not less than 25 % lemonene, 25 % cineole, and 6.7 % (+)-α-pinene.

There is no information in the pharmaceutical literature on the botanical origin of the ingredients.

The chemical composition of myrtol suggests that its actions, adverse effects, and toxicologic properties are very similar to those of cineole and eucalyptus oil. No data are available on the pharmacokinetics of myrtol after oral administration. It is reasonable to assume that the monoterpenes of myrtol are rapidly absorbed from the gastrointestinal tract and that maximum blood levels are reached in 1–2 h. Some of the absorbed cineole and other monoterpenes are excreted via the lungs, a pathway that again brings them into contact with the bronchial mucosa.

4.4.3.4
Anise Oil and Anethole
Anise oil as described in German Pharmacopeia 9 is the essential oil obtained from the ripe fruits (often called seeds) of *Pimpinella anisum* (family Apiaceae, Fig. 4.4) or *Illicium verum* (family Illiciaceae). The principal component (80–90 %) of anise oil is anethole which is obtained from anise oil by freezing.

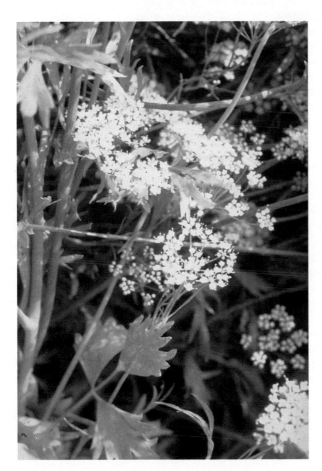

Fig. 4.4.
Anise *(Pimpinella anisum).*

Anise oil is a clear, colorless liquid with a spicy odor and a sweet, aromatic taste that solidifies to a white crystalline mass when refrigerated. Anethole forms white crystals that melt at 20–22 °C.

The expectorant effects of anise oil and anethole are presumably based on their ability to stimulate the ciliary activity of the bronchial epithelium. Moreover, antispasmodic and antibacterial actions have been demonstrated in vitro.

Anethole is rapidly absorbed from the gastrointestinal tract of healthy subjects and is just as rapidly eliminated with the urine (54–69 %) and expired air (13–17 %). Its principal metabolite is 4-methoxyhippuric acid (approximately 56 %); additional metabolites are 4-methoxybenzoic acid and three other metabolites that have yet to be identified (Caldwell and Sutton, 1988; Sangister et al., 1987). Changing the dose does not alter the pattern of metabolite distribution in humans, contrary to findings in the mouse and rat (Sangister et al., 1984). These results do not support the assumption based on animal experiments that higher doses of anethole in humans could block the enzyme system responsible for its degradation.

Adverse effects consist of occasional allergic skin reactions (Opdyke, 1973). The LD_{50} in different animal species (rat, mouse, guinea pig) ranges from 2090 to 3050 mg/kg b. w. for trans-anethole. The cis derivative is at least 15 times more toxic. At present there are no regulations specifying a maximum allowable content of cis-anethole in anethole or anise oil. Animal studies have refuted speculations about a carcinogenic effect (Drinkwater et al., 1976; Miller et al., 1983; Newberne et al., 1989; Truhaut et al., 1989).

The indications for the internal and external use of anise oil and anethole are catarrhal diseases of the upper respiratory tract. The recommended single oral dose is 0.1 g (4 drops) for anise oil. It should be taken in diluted form.

4.4.4
Licorice Root

Licorice root consists of the dried rhizome and roots of *Glycyrrhiza glabra* (family Fabaceae). The genus name *Glycyrrhiza* is derived from the ancient Greek word for licorice (Gr. glykos sweet + rhiza root), which was later latinized to liquiritia and eventually modified to licorice.

The cut, dried herb consists of rough, fibrous, yellowish segments having a somewhat vermiform appearance. Licorice has a faint but characteristic odor and a sweet taste. It contains at least 4 % glycyrrhizin, which is a mixture of the potassium and calcium salts of glycyrrhizic acid.

Licorice root and its preparations are proven expectorants that have mucolytic and secretagogic properties. It is also postulated that glycyrrhizin, like saponins and emetine, increases the bronchial secretion and transport of mucus via a reflex pathway originating in the stomach (Schmid, 1983). This mechanism presumes that glycyrrhizin causes local irritation of the mucosa, but glycyrrhizin does not appear to have this property; indeed, its value in the treatment of peptic ulcers is based on its soothing, demulcent effect on the gastric mucosa.

Perhaps licorice root preparations are more correctly regarded as antitussive agents rather than mycolytics, comparable to the sugar in cough syrups and cough drops. Sweet-tasting substances can influence the urge to cough, and voluntary swallowing can suppress an impending cough. Syrups, teas sweetened with honey or sugar, sweet cough syrups, and cough drops stimulate salivation and elicit more frequent reflex swallowing (Walther, 1979). The indirect antitussive effect of licorice root preparations may involve a degree of central suppression. Glycyrrhizic acid produced an antitussive action comparable to that of codeine when administered to laboratory animals (Anderson and Smith, 1961); further studies are needed to confirm this finding.

Licorice root preparations are useful as flavor correctives in medications that contain bad-tasting or nausea-inducing drug substances. The sweet taste of licorice is due entirely to glycyrrhizin, not to its aglycone, glycyrrhizic acid. Glycyrrhizin is 50 times sweeter than sugar ($f_{sac} = 50$), meaning that the concentration of an aqueous glycyrrhizin solution is equivalent in sweetness to a solution containing 50 times that amount of sugar.

Adverse effects are not a problem when licorice is properly used. Overdosing can lead to a toxic condition that is clinically similar to primary aldosteronism. Martindale (1982) described the case of a 53-year-old man who had eaten 700 g of licorice in one week and developed aldosteronism manifested by cardiac complaints, hypertension, edema, headache, and general weakness. Another man was hospitalized for similar complaints after eating 70 g of licorice sticks daily for a period of two months.

The usual therapeutic dose is 1–2 g of dried licorice root, or equivalent amounts of its preparations, taken three times daily.

4.4.5
Suggested Formulations

Ipecac novum infusion according to DRF (German Prescription Formula Index)

```
Rx    Ipecac root infusion        0.5:170.0
      Ammonium chloride               5.0
      Anise spirit (5%)               5.0
      Marshmallow syrup     to make 200.0
      Directions: Take 1 tablespoon ful every 2 h.
      Shake before using.
```

Explanations: Ipecac root is emetic when given in the proper dosage, owing to its content of the alkaloids emetine and cephaeline. The expectorant dose is one-fifth of the emetic dose. Ipecac, like ammonium chloride, belongs to the class of reflex bronchomucolytics.

Ammonium chloride is a colorless, odorless, crystalline substance with a strong salty taste. The ammonium ion has been recognized as an expectorant for centuries. Presumably it increases bronchial mucus secretion reflexly via the vagus nerve by irritating the gastric mucosa. Marshmallow syrup functions mainly as a flavor corrective. Some effort may be needed to find a pharmacist who is willing to compound a complex individual prescription. An alternative is to prescribe ipecac root in the form of a tincture.

```
Rx    Ipecac tincture             20.0 mL
      Directions: Take 10–20 drops with some liquid 3–5 times daily.
```

Tea Formulas

Indications: bronchitis symptoms and catarrhal diseases of the upper respiratory tract.

Preparation and directions: Pour boiling water (about 150 mL) over 1 tablespoon of tea, cover and steep for about 10 min, and pass through a tea strainer. Drink one cup of freshly brewed tea slowly several times daily, preferably while the tea is still hot.

Antitussive tea according to German Standard Registration

Rx		
	Marshmallow root	25.0
	Fennelseed	10.0
	Iceland moss	10.0
	English plantain	15.0
	Licorice root	10.0
	Thyme	30.0
	Directions (see above)	

Chest tea according to German Pharmacopeia 6*)

Rx		
	Marshmallow root	40.0
	Marshmallow leaves	20.0
	Licorice root	15.0
	Mullein flowers	10.0
	Violet root	5.0
	Aniseed, crushed	10.0
	Directions (see above)	

Chest tea according to Swiss Pharmacopeia 6*)

Rx		
	Marshmallow root	10.0
	Licorice root	10.0
	Marshmallow leaves	10.0
	Mullein flowers	15.0
	Cornflower	5.0
	Helichrysum flowers	10.0
	Mallow flowers	10.0
	Aniseed, crushed	15.0
	Senega root	10.0
	Wild thyme flowers	10.0

Cough and bronchial tea I according to German Standard Registration

Rx		
	Fennelseed	10.0
	English plantain	25.0
	Licorice root	25.0
	Thyme	20.0
	Marshmallow leaves	5.0
	Cornflower	5.0
	Mallow flowers	5.0
	Pimrose flowers	5.0

Cough and bronchial tea II according to German Standard Registration

Rx		
	Aniseed	10.0
	Linden flowers	40.0
	Thyme	20.0
	Iceland moss	5.0
	Mallow flowers	5.0
	Pimrose flowers	5.0
	Heartsease	5.0

Pectoral tea according to Hager (1893)*)

Rx	Marshmallow leaves	20.0
	Nettle leaves	10.0
	Horsetail	10.0
	English plantain	5.0
	Mallow flowers	5.0
	Linden flowers	5.0
	Fennelseed, crushed	5.0
	Mullein flowers	2.5
	Fenugreek seeds, crushed	2.5

*) Original formula modified by substituting marshmallow leaves for coltsfoot leaves.

4.5
Phytotherapy of Sinusitis

First among the 100 most commonly prescribed herbal medications in Germany (see Appendix) is a combination product, Sinupret, approved by Commission E in 1994 for use in the treatment of "acute and chronic inflammations of the paranasal sinuses." A liquid form of the product has been available since 1934, and the coated tablet was introduced in 1968. The active ingredient in the tablet is a mixture of five powdered herbs: 6 mg of gentian root and 18 mg each of pimrose flowers, sorrel, elder flowers, and European vervain. The liquid preparation contains a water-and-alcohol extract from the same herbs, also in proportions of 1:3:3:3:3. The Commission E monographs on these five herbs state that their actions are chiefly mucolytic, so Sinupret comes under the official heading of herbal expectorants.

Table 4.5. Double-blind studies comparing Sinupret (S) with a placebo (P). The comparison of the statistical results is based on the number of patients in the first two studies and on the percentage of patients in the last study.

First author, year	Number of cases (n)	Indication	Duration of treatment (days)	Study criteria: statistical result
Richstein, 1980	31	Chronic sinusitis	7	Headache: "relieved" + "improved" S vs. P = 12 vs. 6 (p = 0.03); X-ray findings: S vs. P p = 0.035
Lechler, 1986	39	Acute sinusitis (adolescent asthmatics)	?	X-ray findings: "normal" + "improved" S vs. P = 16 vs. 9 (p < 0.05)
Berghorn, 1991	139	Acute sinusitis	14	Total symptom score: outcome tended to be better with S than P, but difference was not statistically significant.
Neubauer, 1994	177	Acute sinusitis (160), chronic sinusitis (17)	14	X-ray findings: "normal" + "improved" S vs. P = 87% vs. 70% (p < 0.05). Patient self-rating "relieved" + "improved", S vs. P = 96% vs. 75%.

A monograph published by the manufacturer (Bionorica, 1994) cites more than a dozen pharmacologic and toxicologic studies dealing with the combination product. Of the 12 controlled clinical therapeutic studies, 4 compared Sinupret with a placebo (Table 4.5) and 8 compared it with reference drugs (ambroxol, myrtol, acetylcysteine, and bromhexine).

In the study by Neubauer (1994) in Table 4.5, there was an average difference of only 17% between the outcomes with Sinupret versus a placebo in patients on a basic regimen of antibiotics and decongestant nosedrops. But because three of the four placebo-controlled studies demonstrated a statistically significant superiority of sinupret, it is reasonable to conclude that the product is therapeutically effective. Unfortunately, the low individual doses (156 mg of the herbal mixture or 76 mg of the liquid extract) do not conform to the dosages normally used in traditional herbal medicine (Sect. 1.5.4). Given this fact and the relatively small differences in outcomes between the placebo and the true drug, there is a pressing need for placebo-controlled double-blind studies to furnish additional proof of therapeutic efficacy.

4.6
Drug Products

The category of "Antitussives/Expectorants" in the *Rote Liste 1995* contains more than 100 herbal products, mostly fixed combinations of active ingredients, and numerous products that contain a single active ingredient (Tables 4.1–4.4). The 100 most commonly prescribed phytomedicines include 22 antitussive/expectorant medications, consisting of 8 single-herb products and 14 combination products.

References

Anderson J, Smith WG (1961) The antitussive activity of glycyrrhetinic acid and its derivatives. J Pharm Pharmacol 13: 396–404.

Aviado DM (1972) Antitussives with peripheral actions. In: Pharmacological Principles of Medical Practice. The Williams & Wilkins Co, Baltimore, pp 405–407.

Bauer L (1973) Die Feinstruktur der menschlichen Bronchialschleimhaut nach Behandlung mit Ozothin. Klin Wochenschr 51: 450–453.

Bionorica (1994) Sinupret Tropfen, Sinupret Dragees. Wissenschaftliche Dokumentation zu Klinik, Pharmakologie und Toxikologie.

Boyd EM, Sheppard E (1969) Expectorant action of inhaled alcohol. Arch Otolaryng 90: 138–143.

Boyd EM, Sheppard E (1970 a) The effect of inhalation of citral and geraniol on the output and composition of respiratory tract fluid. Arch Intern Pharmacodyn Ther 188: 5–13.

Boyd EM, Sheppard E (1970 b) Inhaled anisaldehyde and respiratory tract fluid. Pharmacol 3: 345–352.

Bromm B, Scharein E, Darsow U, Ring J (1995) Effects of menthol and cold on histamine-induced itch and skin reactions in man. Neuroscience Lett 187: 157–160.

Burrow A, Eccles R, Jones AS (1983) The effects of camphor, eucalyptus and menthol vapor on nasal resistance to airflow and nasal sensation. Acta Otolaryng (Stockholm) 96: 157–161.

Caldwell J, Sutton JD (1988) Influence of dose size on the disposition of trans-[methoxy-^{14}C] anethole in human volunteers. Food Chem Tox 26: 87–91.

Demling L, Gromotka R, Bünte H (1956) Über den Einfluß peripherer Temperaturreize auf die Durchblutung der Nasen- und Zungenschleimhaut gesunder Versuchspersonen. Z Kreislaufforsch 48: 225–230.

Dickinson A (1996) FDA Food Advisory Committee meeting on ephedra-containing dietary supplements – summary and commentary. Council for Responsible Nutrition Washington DC: 1–29.

Dorow P (1984) Pharmakotherapie der Atmungsorgane. In: Kuemmerle HP, Hitzenberger G, Spitzy KH (eds) Klinische Pharmakologie, Chap. IV-4.5, Ecomed, Landsberg Munich

Dorow P, Weiss Ph, Felix R, Schmutzler II (1987) Einfluß eines Sekretolytikums und einer Kombination von Pinen, Limonen und Cineol auf die mukoziliäre Clearance bei Patienten mit chronisch obstruktiver Atemwegserkrankung. Arzneim Forsch (Drug Res) 37: 1378–1381.

Dorow P (1989) Welchen Einfluß hat Cineol auf die mukoziliare Clearance? Therapiewoche 39: 2652–2654.

Drinkwater NR, Miller EC, Miller JA, Pitot HC (1976) Hepatocarcinogenicity of estragole and 1'-hydroxyestragole in the mouse and mutagenicity of 1-acetoxystragole in bacteria. J Natl Canc Inst 57: 1323–1331.

Eccles R, Jones AS (1982) The effects of menthol on nasal resistance to airflow. J Laryngology Otology 97: 705–709.

Eccles R, Lancashire B, Tolley NS (1987) Experimental studies on nasal sensation of airflow. Acta Otolaryngol (Stockholm) 103: 303–306.

Eccles R, Morris S, Tolley NS (1988) The effects of nasal anaesthesia upon nasal sensation of airflow. Acta Otolaryngol (Stockholm) 106: 152–155.

Endres P, Ferlinz R (1988) Bronchitisches Syndrom. In: Riecker G (ed) Therapie innerer Krankheiten. Springer Berlin Heidelberg New York, pp 137–142.

Fox N (1977) Effect of camphor, eucalyptol and menthol on the vascular state of the mucous membrane. Arch Otolaryngol 6: 112–122.

Germer WD (1985) Erkältungskrankheit. In: Hornbostel H, Kaufmann W, Siegenthaler W (eds) Innere Medizin in Praxis und Klinik. Thieme, Stuttgart, Vol. III, pp 1350–1353.

Göbel H, Schmidt G, Dworschak M, Stolze H, Heuss D (1995) Essential plant oils and headache mechanisms. Phytomedicine 2: 93–102.

Gysling E (1976) Behandlung häufiger Symptome. Leitfaden zur Pharmakotherapie. Huber, Bern Stuttgart Vienna, p 86.

Hager HHJ (1893) Hagers Handbuch der Pharmazeutischen Praxis, 3rd Ed., quoted in Wurm G (ed) (1990) Hagers Handbuch der Pharmazeutischen Praxis, 5th Ed., Vol. 1: Waren und Dienste, Springer, Berlin Heidelberg New York, p 662.

Hahn HL (1987) Husten: Mechanismen, Pathophysiologie und Therapie. Dtsch Apoth Z 127 (Suppl 5): 3–26.

Hamann KF, Bonkowsky V (1987) Minzölwirkung auf die Nasenschleimhaut von Gesunden. Dtsch Apoth Z 125: 429–436.

Hildebrandt G, Engelbrecht P, Hildebrandt-Evers G (1954) Physiologische Grundlagen für eine tageszeitliche Ordnung der Schwitzprozeduren. Z Klin Med 152: 446–468.

Hosoya E (1985) Studies of the construction of prescriptions in ancient Chinese medicine. In: Chang HM, Yeung HW, Tso WW, Koo A (eds) Advances in Chinese Medicinal Material Research. World Scientific Publ, Singapore, pp 73–94.

Iravani J (1972) Wirkung eines Broncholytikums auf die tracheobronchiale Reinigung. Arzneim Forsch (Drug Res) 22: 1744–1746.

Irwin RS, Rosen MJ, Bramann SS (1977) Cough, a comprehensive review. Arch Int Med 137: 1186–1191.

Jackson J (1989) Aromatherapie. Kabel Verlag, Hamburg, pp 175–177.

Jork K(1979) Erkältungskrankheiten – Pathomorphologie und Therapie. Medizin in unserer Zeit 3: 15–19.

Kurz H (1989) Antitussiva und Expektoranzien. Wissenschaftliche Verlagsgesellschaft Stuttgart.

Leiber B (1967) Dieskussionsbemerkung. In: Dost FH, Leiber B (eds) Menthol and Menthol-Containing External Remedies. Thieme Stuttgart, p 22.

Linsenmann P, Swoboda M (1986) Therapeutische Wirksamkeit ätherischer Öle bei chronisch-obstruktiver Bronchitis. Therapiewoche 36: 1162–1166.

Linsenmann P, Hermat H, Swoboda M (1989) Therapeutischer Wert ätherischer Öle bei chronisch obstruktiver Bronchitis. Atemw Lungenkrankh 15: 152–156.

Lorenz J, Ferlinz R (1985) Expektoranzien: Pathophysiologie und Therapie der Mukostase. Arzneimitteltherapie 3: 22–27.

Martindale (1982) The Extrapharmacopoeia (Reynolds JEF, ed) The Pharmaceutical Press London, p 691.

Medici TC (1980) Expektorantien: sinnvoll oder sinnlos? Pharmakritik 2: 21–24.

Merigan TC, Hall TS, Reed SE, Tyrell DAJ (1973) Inhibition of respiratory virus infection by locally applied interferon. Lancet 1: 563–567.

Miller EC, Swanson AB, Phillips DH, Fletcher TL, Liem A, Miller JA (1983) Structure-activity studies of the carcinogenicities in the mouse and rat of some naturally occuring and synthetic alkylbenzene derivates related to safrole and estragole. Cancer Res 34: 1124–1134.

Mims CA (1976) Infektion und Abwehr. Auseinandersetzung zwischen Erreger und Makroorganismus. Witzstrock, Baden-Baden Cologne New York, p 35.

Neubauer N, März RW (1994) Placebo-controlled, randomized double-blind clinical trial with Sinupret® sugar coated tablets on the basis of a therapy with antibiotics and decongestant nasal drops in acute sinusitis. Phytomedicine 1: 177–181.

Newberne PM, Carlton WW, Brown WR (1989) Histopathological evaluation of proliferative lesions in rats fed with trans-anethol in chronic studies. Food Chem Tox 27: 21–26.

Nöller HG (1967) Elektronische Messungen an der Nasenschleimhaut unter Mentholwirkung. In: Menthol and Menthol-Containing External Remedies. Thieme, Stuttgart, pp 146–153, 179.

Nolte D (1980) Expektoranzien, Mukolytika und Antitussiva. In: Nolte D (ed) Asthma. Urban & Schwarzenberg, Munich Vienna Baltimore, pp 155–159.

Pöllmann (1987) Temperaturänderungen der Schleimhaut des Mundes und des Rachens während kalter und warmer Fußbäder. Klin Wschr 65: 281–286.

Opdyke DLJ (1973) Food cosmet toxicol 11, 865 quoted in Leung AY Encyclopedia of Common Drugs and Cosmetics. Wiley, Chichester Brisbane Toronto 1980, pp 31–33.

Patel S, Wiggins J (1980) Eucalyptus oil poisoning. Arch Dis Childh 55: 405–406.

Römmelt H, Schnizer W, Swoboda M, Senn E (1988) Pharmakokinetik ätherischer Öle nach Inhalation mit einer terpenhaltigen Salbe. Z Phytother 9:14–16.

Sangister SA, Caldwell J, Smith RL (1984) Metabolism of anethole. II. Influence of dose size on the route of metabolism of trans-anethole in the rat and mouse. Food Chem Tox 22: 707–713.

Sangister SA, Caldwell J, Hutt AJ, Antony A, Smith RL (1987) The metabolic desposition of methoxy-14C-labeled trans-anethole, estragole and p-propylanisole in human volunteers. Xenobioticy 17: 1223–1232.

Schmid W (1983) Geschälte Süßholzwurzel. In: Böhme H, Hartke K (eds) Deutsches Arzneibuch 8. 1978 Edition, Commentary 2, newly revised edition, Wissenschaftliche Verlagsgesellschaft Stuttgart and Govi-Verlag Frankfurt, p 798.

Schmidt P, Kairies A (1932) Über die Entstehung von Erkältungskatarrhen und eine Methode zur Bestimmung der Schleimhaut-Temperatur. Fischer Jena, pp 1–70.

Schwaar J (1976) Klimaanlagen und Erkältungskrankheiten bei Schiffsreisen in den Tropen. Umschau 76: 719–720.

Stafunsky M, Manteuffel GE, Swoboda M (1989) Therapie der akuten Tracheobronchitis mit ätherischen Ölen und mit Soleinhalationen – ein Doppelblindversuch. Z Phytother 10: 130–134.

Truhaut R, LeBourhis B, Attia M, Glomot R, Newman J, Caldwell J (1989) Chronic toxicity/carcinogenicity study of trans-anethole in rats. Food Chem Tox 27: 11–20.

Walther H (1979) Klinische Pharmakologie. Grundlagen der Arzneimittelanwendung. Volk und Gesundheit, Berlin, pp 360–364.

Zänker KS, Blümel G (1983) Terpene-induced lowering of surface tension in vitro. In: A rationale for surfactant substitution. Resp Exp Med 182: 33–38.

Zänker KS, Blümel G, Probst J, Reiterer W (1984) Theoretical and experimental evidence for the action of terpens as modulators in lung function. Prog Resp Res 18: 302–304.

Ziment I (1985) Possible mechanism of action of traditional oriental drugs for bronchitis. In: Chang HM, Yeung HW, Tso WW, Koo A (eds) Advances in Chinese Medicinal MaterialsResearch. World Scientific Publ, Singapore, pp 193–202.

5 Digestive System

This chapter deals with herbal agents beneficial in the treatment of gastrointestinal disorders. A number of diverse symptoms, including anorexia, dyspepsia, flatulence, and constipation, fall within the domain of herbal medicine. Most herbal gastrointestinal remedies are used to treat functional complaints. Only certain of these medications are covered by health insurance in Germany. Many remedies, such as laxatives, are not covered by insurance and are subject to over-the-counter purchase and use. In all cases the family physician has a responsibility to offer appropriate counseling and guidance, even to patients who self-medicate their gastrointestinal problems.

5.1
Anorexia and Dyspepsia

5.1.1
Introduction

While the symptom of anorexia simply involves lack of appetite, the term dyspepsia can have various interpretations. In pediatrics, it refers to acute nutritional disturbances in infants occurring as a result of diarrhea. In natural healing, it refers to a syndrome featuring nausea, epigastric pressure, bloating, flatulence, and crampy abdominal pains, presumably due to the deficient secretion of gastric juice, deficient bile production, impaired filling and emptying of the gallbladder (biliary dyskinesia), or the deficient secretion of pancreatic juice (exocrine pancreatic insufficiency) (Fintelmann et al., 1993). Effective herbal remedies may be selected from the categories of bitters, cholagogics, or carminatives, depending on whether the dysfunction involves the stomach, biliary tract, or bowel. In practical terms, however, categorical distinctions of this kind cannot be consistently drawn from either a diagnostic or therapeutic standpoint.

Lack of appetite may be a symptom of organic disease (infectious diseases, gastrointestinal disorders, malignant tumors), or it may be psychosomatic (anorexia nervosa, emotional stress) or drug-induced (cancer chemotherapy, antibiotics). In psychophysiologic terms, appetite is an instinctive mechanism whose main locus of control resides in the hypothalamus (limbic system) (Adler, 1979). Mechanisms involved in the anticipatory-metabolic taste reflexes may be even more important in understanding the effects of appetite-stimulating and secretagogic agents, including herbal cholagogues (Nicolaidis, 1969).

5.1.2
Bitter Herbs (Bitters)

Two different interpretations, each supported by experimental data, can be found in the pharmacologic literature regarding the mechanism of action of bitters. Both interpretations agree that stimuli originating in the mouth can reflexly induce gastric secretions. A bitter in the form of an aperitif or stomach bitter, taken in a moderate amount 20–30 min before eating, can stimulate gastric and biliary secretions, increasing the acidity of the gastric juice and aiding digestion (Bellomo, 1939). In one study, 200 mg of gentian root or 25 mg of wormwood herb significantly increased the production of gastric juice even in healthy subjects. The authors concluded that bitters can increase gastric and biliary secretions in healthy subjects compared with the normal volume of secretions induced by food stimuli (Glatzel and Hackenberg, 1967).

These findings are contradicted by other studies showing that bitters taken by healthy subjects with a normal appetite do not increase digestive secretions beyond the reflex secretions that normally occur during the cephalic phase of digestion. The secretory mechanism as a whole is already functioning at an optimum level, and the administration of bitters cannot produce any significant change. In conditions where the reflex secretion of gastric juice is inhibited, however, the administration of bitters can initiate the necessary reflex, leading to gastric secretion of the same intensity and duration (2–3 h) as normal reflex secretion.

There is a definite psychological component to the efficacy of bitters. This was demonstrated by a study in which bitters markedly improved appetite in patients with gastric achylia, despite the fact that increased gastric acid secretion cannot be induced in these patients (Møller, 1947).

Bitters do not invariably act as appetite stimulants. Animals, for example, tend to prefer sweet-tasting foods and avoid bitter-tasting ones (Nachmann and Cole, 1971). Humans are ambivalent toward bitter-tasting foods and beverages, tending to prize the flavor of artichokes, beer, grapefruit, liquors, etc. while disliking the sour taste of pickles and heat-preserved citrus juices. There is a psychological tendency, moreover, to associate a bitter taste with the bitterness of an unpleasant experience.

Bitter herbs can be ranked according to the intensity of their bitter taste (Table 5.1). Bitters that are used medicinally to stimulate appetite and digestive secretions are not merely herbs with a bitter taste; they are herbs that can produce a

Table 5.1.
Relative bitterness of the principal bitter herbs according to the *Deutsches Arzneibuch* (German Pharmacopeia).

Herbs	Relative bitterness
Quassia	40,000–50,000
Gentian	10,000–30,000
Wormwood	10,000–20,000
Condurango bark	10,000–15,000
Devil's claw	ca. 6,000
Lesser centaury	2,000–10,000
Bitter orange peel	600– 2,500
Blessed thistle	800– 1,500
Cinchona bark	ca. 1,000

Table 5.2. Decrease in cardiac stroke volume after swallowing the bitter immediately and after leaving it in the mouth (for 30 seconds). Decrease is shown as a percentage of the pretreatment value (Glatzel, 1968).	Bitter	Stroke volume: percentage decrease	
		Swallowed at once	Left in Mouth for 30 s
	Gentian	8	12
	Hops	7	11
	Bitter orange	5	13
	Rhubarb	4	10
	Wormwood	2	21

pleasant taste sensation in conjunction with their bitter flavor. Another criterion is that medicinal bitters must cause no systemic side effects when used in the proper concentration. Large amounts of bitters reduce gastric secretions, partly by their direct action on the gastric mucosa, and cause appetite suppression. Very strong wormwood tea, for example, can spoil the appetite. Other constituents in bitter herbs are important determinants of taste, and several types of bitter herb are differentiated on that basis:

- Simple bitters such as gentian, bogbean, and centaury.
- Aromatic bitters that contain volatile oils, such as angelica root, blessed thistle, bitter orange peel, and wormwood.
- Astringent bitters that contain tannins, such as cinchona bark and condurango bark.
- Acrid bitters such as ginger and galangal.

Besides their action on the digestive glands, bitter principles act reflexly on the cardiovascular system, causing a decrease in heart rate and cardiac stroke volume (Table 5.2). Taking bitters for several weeks can engender an aversion to certain bitter herbs, accompanied by loss of appetite. The taste of bitter herbs cannot be corrected with raw sugar or other sweeteners. As for adverse effects, bitters occasionally cause headache in susceptible users, and overdoses can induce nausea or vomiting. Because bitters stimulate digestive secretions, they are contraindicated in patients with gastric or duodenal ulcers.

5.1.2.1
Wormwood (Absinth)

The crude drug consists of the dried aerial parts of *Artemisia absinthium* (of the aster family, Fig. 5.1), a perennial shrub native to arid regions of Eurasia and naturalized in North and South America and New Zealand. The leaves and flowering tops are harvested from wild and cultivated plants. Wormwood has a penetrating, aromatic odor and a spicy, strongly bitter taste. The bitter principles contained in the aerial parts of the plant are classified chemically as sesquiterpene lactones, which occur as monomers such as artabsin or dimers such as absinthin. Wormwood contains about 0.3–0.5% volatile oil, up to 70% of which consists of the two stereoisomeric forms of thujone, designated as (−)-thujone and (+)-isothujone; these compounds give the herb its pleasant, fresh, spicy odor.

When the herb is taken in small doses (e.g., 1.0 g in an infusion or tincture), it acts as an aromatic bitter. As the dosage is increased, the toxic effect of the thujone

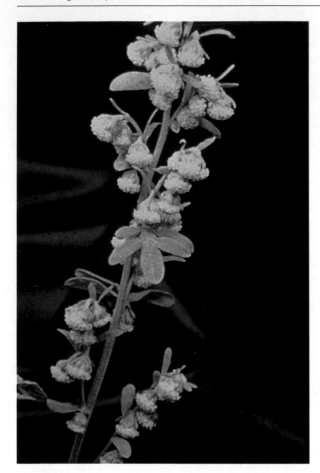

Fig. 5.1.
Wormwood (Artemisia absinthium).

becomes more pronounced, leading to increased salivation and hyperemia of the
mucous membranes and pelvic viscera. The production of pure wormwood liquors
is prohibited by law due to the risk of absinth addiction. Thujone heightens and al-
ters the effects of alcohol, and chronic thujone poisoning leads to cerebral dysfunction with epileptiform seizures, delirium, and hallucinations. Roman wormwood
(Artemisia pontica) is best for making vermouth wines, as this species has a finer
aroma and a much lower thujone content for better tolerance. The leaves of the maritime absinth *(Artemisia maritima)* are also used in making vermouth.

The 1984 Commission E monograph on wormwood states that the crude drug
(dried aerial parts) should have a minimum content of 0.3 % volatile oil and a relative bitterness of at least 15,000. The monograph cites as indications poor appetite,
dyspeptic complaints, and biliary dyskinesia, recommending an average daily dose
of 2–3 g of the crude drug.

5.1.2.2
Other Bitter Herbs

Quassia (bitterwood) is a collective term for two herbs: Jamaican quassia obtained from *Picrasma excelsa*, a stately tree native to the Caribbean, and Surinam quassia obtained from *Quassia amara*, a shrub or small tree native to northern South America. Quassia has a lingering, purely bitter taste. Large amounts of quassia tea irritate the gastric mucosa and induce nausea. A mixture of the bitter principles quassin, neoquassin, and 18-hydroxyquassin (0.1–0.2%) is terpenoid in nature. Quassia is reputed to have value in the treatment of dyspeptic complaints accompanied by constipation. The recommended daily dose is 2–10 mL of a 1:10 tincture.

Gentian root consists of the roots and rhizomes of the yellow gentian, an herbaceous perennial growing to 1 m and native to the mountainous regions of central and southern Europe. It grows in the wild and is also cultivated. Gentian root has a distinctive odor, an initial sweet taste, and a persistent, very bitter aftertaste. Gentiopicroside (known also as gentiopicrin) is the most abundant of the bitter principles (2–3%), but the main active ingredient is amarogentin (about 0.05%), which is 5000 times more bitter than gentiopicroside. The Commission E monograph states that gentian root is indicated for poor appetite, flatulence, and bloating; it is contraindicated by gastric and duodenal ulcers. The average single dose is 1 g of the crude drug, and the average daily dose is 3 g.

Bogbean leaves are obtained from *Menyanthes trifoliata* (family Menyanthaceae, closely related to gentian), a perennial aquatic plant that grows in swampy areas of the northern temperate zone. The leaves are gathered in May or June while the plant is in flower and before the leaves turn dry and brittle later in the summer. Bogbean is odorless and has a strongly bitter taste. The bitter principles of bogbean leaves, like those of gentian root, belong to the class of secoiridoid glycosides.

Hop strobiles, the female flowers of *Humulus lupulus*, are grown commercially and are carefully shielded from pollination by weeding out nearby male plants. This results in larger flowering tops that have strong bitter principles and a powerful aroma. The dried strobile has an aromatic odor and a slightly bitter, acrid taste. The odor changes with prolonged storage, and old hops have the unpleasant smell of isovaleric acid. The bitter taste of hops is due to the presence of so called alpha acids such as humulone, cohumulone, and adhumulone in the hop resin. The bitter principles are susceptible to oxidation and undergo marked chemical changes during storage. Beer no longer contains humulones and lupulones in their original form as the brewing process converts them into water-soluble derivatives. Hops are used in phytotherapy for their calmative properties (Sect. 2.4.2).

Blessed thistle tops are obtained from *Carduus benedictus* (family Asteraceae), an herbaceous plant with spiny leaves native to the Mediterranean region. The dried leaves and flowering tops are almost odorless but have a strongly bitter taste. The bitter principles consist of cninin and lesser amounts of other sesquiterpene lactones.

Condurango bark consists of dried bark from the stems and branches of *Marsdenia condurango,* a climbing vine that grows on the western slopes of the Cordillera range in South America. Condurango bark has a faintly sweet aromatic odor and a slightly bitter, acrid taste. Its main bitter principle is condurangin.

Bitter orange peel is obtained from the fruit of the bitter orange tree *Citrus aurantium*. Most of the white, spongy parenchyma is removed during preparation of the crude drug. Bitter orange peel is an aromatic bitter with a spicy, aromatic odor and a spicy, bitter taste. The flavanone glycosides naringin and neohesperidin are responsible for the bitter flavor. The aroma and spicy taste are based on the 1–2 % content of volatile oils, mostly limonene; other constituents such as jasmone, linalyl acetate, geranyl acetate, and citronellal also contribute to the aroma. A dwarf variety of the bitter orange, the chinotte, has an exceptionally bitter peel that is used to aromatize a popular Italian bitter soft drink (Chinotto).

Centaury (Fig. 5.2), a member of the gentian family, is indigenous to Europe (particularly the Mediterranean region) and northern Africa; it has also become naturalized in North America. The crude drug consists of the dried aerial parts of the plant.

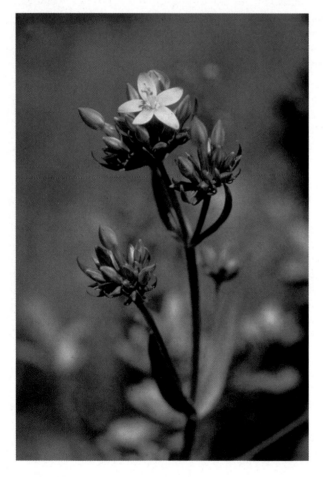

Fig. 5.2.
Centaury *(Centaurium minus)*.

Centaury is nearly odorless and has a strong bitter taste. Some of its bitter principles are identical to those in gentian (gentiopicroside), and some are very closely related chemically (sweroside, centapicrin, swertiamarin).

5.1.3
Biliary Remedies (Cholagogues)

Gallstones are the most frequent cause of biliary tract disease and discomfort. Cases marked by pain and inflammation require short-term treatment with analgesics, antispasmodics, and suitable antibiotics. Other types of pharmacotherapy are appropriate only if surgical treatment is not possible or the patient refuses surgery. The term Cholagogues in this context is a generic one for choleretics (agents that stimulate bile production in the liver) and cholekinetics (agents that promote emptying of the gallbladder and extrahepatic bile ducts).

A number of alkaloidal and aromatic herbs have demonstrated antispasmodic, choleretic, and cholekinetic properties in experimental studies (Table 5.3). While definitive clinical proof of efficacy is lacking, there is ample empirical basis for regarding these herbs as effective, and most have been positively evaluated by Commission E of the former German Fedral Health Agency. Cholagogues in particular are widely prescribed by family practitioners in Germany. According to Weiss (1991), biliary tract dysfunction is a very common problem in family medicine, characterized by vague upper abdominal discomfort that is more pronounced on the right side and often radiates to the back and to the right shoulder. It is not unusual for complaints to be exacerbated by fatty meals. Weiss states that cholagogic herbs are appropriate in cases where a thorough examination fails to disclose an organic illness.

Reasoning by analogy with kidney stones and recurrent urinary tract infection, it is plausible that increasing the bile flow would help to cleanse the biliary tract of

Table 5.3. Herbs used as biliary remedies owing to their choleretic, cholekinetic, or antispasmodic properties.

Herb (Latin name)	Key constituents	Daily dose
Artichoke leaf (Cynarae folium)	Cynarin and bitter principales (e.g., cynaropicrin)	6 g of crude drug
Boldo leaf (Boldo folium)	>0.1% Alkaloids (main active principle: boldine), 2% volatile oils	3 g of crude drug
Fumitory (Fumariae herba)	>0.1% Fumarine and other isoquinoline alkaloids	6 g of crude drug
Tumeric rhizome (Curcumae rhizoma)	>3% Curcumin and desmethoxycurcumin, >3% volatile oils	1.5–3 g of crude drug
Dandelion root and leaf (Taraxici radix cum herba)	Mixture of bitters designated taraxicin, also phytosterols	3–4 g of crude drug
Greater celandine (Chelidonii herba)	>6% Total alkaloids, calculated as chelidonine	2–5 g of crude drug or 12–30 mg total alkaloids

crystallization nuclei and bacteria that have entered the tract by the retrograde route, but such an assumption is difficult to prove experimentally (Ritter, 1984). Of course, lithiasis might be considered a contraindication to cholagogic therapy since stimulating bile flow or gallbladder contractions could cause a gallstone to become impacted. But bitters can induce a mild, almost physiologic stimulation of bile secretion and biliary tract motility (Sect. 5.1.2) (Glatzel, 1968), and generally a strict distinction cannot be drawn between the classes of bitter and cholagogic remedies in practical therapeutic use. Available information suggests that all these remedies have primarily a subjective mode of action. From a practical standpoint, this means that herbal bitters and cholagogues should not contain any ingredients that might be harmful if used on a long-term basis.

5.1.3.1
Some Specific Herbs

Table 5.3 lists six specific herbs whose preparations are often contained in cholagogic remedies. Most of the commercial products available in Germany are made from extracts. If we assume for simplicity that these products have an extract content on the order of about 20 % (approximately 5 : 1 herb-to-extract ratio), the dosage of extract would be in the range of about 300–1200 mg daily. In the case of herbs that are consumed in powdered form, the active daily dose would be as high as 1.5–6 g/day. These figures suggest that some 50 % of the most common single-herb biliary remedies sold in Germany, and virtually all the combination products, are underdosed.

Artichoke leaves, consisting of the fresh or dried foliage leaves of Cynara scolymus, reportedly have choleretic properties in addition to antihepatotoxic and lipid-reducing actions. The choleretic effects are the best documented. For example, two place-

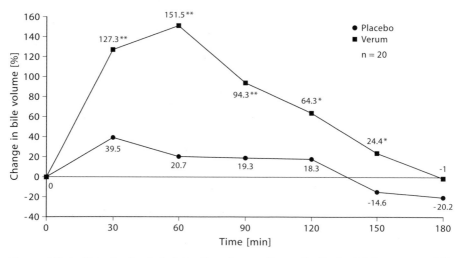

Fig. 5.3. Effect of intraduodenal administration of 1.92 g of a standardized artichoke extract on bile flow. Mean values were measured in 20 healthy subjects. The differences relative to the placebo at 120 and 150 min were statistically significant (* = $p < 0.05$; ** = $p < 0.01$, after Kirchhoff et al., 1994).

bo-controlled studies in humans (Kupke et al., 1991; Kirchhoff et al., 1994) showed respective increases of 127 % and 152 % in bile flow 30 min and 60 min after the intraduodenal administration of 1.92 g of a standardized artichoke extract (Fig. 5.3). The differences relative to a placebo were statistically significant ($p < 0.05$). These findings led the authors to conclude that artichoke extract is beneficial in the treatment of dyspeptic complaints, especially in patients with a suspected dysfunction of bile secretion (Kirchhoff et al., 1994). The Commission E monograph states that artichoke preparations are indicated for dyspeptic complaints and are contraindicated by allergies to artichokes and by biliary tract obstruction.

Boldo leaves are obtained from the evergreen shrub Peumus boldus, a relative of the laurel tree that is native to arid regions of Chile. The crude drug has a burning, aromatic taste and odor caused by its content of volatile oil. Its true active principle is boldine, an aporphine alkaloid. Because the herb contains substances that are potentially toxic (Duke, 1985), it is not recommended for long-term use and should not be taken during pregnancy.

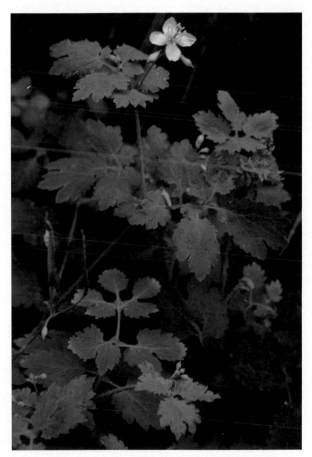

Fig. 5.4.
Greater celandine *(Chelidonium majus)*.

Fumitory *(Fumaria officinalis)* is a traditional native European herb whose extracts reportedly relieve spasms of the sphincter of Oddi and exert a general regulatory effect on biliary functions (Fiegel, 1971).

Turmeric *(Curcuma longa)* **extract** is reported to have choleretic and cholecystokinetic properties (Maiwald and Schwantes, 1991). These are due partly to the presence of curcumins, although whole extracts are thought to be more potent than individual fractions. Curcuma is also described as an anti-inflammatory agent (Ammon and Wahl, 1990).

Dandelion *(Taraxacum officinalis)* **extract** reportedly leads to an increase in bile flow (Böhm, 1959; Pirtkien et al., 1960). This action may be based on bitter principles contained chiefly in the dandelion root.

Extract of greater celandine *(Chelidonium majus,* Fig. 5.4), when administered to experimental animals, causes a slow but steady increase in bile flow that is believed to result more from choleretic than cholekinetic effects (Baumann, 1975). The crude drug, consisting of the dried aerial parts of Chelidonium majus (family Papaveraceae) harvested while the plant is in bloom, contains 0.1–1 % total alkaloids including chelidonine, a papaverine-related compound that reportedly acts as an antispasmodic and a weak central analgesic. Overdoses of greater celandine or its preparations can cause stomach pain, intestinal colic, urinary urgency, and hematuria accompanied by dizziness and stupor. Tea preparations are difficult to dose properly, so greater celandine should not be taken in that form. Commercial products generally contain extracts standardized to a specified alkaloid content and should cause no adverse effects when taken in the recommended dosage.

5.1.4
Digestive Enzymes

Replacement therapy with digestive enzymes may be utilized in an attempt to relieve the complaints resulting from excretory pancreatic insufficiency with associated indigestion. This involves the use of combination products containing lipase, amylase, and proteases. Most of these products contain preparations made from animal pancreatic tissue. Some combination products (e.g., Esberizym) also contain plant proteases – bromelain, which is derived from the fresh juice of the pineapple plant *(Ananas comosus),* and papain, which is obtained from the latex of the fleshy, unripe fruit of the papaya *(Carica papaya).* Since there is no clinical syndrome that would warrant protease replacement as an isolated therapy, and there seems to be no rationale for combining the proteases bromelain and papain with other preparations in this group, Commission E of the former German Federal Health Agency did not sanction the use of bromelain and papain for the replacement therapy of digestive insufficiency.

5.1.5
Suggested Formulations

A) For stomach tinctures and teas
Indications: poor appetite, dyspeptic complaints with bloating and fullness.
Contraindications: gastric and duodenal ulcers.
Adverse effects: occasional headache in patients sensitive to bitters.

Rx   Bitter tincture according to German Pharmacopeia 6.
Directions: Take 10–20 drops in one-half glass of water before meals.
Tonic-aromatic stomach remedy for dyspeptic conditions according to Weiss (1982).

Rx		
Gentian tincture	10.0
Wormwood tincture	10.0
Peppermint tincture	10.0
Directions: (same as above).	

Bitter tea according to Austrian Pharmacopeia*)

Rx		
Wormwood	20.0
Centaury	20.0
Bogbean leaves	15.0
Gentian root	15.0
Bitter orange peel	20.0
Cinnamon bark	10.0
Mix to make tea	

Directions: Take 2 teaspoonsful in 1 cup as an
infusion 30 min before meals several times daily.
*) Modified to omit calamus root.

Stomach tea I according to German Standard Registration

Rx		
Gentian root	20.0
Bitter orange peel	20.0
Centaury	25.0
Wormwood	25.0
Cinnamon bark	10.0

Stomach tea II according to German Standard Registration

Rx		
Angelica root	25.0
Yarrow	25.0
Centaury	15.0
Wormwood	15.0
Aniseed	5.0
Cornflower	5.0
Orange blossoms	5.0
Rosemary	5.0

Stomach tea III according to German Standard Registration

Rx		
Wormwood	25.0
Yarrow	25.0
Balm leaves	25.0
Blackberry leaves	5.0
Cornflower	5.0
Orange blossoms	5.0
Calendula flowers	5.0
Sage leaves	5.0

Stomach tea IV according to German Standard Registration

Rx	Gentian root	20.0
	Dandelion leaves and root	35.0
	Centaury	30.0
	Basil	5.0
	Calendula flowers	5.0
	Sage leaves	5.0

Note: Each formula should include (1) mix to make tea and (2) the same directions stated for the Austrian Pharmacopeia tea.

B) Suggested formulations for bile teas

Indications: supportive treatment of noninflammatory gallbladder complaints involving a disturbance of bile flow, also gastrointestinal complaints that involve bloating and digestive problems.

Contraindications: inflammation or obstruction of the bile ducts; bowel obstruction.

Directions to patient: Infuse 1 teaspoonful in 1 cup of water (about 150 mL); drink 1 fresh cup 30 min before meals 3 or 4 times daily.

Bile tea I according to German Standard Registration

Rx	Dandelion leaves and root	30.0
	Javanese turmeric rhizome	20.0
	Peppermint leaves	20.0
	Milk thistle fruit	20.0
	Caraway fruit	10.0

Bile tea II according to German Standard Registration

Rx	Dandelion leaves and root	15.0
	Javanese turmeric rhizome	20.0
	Peppermint leaves	20.0
	Yarrow	20.0
	Fennelseed	5.0
	Chamomile	5.0
	Calendula	5.0
	Licorice root	5.0
	Wormwood	5.0

5.1.6
Drug Products

Liquid preparations are the recommended dosage form for administering bitters. Teas can be prepared at home as an alternative to ready-made products, provided this can be done with an acceptable therapeutic risk (see wormwood). There is a welcome trend among manufacturers to produce single-herb cholagogic remedies in adequate dosage, yet physicians continue to prescribe mostly combination products. Combinations that include a laxative are best avoided. This type of product is based on the old pharmacodynamic fallacy that the bowels have a kind of suction effect on sluggish bile flow (Guttenberg, 1926) and that increased peristalsis in the small bowel can "milk" bile from the common bile duct (Kohlstaedt, 1947). But the most commonly used anthranoid laxatives act only on the large bowel, and only preparations such as castor oil or podophyllin could produce this kind of effect in the small bowel. A more plausible explanation is that certain groups of patients (e.g., those who have undergone cholecystectomy) are more likely to develop constipation. Another reason for the popularity of cholagogue-laxative combinations may simply be that laxative products are not covered by health insurance, so a biliary remedy is prescribed as a substitute (Bode, 1995).

References

Adler M (1979) Physiologische Psychologie, Part II: Spezielle Funktionssysteme, Enke Stuttgart, pp 177–185.

Ammon HPT, Wahl MA (1990) Pharmacology of Curcuma longa. Planta Med 57: 1–7.

Baumann J (1975) Über die Wirkung von Chelidonium, Curcuma, Absinth und Carduus marinus auf die Galle- und Pankreassekretion bei Hepatopathien. Med Mschr 29: 173.

Bellomo A (1939) Richerche cliniche. Giorn cad Med Torino 52: 181.

Bode JC (1995). Leber- und Gallenwegstherapeutika. In: Schwabe U, Paffrath D (eds) Arzneiverordnungs-Report '95. Gustav Fischer Verlag, Stuttgart Jena, pp 272–280.

Böhm K (1959) Untersuchungen über choleretische Wirkungen einiger Arzneipflanzen. Arzneim Forsch/Drug Res 9: 376.

Duke HA (1985) CRC Handbook of Medicinal Herbs. CRC Press, Boca Raton, pp 358–359.

Fiegel G (1971) Die amphocholeretische Wirkung der Fumaria officinalis. Z Allg Med 34: 1819.

Fintelmann V, Menssen HG, Siegers CP (1993) Phytotherapie Manual. Pharmazeutischer, pharmakologischer und therapeutischer Standard. 2nd Ed. Hippokrates Verlag Stuttgart.

Glatzel H, Hackenberg K (1967) Röntgenuntersuchungen der Wirkungen von Bittermitteln auf die Verdauungsorgane. Planta Med 15: 223–232.

Glatzel H (1968) Die Gewürze. Ihre Wirkungen auf den Menschen. Nicolaische Verlagsbuchhandlung, Herford, p 170.

Guttenberg A (1926) Das Cholagogum Curcumen. Klin Wschr 5: 1998–1999.

Kirchhoff R, Beckers Ch, Kirchhoff GM, Trinczek-Gärtner H, Petrowicz O, Riemann HJ (1994) Increase in choleresis by means of artichoke extract. Phytomedicine 1: 107–115.

Kohlstaedt E (1947) Choleretika, Cholekinetika und Cholagoga. Pharmazie 2: 529–536.

Kupke D, Sanden H, Trinczek-Gärtner H, Lewin J, Blümel G, Reimann HJ (1991) Prüfung der choleretischen Aktivität eines pflanzlichen Cholagogums. Z Allg Med 67: 1046–1058.

Maiwald I, Schwantes PA (1991) Curcuma xanthorrhiza Roxb., eine Heilpflanze tritt aus dem Schattendasein. Z Phytother 12: 35–445.

Möller K (1947) Pharmakologie, Benno Schwabe & Co Verlag, Basel, pp 133–136.

Nachmann M, Cole LP (1971) Role of taste in specific hungers. In: Beidler LM (ed) Handbook of Sensory Physiology, Vol IV, Chemical Senses 2, Taste. Springer Berlin Heidelberg New York, pp 337–362.

Nicholaidis S (1969) Early systemic responses in the regulation of food and water balance: functional and electrophysiological data. In: Neural regulation of food and water intake. Ann NY Acad Sci 157: 1176–1203.

Pirtkien R, Surhe E, Seybold G (1960) Vergleichende Untersuchungen über die choleretischen Wirkungen verschiedener Arzneimittel bei der Ratte. Med Welt 1: 1417.

Ritter U (1984) Therapie mit Choleretika und Cholekinetika. Med Mo Pharm 7: 99–104.

Weiss RF (1982) Lehrbuch der Phytotherapie. 5th Ed. Hippokrates Verlag Stuttgart.

5.2
Bloating and Flatulence

Bloating and flatulence are among the most common symptoms encountered by the general practitioner. Their causes are diverse and range from inflammatory gastrointestinal disorders and biliary/pancreatic secretory dysfunction to atherosclerotic lesions of the mesenteric blood vessels. Most cases are thought to be based less on excessive gas formation than on deficient gas absorption. Although bloating and flatulence generally are not painful, they can be very troublesome for the patient. They not only affect mood, appetite, and sleep but can have adverse circulatory effects corresponding to the gastrocardiac symptom complexes described by Roemheld at the turn of the century.

5.2.1
Definition and Actions of Carminatives

Herbal preparations play a special role in the treatment of flatulence. Herbs that are useful in expelling gas to relieve flatulence are called carminatives (from the Latin carminare, to cleanse). The pharmacologic literature (Gunn, 1920; Sigmund and McNally, 1969) defines carminatives as preparations, originally taken with food, that produce a warm sensation when ingested and promote the postprandial elimination of digestive gas by flatus or eructation. These products include essential oils as well as herbal preparations and plant extracts that have a high content of volatile oils, most notably caraway, fennel, and anise as well as peppermint, chamomile, lemon balm, and angelica root.

It has been well established, at least in vitro, that many of the essential oils used as carminatives have antispasmodic actions (Schwenk and Horbach, 1978; Forster, 1983; Reiter and Brandt, 1985). This particularly applies to peppermint oil (Taylor et al., 1983; Hills and Aaronson, 1991). Studies in human subjects have shown that the administration of peppermint oil can relax the lower esophageal sphincter in minutes, equalizing the intraluminal pressures between the stomach and esophagus (Sigmund and McNally, 1969). It has been found that alcoholic extracts of the typical carminative herbs caraway, fennel, and anise have antispasmodic activity, but their essential oils do not (Forster, 1983); indeed, the latter substances tend to heighten muscle tonus and stimulate bowel motility (Brandt, 1988). Thus, while carminatives are unquestionably effective from the standpoint of the user, the mechanisms that underlie their efficacy are not yet fully understood.

5.2.2
Typical Carminative Herbs

Caraway (*Carum carvi*, Fig. 5.5): The dried ripe fruits (often called seeds) of this plant of the family Apiaceae are considered the most typical and effective of the carminative herbs. Caraway is a biennial plant that grows wild in Europe and Asia, but the herb used for medicinal and seasoning purposes is obtained almost exclusively by cultivation. Caraway fruits contain 2–7 % volatile oil and about 10–20 % fatty oil. The volatile oil consists mainly of carvone (50–60 %) and limonene. Alcoholic caraway extracts have been used for centuries as stomachics.

Fennel (*Foeniculum vulgare*), also a member of the family Apiaceae, grows to 1–2 m and is native to southern Europe. Its fruits (seeds) are used medicinally and contain 2–6 % volatile oil and 9–12 % fatty oil. Fennel volatile oil consists mostly of fenchone and anethole. The fruits are mainly carminative but also act as a mild expectorant,

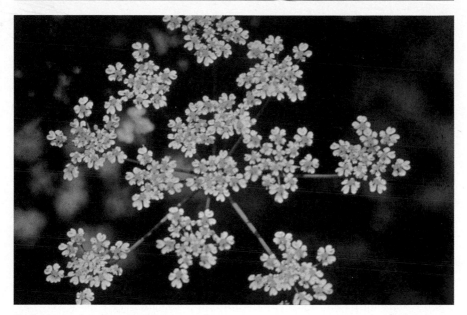

Fig. 5.5. An umbel of caraway *(Carum carvi)*.

especially in children. Fennel also makes an excellent flavor corrective for carminative tea mixtures. Additionally, fennel tea is a common European remedy for infants with dyspepsia and diarrhea. Allowing only fennel tea during the initial fasting period not only supplies the infants with fluid but also provides a carminative effect that reduces flatulence and eases intestinal spasms.

Anise *(Pimpinella anisum)* is native to the Orient but is also grown in certain regions of Germany. Like caraway and fennel, anise is a member of the family Apiaceae. It has a pungent odor and grows to a height of about $^1/_2$ m. Aniseed (technically a fruit) contains 2–3 % volatile oil and about 10 % fatty oil. The main constituent of the volatile oil is anethole. Anise is a less potent carminative than caraway but reportedly has a stronger expectorant action. Weiss (1991) ranks the umbelliferous herbs as follows in order of decreasing carminative effect and increasing expectorant effect: caraway, fennel, anise.

Other herbs considered to have carminative actions are chamomile, peppermint, lemon balm, angelica root, and coriander seeds. Angelica root has an unpleasant odor and a spicy, bitter taste. It contains about 0.4–0.8 % volatile oil. The fruits of coriander, native to the Mediterranean region, have a spicy aromatic odor and a slightly burning taste. Their odor and taste are due to the content of volatile oil, consisting mainly of linalool (60–70 %). The aerial parts of marjoram are also said to have a weak carminative action but are used mainly as a culinary spice.

5.2.3
Suggested Formulations

Indications: complaints such as bloating, flatulence, and mild gastrointestinal cramping; also nervous gastrointestinal complaints.

Compound caraway tincture according to German Prescription Formula Index

Rx	Caraway volatile oil	2.0
	Valerian tincture	to make 20.0
	Directions: Take 30 drops in water 3 times daily.	

Carminative rub according to Fintelmann.

Rx	Caraway volatile oil	2.0
	Olive oil	to make 20.0
	Directions: Use externally for bloating; rub several drops into the periumbilical area.	

Tea Mixtures
Preparation and use: Pour boiling water (about 150 mL) over 1–2 teaspoons of the tea mixture, steep for 10 min, and strain. Drink 1 cup warm after every meal.

Carminative tea according to German Prescription Formula Index (DRF, 1950)

Rx	Chamomile	
	Peppermint	
	Valerian root	
	Caraway fruit	
	Aniseseed	aa, to make 100.00
	Directions (see above).	

Gastrointestinal tea I according to German Standard Registration

Rx	Valerian root	
	Caraway fruit	
	Peppermint	
	Chamomile	aa, to make 100.0
	Directions (see above).	

Gastrointestinal tea III according to German Standard Registration

Rx	Fennelseed	30.0
	Coriander fruit	30.0
	Calendula flowers	5.0
	Cornflower	5.0
	Directions (see above).	

Gastrointestinal tea IX according to German Standard Registration

Rx	Aniseseed	
	Fennelseed	
	Caraway fruit	
	Chamomile	
	Yarrow	aa, to make 100.0
	Directions (see above).	

Gastrointestinal tea XII according to German Standard Registration

Rx   Chamomile   30.0
     Licorice root   30.0
     Yarrow   20.0
     Mallow flowers   5.0
     Balm leaves   5.0
     Calendula flowers   5.0
     Cinnamon bark   5.0
     Directions (see above).

References

Brandt W (1988) Spasmolytische Wirkung ätherischer Öle. In: Phytotherapie. Hippokrates Stuttgart, pp 77–89.
DRF (1950) Deutsche Rezeptformeln. Duncker & Humblot, Berlin.
Forster H (1983) Spasmolytische Wirkung pflanzlicher Carminativa. Allgemeinmedizin 59: 1327–1333.
Gunn JWC (1920) The carminative action of volatile oils. J Pharmacol Exp Ther 6: 93–143.
Hills JM, Aaronson PI (1991) The mechanisms of action of peppermint oil on gastrointestinal smooth muscle. Gastroenterol 101: 55–65.
Reiter M, Brandt W (1985) Erschlaffende Wirkungen auf die glatte Muskulatur von Trachea und Ileum des Meerschweinchens. Arzneim-Forsch/Drug Res 35: 408–415.
Schwenk HU, Horbach L (1978) Vergleichende klinische Untersuchung über die Wirksamkeit von Carminativum-Hetterich bei Kindern mittels wiederholter Sonographie des Abdomens. Therapiewoche 28: 2610–1615.
Sigmund CJ, McNally EF (1969) The action of a carminative on the lower esophageal sphincter. Gastroenterol 56: 13–18.
Taylor BA, Luscombe DK, Duthie HL (1983) Inhibitory effect of peppermint on gastrointestinal smooth muscle. Gut 24, A 992 T (abstract).
Weiss RF (1991) Lehrbuch der Phytotherapie. 7th Ed. Hippokrates Verlag Stuttgart.

5.3
Gastritis and Ulcer Disease

Inflammations of the gastric mucosa, ranging from relatively mild forms of gastritis to peptic ulcer disease, are treated pharmacologically with acid-neutralizing agents (antacids), agents that inhibit acid secretion (anticholinergics, H_2-antagonists), and with demulcent and anti-inflammatory remedies. Phytotherapy has made a significant contribution to anticholinergic therapy, at least from an historical perspective, in that the alkaloids derived from the deadly nightshade (*Atropa belladonna*), atropine and scopolamine, are the prototypes of all anticholinergic drugs. Due to their narrow therapeutic range, however, preparations made from the leaves of deadly nightshade or henbane (0.2–0.3 % hyoscyamine and scopolamine) cannot be recommended today.

Some mucilaginous herbs have demulcent properties that can reduce local irritation in acute gastritis, particularly linseed, marshmallow leaves and roots, and common mallow leaves. A proven home remedy in this regard is linseed, which should be presoaked in water for about 30 min, similar to its mode of use as a laxative (Sect. 5.8.2.1). Linseed can also be combined with chamomile preparations.

The main phytomedicines in use today for gastritis relief are chamomile and its preparations and licorice root preparations. Their effects are assumed to be based on anti-inflammatory and demulcent actions.

5.3.1
Chamomile

German chamomile *(Matricaria recutita)* is one of the best known and most versatile medicinal plants. Its many dermatologic uses are reviewed in Chap. 8.

Today it is believed that chamomile owes its therapeutic properties to three groups of active principles. First, there are the terpenoid volatile oils (content 0.25–1%), especially bisabolol and chamazulene, both of which show a mild anti-inflammatory action in experimental animals (Isaak, 1980). Next come the flavonoids (content about 2.4%), with apigenin showing particular activity as an antispasmodic agent. Finally, chamomile flowers have a 5–10% content of pectin-like mucilages. It is assumed that these substances are preferentially released during the infusion process and act swiftly to soothe irritation of the gastric mucosa.

Chamomile flowers prepared as an infusion or contained in an extract-based product have mild anti-inflammatory and antispasmodic activity. This lends credence to physicians' observations that the therapeutic use of chamomile in acute flareups of chronic ulcer disease promotes ulcer healing. Chamomile no longer has a role in the treatment of chronic gastritis, Crohn's disease, or ulcerative colitis. It should be noted that the pharmacologic actions of various commercial products are affected by the solvent that was used in making the product. For example, while an aqueous infusion will extract no more than 15% of the volatile oil contained in the dried herb, this process will extract almost all of certain flavonol glycosides and mucilaginous principles. Alcoholic extracts, in turn, are associated with a different spectrum of constituents. Thus, the results of several clinical studies in the late 1950s documenting the efficacy of a certain chamomile extract in acute gastritis and parapyloric ulcer disease (surveyed in Schilcher, 1987) cannot be readily applied to other types of preparation.

5.3.2
Licorice Root

Licorice root consists of the dried rhizome and roots of Glycyrrhiza glabra (Fig. 5.6). The genus name is derived from the Greek glykos (sweet) and rhiza (root). The crude drug contains two types of active principles: glycyrrhizin (5–15%) and the flavonoids liquiritin and isoliquiritin. Orally administered glycyrrhizin is believed to relieve gastric inflammation by its inhibition of prostaglandin synthesis and lipoxygenase (Inoue et al., 1986; Tamura et al., 1979). Because of the mineralocorticoid-like action of glycyrrhizin, the average daily dose should not exceed 5–15 g of the dried herb (equivalent to 200–600 mg glycyrrhizin), and the course of treatment should not exceed 4–6 weeks. A higher dosage or longer use could lead to adverse effects consisting of sodium and water retention, blood pressure elevation, potassium loss, and edema. These side effects should be absent or minimal with licorice root extracts that have a low glycyrrhizin content.

Licorice root preparations are contraindicated by cholestatic liver disorders, cirrhosis of the liver, hypertension, hypokalemia, severe renal failure, and pregnancy.

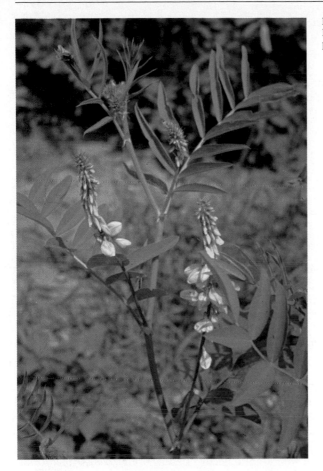

Fig. 5.6.
Flowering tops of the licorice
plant *(Glycyrrihiza glabra).*

Given the risks and the other pharmacologic options currently available for the treatment of peptic ulcers (anticholinergics, H_2-antagonists antibiotics), licorice root preparations have become largely obsolete for this type of indication.

5.3.3
Drug Products

Chamomile
A comprehensive review of the most important chamomile preparations is given in Chap. 8. Two types of preparation are adequate for medicinal purposes in the treatment of gastritis and ulcer disease:

- Chamomile flowers, provided they conform to the pharmacopeia standard. To make an infusion: Cover 1 teaspoon with hot water (about 150 mL) and steep for 5–10 min. Dosage: 1 fresh cup 3 or 4 times daily; drink slowly.

- Liquid extracts and comparable commercial products. For internal use: 30 drops in 1 cup of warm water.

Licorice Root

The *Rote Liste 1995* contains two pharmaceutical products that deliver single doses of 280–350 mg and 300 mg of licorice root extract.

References

Inoue H, Saito K, Koshihara Y, Murota S (1986) Inhibitory effect of glycyrrhetinic acid derivatives of lipoxygenase and prostaglandin synthetase. Chem Pharm Bull 34: 897.
Isaac D (1980) Die Kamillentherapie – Erfolg und Bestätigung. Dtsch Apoth Ztg 120: 567–570.
Jenss H (1985) Zur Problematik funktioneller Magen-Darm-Krankheiten am Beispiel des Colon irritabile. In: Oepen I (ed) An den Grenzen der Schulmedizin, eine Analyse umstrittener Methoden. Deutscher Ärzte-Verlag Cologne, pp 197–212.
Schilcher H (1987) Die Kamille. Handbuch für Ärzte, Apotheker und andere Naturwissenschaftler. Wissenschaftliche Verlagsgesellschaft, Stuttgart.
Tamura Y, Nishikawa T, Yamada K, Yamamoto M, Kumagai A (1979) Effects of glycyrrhetinic acid and its derivatives on Δ-5 α- and 5 β-reductase in rat liver. Arzneimittel Forsch/Drug Res 29: 647.
Weizel A (1980) Colon irritabile. Therapiewoche 30: 3898–3900.

5.4
Irritable Bowel Syndrome

5.4.1
Symptoms and Approaches to Treatment

Approximately 20% of all gastrointestinal disorders seen in the physician's office are functional complaints that are largely synonymous with irritable colon or spastic colon. The syndrome is characterized by varying and ambiguous complaints involving the mid- and lower abdomen with scant objective findings (e.g., a distended colon segment palpable as a tender, cylindrical mass). The cardinal symptoms, besides chronic recurring abdominal cramping, are a change in bowel habits (constipation and/or diarrhea), anorexia, nausea, bloating, and flatulence. The severity of complaints is influenced by individual factors and particularly by emotions (Weizel, 1980; Jenss, 1985). A diagnosis of irritable bowel syndrome should be made only after organic colon disease (carcinoma!) has been definitely excluded. X-ray findings are nonspecific and consist of narrowed segments of the sigmoid and descending colon that may alternate with areas of dilatation.

Because the complaints are chronic in nature and available therapeutic options are often less than successful, patients with irritable bowel are prone to trials with self-medication, particularly the long-term use of stimulant laxatives. In this situation the physician may have the unenviable task of weaning the patient away from laxative abuse. Bulk-forming agents (Sect. 5.6.2) are essential for establishing regular bowel habits in these patients. An important factor in selecting a preparation is its potential to cause bloating, since laxative withdrawal is often made difficult by the fullness and bloating that occur during the initial weeks after introducing a bulk additive. Bloating potential appears to be related to the pentosan content of the bulk material. Rösch and Hotz (1987) prefer mucilages, which cause less bloating than pentosan-rich bran, for example, and whose water-binding capacity makes them useful for the symptomatic treatment of episodes of diarrhea.

Anticholinergics can normalize the postprandial increase in colonic motility, but they do not improve the patient's subjective symptoms (Bär, 1987). They can be particularly useful in the spastic form of irritable colon, but none of the synthetic anticholinergics is considered superior to atropine (Ivey, 1975). A 1975 review of publications dealing with more than 18 commonly used anticholinergics gave a basically negative appraisal (Schmidt, 1983), and drugs like hyoscine butylbromide, methixene, oxyphenonium bromide, and propantheline bromide are considered to have unacceptably high rates of adverse side effects (Bär, 1987; Rösch, 1986).

Some products that claim to be beneficial for irritable colon contain digestive enzymes. But because there is no deficiency of digestive enzymes in irritable bowel syndrome, there is no rationale for the therapeutic use of these products (Bär, 1987). On the other hand, a strong rationale exists for the use of muscle relaxants of the mebeverine type that act principally on the colonic smooth muscle (Kraft et al., 1960). Peppermint oil has a comparable mechanism of action. Useful adjuncts include herbal carminatives and physical measures such as warm, moist compresses, which can act through viscerocutaneous reflexes to ease spasms of the intestinal smooth muscle.

5.4.2
Peppermint

Medicinal peppermint (*Mentha piperita;* family Lamiaceae) is a hybrid that was first cultivated in late seventeenth-century England; it does not grow in the wild. Cultivation has yielded a number of varieties distinguished by their habit, growth vigor, resistance, and content of volatile oil. Still the most important variety is Mitcham mint, first grown in England more than 200 years ago.

Peppermint is a perennial plant that grows to about 30–80 cm and sends off numerous underground and surface runners. Related plants that grow in the wild (e.g., water mint, curly-laeved mint) are much inferior to peppermint in their fragrance, taste, and volatile oil content.

5.4.2.1
Crude Drug and Constituents
All the aerial parts of peppermint are machine-harvested shortly before the plant blooms (Fig. 5.7) and are dried at a low temperature. The crude drug should contain at least 1.2 % volatile oil. It also contains 6–12 % tannins along with flavonoids, triterpenes, and bitter principles (Wichtl, 1989). Dried peppermint leaves are used in making teas.

5.4.2.2
Peppermint Oil
Peppermint oil, obtained by steam distillation of the dried herb, is a colorless to pale green liquid with a pungent odor of peppermint. It has an initially burning taste and cool aftertaste, especially when air is drawn in through the mouth. To date, 85

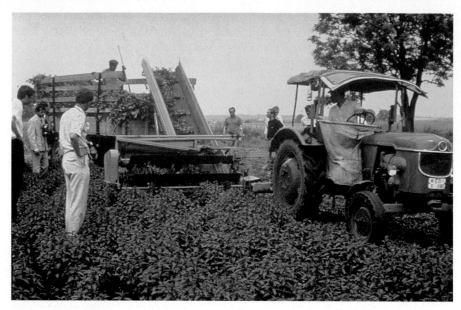

Fig. 5.7. Harvesting peppermint.

chemical compounds have been isolated from peppermint oil. The main constituent (about 50–60 %) is menthol, which partially crystallizes at low temperatures. Peppermint oil also contains menthone (5–30 %), a number of esters (about 5–10 %), and small amounts of cineole and other terpenes.

5.4.2.3
Pharmacokinetics

Human studies have been conducted on the key constituent, menthol (Sommerville et al., 1984; White et al., 1987). Absorbed menthol is excreted by the renal and biliary routes in the form of its glucuronide. Within 24 h, 35–50 % of the orally ingested menthol dose is excreted in the urine. Absorption and elimination depend on the formulation. Oil that is not adsorbed onto a carrier is mostly released in the upper gastrointestinal tract. Menthol excretion is maximal 3 h after ingestion and declines sharply thereafter. Menthol administered in oil that has been adsorbed onto a carrier is released over a much longer period of time; menthol excretion continues for 3–9 h, suggesting that some amount of unabsorbed menthol enters the colon.

5.4.2.4
Pharmacology

Peppermint oil has an antispasmodic action on isolated segments of ileum (rabbits and cats) at dilutions no greater than 1:20,000. This effect, which is reversible, is marked by a decline in the number and amplitude of spontaneous contractions, in some cases to the point of complete paralysis. Peppermint oil antagonizes the spasmogenic action of barium chloride, pilocarpine, and physostigmine (Gunn, 1920).

It relaxes ileal longitudinal muscle, though it is less potent in this action than papaverine (Brandt, 1988). Peppermint oil acts competitively with nifedipine and blocks Ca^{2+}-exciting stimuli. Thus, the antispasmodic action of peppermint oil is based on properties that are characteristic of Ca^{2+} antagonists (Taylor et al., 1983; Hawthorn et al., 1988).

5.4.2.5
Therapeutic Efficacy

An aqueous suspension of peppermint oil injected along the biopsy tract in 20 patients prevented the colonic spasms that otherwise occur in endoscopic examinations (Leicester and Hunt, 1982). Peppermint oil relaxes the esophageal sphincter when administered orally (15 drops of oil suspended in 30 mL of water), eliminating the pressure differential between the stomach and esophagus and allowing reflux to occur (Sigmund and McNally, 1969). Two double-blind studies confirmed the antispasmodic, pain-relieving action of peppermint oil administered in enteric coated capsules (Rees et al., 1979; Dew et al., 1984). In another study, peppermint oil was unable to relieve pain in 41 patients hospitalized with severe irritable bowel syndrome (Nash et al., 1986). Another study found that a 14-day course of peppermint oil taken in soft gelatin capsules with an enteric coating (Mentacur) was effective in a total of 40 patients with irritable bowel syndrome. The objective parameter in this study, intestinal transit time, was prolonged, and there was significant subjective improvement in the rating scores for fullness, bloating, bowel noises, and abdominal pain (Wildgrube, 1988).

The Commission E monograph also ascribes a cholagogic action to peppermint oil. The analgesic effects of peppermint oil applied externally are discussed in Sect. 8.5.

5.4.2.6
Risks and Side Effects

Even the long-term use of peppermint tea is not associated with risks or significant side effects.

Peppermint oil should not be applied to the nasal area of small children as it can provoke glottic spasms and respiratory arrest. The ingestion of excessive amounts of peppermint oil has been associated with interstitial nephritis and acute renal failure. The estimated lethal dose of menthol for humans is approximately 2–9 g. No mutagenic or carcinogenic effects of peppermint oil have been reported.

An overview of the risks and side effects of peppermint leaves and oil can be found in Bowen and Cubbin (1993).

5.4.2.7
Indications, Dosages, and Contraindications

The two Commission E monographs of 1986 state that peppermint leaves are indicated for "colicky pains in the gastrointestinal region, gallbladder, or biliary tract," and that peppermint oil can be taken internally for "colicky pains in the upper gastrointestinal tract and biliary tract, irritable colon, and catarrhal diseases of the upper respiratory tract." An average daily dose of 3–6 g is recommended for peppermint leaves taken in tea form. An average dose of 6–12 drops daily is recommended for peppermint oil. An average single dose of 0.2 mL, or average daily dose of 0.6 mL, is recommended for the treatment of irritable colon. Patients with this condition should take enteric-coated tablets before meals to ensure that the tablet will not dissolve inside the stomach with the chyme. The Commission states no contraindications to the herb. The oil is contraindicated by biliary tract obstruction, cholecystitis, and severe liver damage, and it should not be applied to the facial region of small children.

References

Bär U (1987) Medikamentöse Therapie des Colon irritabile. In: Holz I, Rösch W (eds) Funktionelle Störungen des Verdauungstrakts. Springer Verlag, Berlin Heidelberg New Work, pp 196–202.

Bowen IH, Cubbin IJ (1993) Mentha piperita and Menta spicata. In: De Smet PAGM, Keller K, Hänsel R, Chandler RF (eds) Adverse Effects of Herbal Drugs 1. Springer Verlag, Berlin Heidelberg New Work, pp 171–178.

Brandt W (1988) Spasmolytische Wirkung ätherischer Öle. In: Phytotherapie, Hippokrates Stuttgart, pp 77–89.

Dew MJ, Evans BK, Rhodes J (1984) Peppermint oil for the irritable bowel syndrome: a multicentre trial. Br J Clin Pract 38: 394–395.

Gunn JWC (1920) The carminative action of volatile oils. J Pharmacol Exp Ther 16: 93–143.

Hawthorn M, Ferrante J, Luchowski E, Rutledge, A, Wei XY, Triggle DJ (1988) The actions of peppermint oil and menthol on calcium channel dependent processes in intestinal, neuronal and cardiac preparations. Aliment Pharmcol Therap 2: 101–118.

Ivey K-J (1975) Are anticholinergics of use in the irritable colon syndrome? Gastroenterol 68: 1300–1307.

Jenss H (1985) Zur Problematik funktioneller Magen-Darm-Krankheiten am Beispiel des Colon irritabile. In: Oepen I (ed) An den Grenzen der Schulmedizin, eine Analyse umstrittener Methoden. Deutscher Ärzteverlag, Cologne, pp 197–212.

Kralt T, Moed HD, Classen V, Hendrickesen TWJ, Lindner A, Selzer H, Brucke F, Hertting G, Gogolak G (1960) Reserpine analogues. Nature (Lond) 183: 1108.

Leicester RJ, Hunt RH (1982) Peppermint oil to reduce colonic spasm during endoscopy. Lancet: 989.

Nash P, Gould SR, Barnardo DE (1986) Peppermint oil does not relieve the pain of irritable bowel syndrome. Br J Clin Pract 40: 292–293.

Rees WDW, Evans BK, Rhodes J (1979) Treating irritable bowel syndrome with peppermint oil. Brit Med J II: 835–838.

Rösch W, Hotz J (1987) Therapie: Zusammenfassung und praktische Konsequenzen. In: Hotz J, Rösch W (eds) Funktionelle Störungen des Verdauungstrakts. Springer, Berlin Heidelberg New York, pp 222–223.

Rösch W (1986) Reizmagen – Reizdarm. Plädoyer für eine differenzierte Therapie. Med Klin 81: 316–319.

Schmidt J (1983) Behandlung des Colon irritabile. Pharmakritik 5: 89–92.

Sigmund CJ, McNally EF (1969) The action of a carminative on the lower esophageal sphincter. Gastroenterol 56: 13–18.

Sommerville KW, Richmond CR, Bell GD (1984) Delayed release peppermint oil capsules (Colpermin) for the spastic colon syndrome: a pharmacokinetic study. Br J Clin Pharmac 18: 638–640.

Taylor BA, Luscombe DK, Duthie HL (1983) Inhibitory effect of peppermint on gastrointestinal smooth muscle. Gut 24: A 992 (abstract).

Weizel A (1980) Colon irritabile. Therapiewoche 30: 3898–3900.

White DA, Thompson SP, Wilson CG, Bel JD (1987) A pharmacokinetic comparison of two delayed-release peppermint oil preparations, Colpermin and Mintec, for treatment of the irritable bowel syndrome. Int J Pharmaceutics 40: 151–155.

Wichtl M (ed) (1989) Teedrogen. Wissenschaftliche Verlagsgesellschaft mbH Stuttgart, pp 372–374.

Wildgrube HJ (1988) Untersuchung zur Wirksamkeit von Pfefferminzöl auf Beschwerdebild und funktionelle Parameter bei Patienten mit Reizdarmsyndrom (Studie). NaturHeilpraxis 41: 2–5.

5.5
Acute Diarrhea

Diarrhea refers to the frequent (more than three times daily) passage of a liquid or semiliquid stool. Acute diarrhea has an abrupt onset, usually lasts only 3–4 days, often has an infectious cause, and tends to be self-limiting. Chronic diarrhea persists longer than 4 weeks and may be symptomatic of a chronic underlying illness such as ulcerative colitis, Crohn's disease, or hyperthyroidism. Causal treatment of the underlying disease is essential in all chronic forms of diarrhea. Brief episodes of acute diarrhea in particular warrant the use of symptomatic measures that may be both dietary and pharmacologic. Phytomedicines have a significant role, both as traditional home remedies and as galenic preparations, in the symptomatic treatment of diarrhea. Three groups of preparations are particularly important: tannin-containing herbs, pectins, and a special strain of live dried yeast.

5.5.1
Tannin-Containing Herbs

Tannins have a protein-precipitating action. When applied to mucous membranes, tannins cause proteins to be deposited on the epithelial surface, the precipitate forming a stable, coherent membrane. Particularly in the intestinal tract, this process could line the bowel lumen with a protective film that would hamper the absorption of toxins, blunt the action of local irritants, and normalize hyperperistalsis (Sollmann, 1948). This classic hypothesis on the mechanism of action of tannins is plausible but still needs to be confirmed by controlled clinical studies.

Table 5.4 reviews the tannin-containing herbs and preparations that are most commonly used in the treatment of acute diarrhea. Most tannins in this series are chemical derivatives of the pentahydroxyflavanol catechin. They are water soluble oligomeric or polymeric products that are resistant to acid hydrolysis. Some herbs contain both catechins and gallotannins. Tannic acid, a mixture of the tannins found

Table 5.4. Tannin-containing herbs and preparations for the treatment of acute diarrhea

Herb or preparation	Active constituents	Average daily dose
Green or black tea	5–20% Tannins 2–5% Caffeine 1% Volatile oil	3–10 g of crude drug[1]
Bilberry	5–10% Tannins 1% Fruit acids	20–60 g of berries[2]
Witch hazel leaf and bark	5–15% Tannins	0.1–1 g of crude drug[3]
Tormentil root	15–20% Tannins	2–6 g of crude drug[1]
Oak bark	10–20% Tannins	2–6 g of crude drug[1]
Albumin tannate	ca. 50% Tannins	2–4 g

[1] prepare as infusion (tea);   [2] dried berries; use about 5 times more fresh berries;   [3] for external use only.

in oak bark, is a pure gallotannin. Pure gallotannins are extensively hydrolyzed in the upper small bowel, so they can produce little if any astringent action in the colon. Reportedly, tannins can be bound to albumin (tannalbin) to make them bioavailable in the colon as well.

5.5.1.1
Green and Black Tea

By far the most pleasant way to take tannins is to ingest them in the form of green or black tea. The tea should be steeped for 15–20 min, however, to release as much of the tannins as possible; this will necessarily impart a bitter taste to the beverage.

Black and green tea are both derived from the tea shrub (Camellia sinensis, formerly known also as Thea sinensis), an evergreen woody plant that is native predominantly to southeastern Asia and can grow to 9 m (Fig. 5.8). The cultivated plant is pruned to a bushy shrub to facilitate harvesting. The leaves are harvested and dried to yield the crude drug. The quality and action of a tea depend on the provenance and age of the tea leaves (young shoots > younger leaves > older leaves) and on their initial processing:

- Green tea consists of leaves that are heated immediately after harvesting, mechanically rolled and crushed, and then dried to prevent enzymatic changes. In this way the natural constituents and color of the tea leaf are essentially preserved. As a result, green tea (haysan, gunpowder, imperial, etc.) has a particularly high tannin content and is strongly astringent.

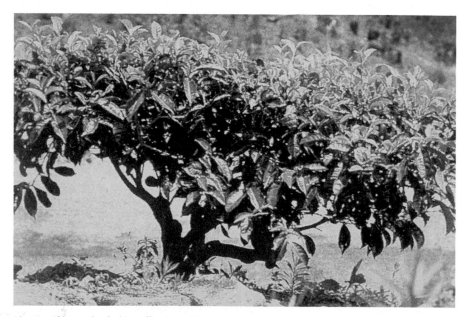

Fig. 5.8. The tea shrub *(Camellia sinensis).*

● Black tea is produced by fermentation. The leaves are wilted before they are rolled and then left in a humid environment for several hours to promote enzymatic changes in the herb, which gradually turns reddish brown. The herb is then dried to yield the black leaf that has a distinctive varietal flavor (e.g., pekoe, souchong, congo).

In 12 healthy test subjects who consumed 2 L of tea daily (containing 8 g of herb), intestinal transit time after 4 days was significantly prolonged relative to a group taking a placebo (Hojgaard, 1981). The excretion of bile acids in the stool was decreased, and increased amounts of oxalic acid were excreted in the urine. In interpreting the results, the authors attributed the constipating action less to the tannin content of the tea than to its theophylline content, reasoning that the increased glomerular filtration led to extracellular dehydration resulting in greater fluid absorption from the bowel. However, the very small amount of theophylline (5–10 mg/L) casts doubt on this interpretation, and it appears more likely that tannins are the key active principle (Table 5.5.1).

When proper attention is given to the caffeine content of tea (Sect. 2.2.1.1), the usage risks are minimal. The tannins could become hepatotoxic if tea were consumed to excess by an individual with preexisting liver damage. For example, one woman who consumed an amount of tea equivalent to 65 g of tea leaves daily for 5 years developed liver dysfunction. But splenomegaly and ascites resolved after the tea was withdrawn (Martindale, 1989).

Ludewig (1995) and Scholz and Bertram (1995) have published up-to-date reviews of the actions and side effects of black and green tea for culinary and medicinal use.

5.5.1.2
Other Tannin-Containing Herbs

Bilberries (European blueberries) are the dried ripe fruit of *Vaccinium myrtillus,* a dwarf shrub of the Ericaceae family. Dried bilberries contain 5–10 % catechins, about 30 % invertose, and small amounts of flavonone glycosides and anthocyanosides, particularly glycosides of malvidin, cyanidin, and delphinidin.

Bilberries are used either by soaking 20–60 g of dried berries (daily dose) in water or red wine, then chewing well and swallowing, or by consuming fresh or freshly preserved berries in an amount 5–10 times the quantity of the dried herb. Bilberries are a home remedy for the treatment of acute, nonspecific diarrhea and are particularly recommended in school-age children.

Tormentil rhizome, known also as *cinquefoil* or *potentilla,* is the dried rhizome of *Potentilla erecta,* an herbaceous plant of the Rosaceae family that is widely distributed in Europe and North America. Tormentil is odorless and has a strongly astringent taste. The herb contains catechins (15–20 %) and tannins (1–2 %), including agrimoniin as the main component (Lund and Rimpler, 1985). It is used chiefly as a tea (2–3 g herb in 1 cup water ≈150 mL). The recommended dose for acute nonspecific diarrhea is 1 cup 2–3 times daily between meals. Nausea or vomiting may occur in sensitive individuals.

Oak bark consists of the dried bark of young twigs of *Quercus robur* harvested in the spring. It contains 10–20 % tannins, including a high content of gallotannins. The

Commission E monograph states that oak bark is used externally for inflammatory skin diseases and internally for nonspecific acute diarrhea; it is also applied locally for mild inflammatory conditions involving the mouth, throat, genitalia, or anal region. Patients with diarrhea should take oak bark for no longer than 3–4 days. Oak bark is reported to have antiviral activity in addition to its astringent properties.

5.5.1.3
Tannic Acid and Albumin Tannate

Tannic acid, obtained from nutgalls, is a heterogeneous mixture of various esters of gallic acid with glucose. The brownish yellow powder, which has a faint but characteristic odor and a puckery taste, disperses readily in water to form a colloid. Tannic acid has an astringent action when applied locally in concentrations of 1:20000 to 1:50,000. Higher concentrations can be cytotoxic, and oral administration may irritate the gastric mucosa and cause vomiting.

Gallotannins are hydrolyzed in the small intestine, forming free gallic acid that does not have an astringent action. Therefore, they are administered therapeutically in the form of albumin tannate, a protein-tannic acid compound with a tannin content of about 50%. Heating the reaction product to 110–120 °C makes it resistant to gastric juices and delays tannin release until the product reaches the alkaline medium of the intestine; there the tannin is released gradually, producing an astringent action in the small intestine and colon. Whereas orally administered tannin does not enter the stool, free tannin is detected in the stool following the administration of albumin tannate. The average single dose is 0.5–1 g; the daily dose for adults is 2–4 g.

5.5.2
Pectins

Pectins are biopolymers with molecular weights of 60000 to 90,000. Their basic structural framework is formed by galacturonic acid molecules. Numerous acid groups give pectins their ability to hold water and form gels. These gels are not attacked by digestive enzymes and pass unchanged into the colon, where they are broken down by colonic bacteria. In the small intestine, pectin gels can form a protective film on the mucosa. But bacterial degradation precludes this type of action in the colon, so a different antidiarrhetic mechanism is required. One hypothesis is that the short-chain fatty acids released from the microbial breakdown of pectins in the colon have an inhibitory action on colonic motility (Yajima, 1985).

Pectins consistently accompany cellulose, so they contribute much to the structural integrity of the cell and of the plant in general. Pectins are present to some degree in all plant products but are particularly abundant in fleshy fruits and storage roots. Rich commercial sources are sugar beet fragments, apple residue, orange and lemon waste products, and carrots. The following "home remedies" and dietary constituents have proven useful in the treatment of diarrhea:

- 1–1.5 kg of raw greated apples, eaten throughout the day;
- bananas, cut into small pieces and eaten as often as desired (particularly recommended for children);

• carrot preparations are suitable for infants and small children, e.g.: boil 500 g of peeled carrots in 1 L of water for 1–2 h, pour through a strainer, and puree in a blender. Add water to make 1 L, and add 3 g of table salt (Schulte and Spranger, 1988).

5.5.3
Live Dried Yeast

While traveling through Indochina in 1923, the French mycologist Henri Boulard noticed that the native population used the skins of tropical fruits as a remedy for diarrhea. Boulard found that a yeast isolated from the surface of these fruits had antidiarrheal properties. The Centraalbureau voor Schimmelcultures in the Netherlands classifies this tropical wild yeast as *Saccharomyces cerevisiae* Hansen CBS 5926, but it is known internationally as *S. boulardii.*

Yeasts occur ubiquitously in nature wherever there are fermentable juices with a high sugar content. The best known variety is brewer's yeast (Saccharomyces cerevisiae). Unlike bacteria, yeasts have a true cell nucleus and are classified as fungi. This makes *S. boulardii* a member of the plant kingdom, so its medicinal use is a form of phytotherapy.

For commercial production the yeast strain is grown in large fluid cultures and freeze-dried; the lyophilization preserves the viability of the cells. The optimum development temperature is 30–40 °C, corresponding to the normal temperature range in the bowel. Lactose is added to the lyophilisate for technical reasons (to allow the precise filling of capsules). Microbiologic and microscopic quality control measures are conducted to check the purity of the cultures and the viability of the cells.

5.5.3.1
Pharmacology and Toxicology

The antidiarrheal action of *S. boulardii* is based on its antagonistic effects on pathogenic microorganisms and its stimulatory effect on the enteric immune system. Ist therapeutic efficacy depends on the viability of the yeast cells (Massot et al., 1982), which must be sustained as the cells pass through the intestinal tract. On entering the colon, however, the cells undergo a bacterial breakdown that leaves only 0.05% of the ingested dose of yeast cells to be excreted in the stool. *S. boulardii* is antagonistic to a number of pathogenic microorganisms, which are damaged or destroyed by the presence of the cells (Böckeler and Thomas, 1989). One study showed that mannose structures on the surface of the yeast cells enable them to bind and entrap fimbriated pathogenic E. coli (Gedek, 1989). *S. boulardii* can also reduce the activity of bacterial toxins (Czerucka et al., 1994). Other experimental studies showed that the yeast has a stimulatory effect on the natural immune system of the bowel (Jahn and Zeitz, 1991).

According to the Commission E monograph of 1994, no toxic reactions were observed in mice and rats given a single oral dose of 3 g/kg. Similarly, doses of approximately 330 mg/kg given to dogs for 6 weeks and doses of 100 g/kg given to rats and rabbits for 6 months caused no adverse changes. The Ames test showed no evidence of mutagenicity.

5.5.3.2
Therapeutic Efficacy

Five double-blind studies were performed between 1983 and 1993 to test the therapeutic efficacy of Perenterol 5, a standardized preparation of *S. boulardii*, in various forms of acute diarrhea.

Tempé et al. (1983) tested the efficacy of *S. boulardii* in preventing nutritionally related diarrhea in 40 patients fed by gavage. When the yeast preparation was added prophylactically to the nutrient solutions, the incidence of diarrhea averaged 8.7% compared with 16.9% in patients given a placebo. The difference between the two treatment groups was statistically significant.

Kollaritsch et al. (1988) tested the efficacy of *S. boulardii* in preventing travel-related diarrhea. In a group of 1231 travelers, 406 were given a placebo, 426 received the yeast preparation in a dose of 250 mg/day, and 399 received a dose of 500 mg/day. The treatment was started 5 days before the subjects began their travels and was continued throughout their stay in tropical or subtropical regions. The incidence of diarrhea was 42.6% in the placebo group, 33.6% in the low-dose treatment group, and 31.8% in the higher-dose treatment group. The reduction in both treatment groups was statistically significant relative to the placebo.

Surawicz et al. (1989) tested the efficacy of *S. boulardii* in preventing antibiotic-associated diarrhea. The 180 patients in the study were divided into two groups, one receiving a placebo and the other receiving 500 mg/day of the yeast preparation during at least a 3-day course of antibiotic therapy. The incidence of diarrhea was 22% in the placebo-treated group versus only 9.5% in the yeast-treated group. Again, the difference between the groups was statistically significant ($p < 0.04$).

Höchter et al. (1990) performed a study in 92 ambulatory patients with acute diarrhea. One group was given a daily dose of 300–600 mg of *S. boulardii,* the other a placebo. The patients treated with S. boulardii showed a significantly greater reduction in their stool-frequency and -quality score (the main study criterion) than the placebo group after 4 days' treatment (respective score changes of –17.2 and –13.6; $p < 0.04$).

Plein and Hotz (1993) conducted a pilot study in 20 patients with Crohn's disease. First, all the patients were given 750 mg of *S. boulardii* daily for 14 days. The average frequency of bowel movements declined during this period from 5 to 4.4 per day. At 14 days, half the patients continued to receive S. boulardii while the other half were switched to a placebo. The frequency of bowel movements continued to decline in the yeast-treated group (to 3.3/day) but returned to the initial value (5/day) in the control group.

5.5.3.3
Indications, Dosages, Risks, and Contraindications

The Commission E monograph of 1994 states that the dried yeast *Saccharomyces boulardii* is used for the symptomatic treatment of acute diarrhea and the prevention and symptomatic treatment of diarrhea associated with travel or feeding by gavage. The monograph also notes its adjunctive use in the treatment of chronic forms of acne.

The recommended dose is 250–500 mg/day, with a daily dose of 500 mg recommended for diarrhea related to feeding by gavage. For the prevention of travel-related diarrhea, treatment should be initiated 5 days before the start of the trip. In cases of acute diarrhea, treatment should be continued for several days after symptoms have abated.

There have been reports of bloating and sporadic intolerance reactions in the form of itching, urticaria, and generalized skin eruptions. Yeast sensitivity is a contraindication. A fall in blood pressure may occur as a drug interaction in patients who are also taking a monoamine oxidase inhibitor.

5.5.4
Other Herbal Antidiarrheals

Opium, the air-dried milky sap obtained from the unripe capsules of the opium poppy *(Papaver somniferum),* has a powerful constipating effect. Opium contains 20–25% alkaloids, including 7–20% morphine, which is chiefly responsible for this action. Opium does not actually immobilize the bowel; it intensifies its contractions (segmental constrictions), producing a state of spastic constipation (Ewe, 1983). Opium and its derivative morphine are not herbal medications in the true sense (see Sect. 1.2) and are outside the scope of this volume.

Calumbo root is obtained from *Wateorhiza palmata,* a woody vine (liana) native to tropical eastern Africa. Pieces of the bulbous, fleshy roots are dug up, washed, sliced, and dried, yielding a crude drug that contains 1–2% berberine-type alkaloids along with bitter principles. As for therapeutic applications, it is interesting to note older pharmacologic results indicating that the herb is similar to morphine in its ability to increase resting tonus. Because the side effects of calumbo root are comparable to those of morphine, the herb is no longer important as an antidiarrheal.

Uzara root is another obtained from *Xysmalobium undulatum,* another herb of African origin that is used by natives as an antidiarrheal. Until a few years ago, preparations made from the uzara root were still marketed in Germany, but the *Rote Liste 1995* no longer contains any of these products. Nor are there any rigorous studies to support the healing claims that have been made for uzara root preparations.

Carob bean or St. John's bread is obtained from the evergreen tree *Ceratonia siliqua,* native to the Mediterranean region. A meal made from carob seeds makes a safe, natural antidiarrheal that is particularly useful in infants, toddlers, and children. A special extraction process is used to produce this meal from portions of the carob seed. Carob seed meal consists of galactomannoglycans (about 88%) and other polysaccharides (5%) in addition to proteins and minerals. Its molecular weight is 310000 daltons, signifying a high degree of polymerization (d. p. ≈ 19000). A branched linear heteropolysaccharide, it has a high water-holding capacity even in low concentrations (50 to 100 times its dry weight). Besides its use as an antidiarrheal, carob seed meal is also used as a component of low-calorie diets.

5.5.5
Suggested Formulations

Antidiarrheal tea

Rx   Black tea leaves   40.0
     Balm leaves   20.0
     Fennelseed, crushed   20.0
     Centaury   20.0
     Mix to make tea
     Directions: Prepare 2 teaspoons in 1 cup as an infusion; steep 10–20 min.

References

Böckeler W, Thomas G (1989) In-vitro-Studien zur destabilisierenden Wirkung lyophilisierter Saccharomyces cereviseae Hansen CBS 5926-Zellen auf Enterobakterien. Läßt sich diese Eigenschaft biochemisch erklären? In: Müller J, Ottenhann R, Seifert J (eds) Ökosystem Darm. Springer Verlag, pp 142–253.

Czerucka D, Roux I, Rampal P (1994) Saccharomyces boulardii inhibits secretagogue-mediated adenosine 3',5'-cyclic monophosphate induction in intestinal cells. Gastroenterology 106: 65–72.

Ewe K (1983) Obstipation – Pathophysiologie, Klinik, Therapie. Int Welt 6: 286–292.

Gedek B, Hagenhoff G (1989) Orale Verabreichung von lebensfähigen Zellen des Hefestammes Saccharomyces cerevisiae Hansen CBS 5926 und deren Schicksal während der Magen-Darm-Passage. Therapiewoche 38 (special issue): 33–40.

Höchter W, Chase D, Hagenhoff G (1990) Saccharomyces boulardii bei akuter Erwachsenendiarrhoe. Münch Med Wschr 132: 188–192.

Hojgaard I, Arffmann S, Jorgenson M, Krag E (1981) Tea consumption: a cause of constipation. Br Med J 282: 864.

Jahn HU, Zeitz M (1991) Immunmodulatorische Wirkung von Saccharomyces boulardii beim Menschen. In: Seifert J, Ottenhann R, Zeitz M, Bockenmühl J (eds). Ökosystem Darm III. Springer-Verlag, pp 159–164.

Kollaritsch HH, Tobüren D, Scheiner O, Wiedermann G (1988) Prophylaxe der Reisediarrhoe. Münch Med Wschr 130: 671–673.

Ludewig R (1995) Schwarzer und Grüner Tee als Genuß- und Heilmittel. Dtsch Apoth Z 135: 2203–2218.

Lund K, Rimpler H (1985) Tormentillwurzel. Dtsch Apoth Z 125: 105–107.

Reynolds JEF (ed) (1989) Martindale. The Extra Pharmacopoeia. 29th Ed. The Pharmaceutical Press, London, p 1535.

Massot J, Desconclois M, Astoin J (1982) Protection par Saccharomyces boulardii de la diarrhée à Escherichia coli du souriceau. Ann Pharm Fr 40: 445–449.

Plein K, Hotz J (1993) Therapeutic effect of Saccharomyces boulardii on mild residual symptoms in a stable phase of Crohn's disease with special reference to chronic diarrhea – a pilot study. Z. Gastroenterol 31: 129–134.

Scholz E, Bertram B (1995) Camellia sinensis (L.) O.Kuntze – Der Teestrauch. Z Phytother 17: 235–250.

Schulte FJ, Spranger J (1988) Lehrbuch der Kinderheilkunde. Fischer, Stuttgart, p 320.

Sollmann T (1948) A Manual of Pharmacology. 7th Ed. Saunders Company, Philadelphia London, p 110.

Surawicz C, Elmer GW, Speelman P, McFarland LV, Chinn J, van Belle G (1989) Die Prophylaxe Antibiotika-assoziierter Diarrhöen mit Saccharomyces boulardii. Eine prospektive Studie. Gastroenterol 96: 981–988.

Tempé JD, Steidel AL, Blehaut H, Hasselmann M, Lutun P, Maurier F (1983) Prévention par Saccharomyces boulardii des diarrhées de l'alimentation entérale à débit continu. La Semaine des Hôpitaux de Paris 59: 1409–1412.

Yajima T (1985) Contractile effect of short-chain fatty acids on the isolated colon of the rat. J Physiol 368: 667–678.

5.6
Constipation

5.6.1
Symptoms, Causes, General Measures

Constipation is characterized by findings and complaints that are based largely on the frequency and difficulty of bowel movements. Constipation is considered to be present when the frequency of bowel movements is less than once in 2–3 days. But constipation assumes pathologic significance by its subjective features, i.e., straining heavily at stool, painful defecation, and a feeling of incomplete evacuation (Table 5.5). Constipation is often accompanied by other types of discomfort such as abdominal cramping, a feeling of fullness, or autonomic dysfunction. Constipation alternating with bouts of diarrhea is a feature of irritable colon (Sect. 5.4).

Constipation of acute onset may have a trivial cause such as a change in diet, travel, or a febrile illness with confinement to bed. Numerous drugs, including antacids and anticholinergics, can also lead to constipation. A new irregularity in bowel habits with no obvious cause should always be investigated due to the risk of malignant disease. But in the great majority of cases, the cause of chronic constipation is functional in nature. The following factors are important in the pathogenesis of constipation:

- a faulty lifestyle (lack of exercise) and poor eating habits (low-fiber diet, hasty or irregular meals);
- psychological factors such as ignoring the urge to defecate due to emotional stress or an exaggerated personal cleanliness;
- fear of disease or self-poisoning leading to pseudoconstipation (Ewe, 1983).

Thus, the treatment of chronic constipation should always start with dietary counseling and, where appropriate, psychotherapeutic counseling. Dietary counseling should include specific recommendations for increasing the intake of dietary fiber, increasing fluid intake (4–6 glasses of water during the morning hours), and the consumption of laxative fruits and vegetables such as prunes, dates, figs, and rhubarb. Physical measures should include an exercise program to strengthen the abdominal muscles, perhaps abdominal-wall massage, and a general recommendation for more exercise. Phytotherapy starts with a recommendation and prescription for bulk-forming agents. Stimulant laxatives, especially anthranoid-containing herbs, are agents of second choice.

Table 5.5. Syndrome of constipation (Ewe, 1988)

Findings and complaints	Explanations
Infrequent passage of stool	Less than three bowel movements a week
Difficult passage of stool	Straining at stool
Passing stools of hard consistency	Small, hard stools
Passing scant stool	Small stool volume (< 50 g)
Subjective sensations	Sense of delayed, difficult, and incomplete evacuation

5.6.2
Bulk-Forming Agents

These products (Table 5.6), consisting of bulking and swelling agents, are gentle, low-risk laxatives that simulate the physiologic effects of a high-fiber diet. Their water-binding capacity also makes them useful for the symptomatic treatment of diarrhea in some patients. Bulk-forming agents are also widely recognized for their value in the long-term management of irritable colon and chronic diverticulitis.

5.6.2.1
Mechanism of Action

The term bulking agent is used synonymously in this chapter with bulk materials and dietary fiber. Bulking agents are normally ingested as components of food. They are composed of indigestible carbohydrates, which may undergo complete (pectins) or partial breakdown (bran) by colonic bacteria. These substances stimulate bowel activity through their bulk-producing action and hasten the transit of fecal material through the intestinal tract. All bulking agents can swell to a degree through the uptake of water, and the distinction from swelling agents is purely quantitative. Swelling agents in the strict sense are more distinguished by their capacity to form mucilages or gels. They are virtually synonymous with the thickening agents used in food processing and with the mucilaginous agents used in pharmacy and medicine (Hutz and Rösch, 1988). Mucilaginous swelling agents usually are not contained in foods but are taken in medicinal form (e. g., psyllium husks) or in the form of a crude herbal product (e. g., karaya gum). Like bulking agents, they are composed of indigestible carbohydrates, but they differ from bulking agents in that they undergo little or no degradation by intestinal flora.

To understand the mechanism of action of bulk-forming agents, it is helpful to know the relationships between stool weight, intestinal transit time, and the quantitative composition of the feces. Intestinal transit time is the period that elapses between the ingestion of food and the excretion of its indigestible components as feces. Transit time is greatly influenced by the content of indigestible food constituents.

Table 5.6.
Herbs used as bulk laxatives for the treatment of constipation

Herbs	Daily dose[1]	Remarks
Linseed	30–50 g	Take in the form of crushed whole seeds.
Wheat bran	20–40 g	Not for use in small children or patients with glutin-induced enteropathy.
Psyllium	5–10 g	Husks have 3 times the fiber content of the seeds (reduce daily dose to 3 g).
Agar	5–10 g	Bulk laxative stimulates peristalsis by increasing the stool volume.

[1] Should be taken with liquid volume equal to about 10 times the dose volume.

Bulk materials have little effect on transit time through the small intestine, but they do affect colonic transit. The heavier the stool weight, the shorter the transit time. Besides their absolute quantity, the composition of indigestible materials is also important. Surprisingly, the increase in fecal bulk caused by water absorption appears to be less crucial to the action of bulk-forming agents than their content of pentosans. For example, 20 g of wheat bran increases stool weight by 127 %, whereas 5 g of guar, despite its high water-binding capacity, increases stool weight by only 20 % (Cummings, 1978).

Therefore it appears that the stimulation of bowel motility caused by an increase in fecal bulk is not the only determinant of efficacy. Another key factor is the modification of the intestinal flora. The colon is inhabited by more than 400 bacterial species, whose precise makeup is determined by the nature of the available substrate. Bacteria constitute more than 50 % of the total dry mass of the feces (Stephen and Cummings, 1980). Bulk materials provide the bacterial flora with a substrate for their proliferation, causing an increase in bacterial mass and stool weight. Because the bacteria are specific to particular substrates, a latent period of 4–6 weeks is needed to establish a more suitable intestinal flora. This concept is supported by studies in healthy subjects in which a 3-week period of increased dietary fiber intake was necessary before significant changes occurred in transit time and stool weight (Cummings et al., 1978).

The celluloses, hemicelluloses, lignins, and pectins contained in bulk-forming agents are resistant to human digestive enzymes so they pass unchanged through the small intestine into the colon. The colonic bacteria can then break down all or part of the bulk materials, mainly releasing short-chain fatty acids (particularly acetic, propionic, and butyric acids) along with methane, carbon dioxide, and molecular hydrogen. It has been suggested that the metabolism of short-chain fatty acids in the colonic mucosa may have a protective role in maintaining normal mucosal function (bibliography in Kasper, 1985). But the main significance of the short-chain fatty acids is their ability to promote the absorption of salts and water (Ruppin et al., 1980) and to provide osmotic stimuli that promote colonic motility (Yajima, 1985) Swelling agents make the stool softer and enable it to pass through the bowel more easily. It has also been postulated that swelling agents stimulate intrinsic intestinal activity by causing distention of the bowel wall.

Gases generated by bacterial breakdown in the lower bowel may cause bloating and flatulence, and constipation may worsen during the first two weeks following initial consumption of bulking agents. Generally these symptoms resolve once a new intestinal flora has been established. It may be useful to start treatment with one-half the normal dosage. A change of product may become necessary in some cases (Fingl, 1980).

It is imperative that bulk-forming agents be taken with sufficient liquid. The amount of liquid depends on the swelling capacity of the agent and generally is 5 to 10 times the dry weight of the agent. Stenotic lesions of the gastrointestinal tract contraindicate the use of bulk-forming agents. Even in the absence of such lesions, treatment with bulking agents may rarely lead to bowel obstruction, underscoring the urgency of an adequate fluid intake. Bulk-forming agents should not be taken at bedtime or while the patient is lying down. They should not be used in conjunction with an antiperistaltic (e.g., loperamide).

5.6.2.2
Linseed

Linseed consists of the dried, ripe seeds of flax (*Linum usitatissimum*, Fig. 5.9), one of the world's oldest cultivated plants. Linseed is grown for its oil-bearing seeds and for its fiber. The seeds of the annual herb are odorless and, when placed in the mouth, slowly acquire a mucilaginous taste. The main constituents are mucilages (7–12 %), fatty oil (about 40 %), protein (about 23 %), as well as crude fiber, minerals, and cyanogenic glycosides (about 1 %).

The key swelling constituents of linseed are the mucilages, which are located in the epidermis of the seed husk. The seed must be ground, or preferably cracked, so that it can absorb fluid and swell. Cracking or crushing allows rapid swelling without releasing large amounts of fatty oil (about 500 kcal in 100 g linseed) for intestinal absorption. The whole seeds have a significantly longer shelf life, for the highly unsaturated fatty acids in linseed meal quickly become rancid when exposed to atmospheric oxygen.

The seeds swell to several times their dry volume. Linseed mucilage retains its colloidal structure even in the acid milieu of the stomach, and its swelling and lubri-

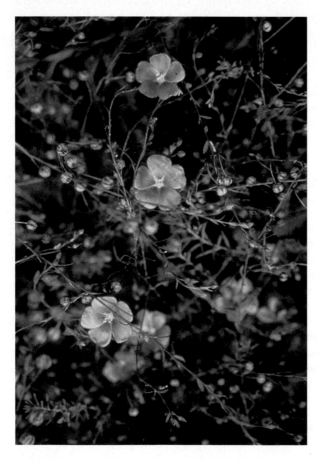

Fig. 5.9.
Flowering tops of linseed
(*Linum usitatissimum*).

cating properties are undiminished by the weakly alkaline medium of the small intestine. The bulk materials are also thought to contribute to the stimulation of peristalsis. Onset of action is preceded by a latent period of several days (Sewing, 1986).

Risk from Hydrogen Cyanide

Due to its content of linamarin, a cyanogenic glycoside, linseed (along with bitter almonds) was long considered a potential source of dietary hydrogen cyanide (HCN) poisoning. One hundred grams of linseed contains approximately 30 mg of HCN (by comparison, 100 g of bitter almonds contains about 250 mg). The lethal dose of HCN for humans is approximately 50–100 mg. But while HCN is absorbed in minutes through the gastric mucosa when administered in, say, cyanogenic salts such as potassium cyanide, only very low blood levels of HCN were found after the ingestion of 100 g linseed. Similarly low levels were detected after the consumption of 10 bitter almonds, but eating 50 bitter almonds produced blood levels that were life-threatening in one test subject (Schulz et al., 1983) (Fig. 5.10).

One reason for the nonlinear absorption and elimination kinetics of HCN in the body lies in the enzyme-dependency of the release of HCN from its glycosidic bond. In the case of linseed, this cleavage is catalyzed by the plant enzyme linamarase; the acidic gastric juice partially inactivates this enzyme, slowing the release of HCN. Once it is absorbed, HCN is subject to transformation by the enzyme rhodanase, which is present in the mitochondria of all somatic cells and rapidly converts small amounts of HCN into the harmless compound thiocyanate. The rhodanase detoxification system has a limited capacity, however. The sudden ingestion of large amounts of HCN can easily overwhelm this system, leading to swift and fatal poisoning (Schulz, 1984).

In a controlled study, 20 healthy subjects ingested 30 or 100 g of cracked linseed acutely followed by 45 g daily over a period of 5 weeks. None of the subjects showed

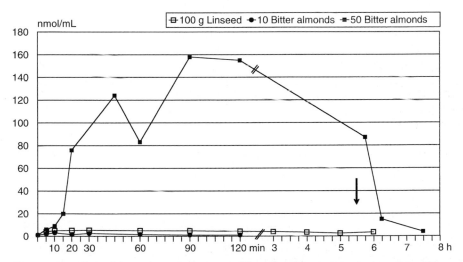

Fig. 5.10. Cyanide level in a volunteer who ingested linseed and bitter almonds. At 5.5 hours (↓), 1 g of sodium thiosulfate was administered by intravenous infusion as an antidote (Schulz et al., 1983).

a significant rise in HCN blood levels. The HCN metabolite thiocyanate did show rising serum levels during the course of the treatment period, accompanied by an average 75% increase in the urinary excretion of thiocyanate, comparable to the elevations typically measured in heavy smokers. This moderate accumulation of thiocyanate did not imply any special risks or contraindications (Schulz et al., 1983).

5.6.2.3
Wheat Bran

Wheat bran is a byproduct formed in the manufacture of wheat flour from the grain of *Triticum aestivum*. It consists mainly of the outer layers of the wheat kernel, including the aleurone layer, i.e., the husk, seed coat, and germ. Because there is no natural demarcation between the starch-containing endosperm and the bran layers, the composition of the bran can vary somewhat, depending on the milling process. A dietary bran for long-term use must meet certain criteria. First, dietary bran must conform to the provisions of food regulations, especially in terms of its pesticide content. It must not be contaminated by actinomyces or other bacteria. Moreover, the size of the bran particles must be defined and standardized, and their water content must be substantially lower than in unprocessed bran. Finally, bran products are deemed acceptable only if the trypsin inhibitors present in unprocessed bran have been inactivated.

The composition of wheat bran is shown in Table 5.7. The protein fraction contains gluten, which is why wheat bran should not be used in patients with gluten-induced enteropathies. The gluten content also contraindicates the use of bran in children younger than 2 years of age. Some bran constituents are digestible, but the calorific value, at 150–175 kcal, is low. The remaining components enter the colon unchanged, where especially the pentosans and other hemicelluloses are broken down by bacteria. The increase in stool bulk is based on three factors: the swelling capacity of the pentosans, the bulk characteristics of indigestible materials (fibers and lignin), and the proliferation of intestinal bacteria. Additionally, short-chain acids are released that cause chemical irritation of the intestinal mucosa.

Bran is also useful for preventing inflammation in patients with diverticulosis. In one study, 70 patients received 12–14 g bran daily as a supplement to their low-fiber diet. Following a latent period of 2–4 weeks, 62 of the patients were free of complaints (Weinreich, 1980). The desired therapeutic effects, especially in terms of shortening intestinal transit time, appear to depend strongly on the particle size of the bran. Coarse particles larger than 1 mm in diameter are the most effective (Smith et al., 1981).

Table 5.7.
Chemical composition of wheat bran (Huth et al., 1980)

Components	%
Water	10
Protein	15
Fat	5
Carbohydrates	55
– Starch	12
– Cellulose	21
– Hemicelluloses	22
Lignin	8
Vitamins and minerals	7

The administration of bran (2×15 g/day) to healthy test subjects for 6 weeks led to significant changes in the relative proportions of bile acids, marked by a decrease in deoxycholic acid and an increase in chenodeoxycholic acid (Kasper, 1980). However, the clinical relevance of this observation is unclear. The use of wheat bran carries a risk of bowel obstruction only if fluid intake is inadequate.

5.6.2.4
Psyllium Seed and Husk

Psyllium seed consits of the ripe seed obtained from several Plantago species. The seeds are elliptical and about 2–3 mm long; they are odorless, bland-tasting, and become mucilaginous when chewed. The mucilaginous husk of the Indian variety separates fairly easily from the rest of the seed, so these husks constitute a separate commercial product (psyllium husk). The important swelling agents (mucilages, hemicelluloses) are located in the epidermis of the husk, making the husks about five times more active than the seeds themselves.

The whole seeds or husks are soaked in water for several hours and are then taken with a copious amount of liquid. The mucilage retains the moisture during gastrointestinal transit, promoting the passage of a soft stool after a transit time of 6–12 h. It has also been suggested that the laxative action involves a purely mechanical irritation of the bowel wall causing a reflex stimulation of peristalsis (USD, 1967).

Rare cases of allergic reactions have been reported. In animal studies, feeding powdered psyllium seeds to rats for 18 weeks and to dogs for 4 weeks led to the deposition of a brownish black pigment in the proximal renal tubules with no associated impairment of renal function. Similar phenomena were not observed following the long-term use of whole psyllium seeds (Leng-Peschlow and Mengs, 1990).

5.6.2.5
Agar and Karaya Gum

Agar (or agar agar) is a dried, hydrophilic, colloidal substance obtained by extracting various species of red algae. The main constituents of the product are two polysaccharides:

- agarose, a long-chain compound in which about 10 % of the chains are esterified with sulfuric acid;
- agaropectin, which differs from agarose in its significantly higher degree of esterification with sulfuric acid. The molecule also contains pyruvic acid in a ketal bond.

Agar is sold commercially in the form of pale yellow strips or pieces or as a yellowish powder. The products are odorless and tasteless. Agar is indigestible and passes through the gastrointestinal tract almost unchanged. It undergoes little if any breakdown by intestinal microorganisms, which may account for its relatively low activity in regulating the bowel. It acts solely by its ability to absorb water and swell within the intestine.

Karaya gum, known also as karaya, sterculia gum, or Indian tragacanth, is a substance that exudes from the incised tree trunks of *Sterculia urens, Cochlospermum gossypium,* and related species of these genera. The crude drug consists of yellow-brown, yellowish, or reddish pieces that have a marked acetic acid smell when pulverized. Karaya gum is also composed of polysaccharides, and its macromolecular structure is similar to that of pectins. The product has a great swelling capacity, and a 10 % solution will expand to form a homogeneous, sticky gelatinous mass.

5.6.3
Osmotic Agents

The prototypes of osmotic laxatives are certain salts that are highly water-soluble but poorly absorbable, such as sodium sulfate and magnesium sulfate. These salts retain water in the bowel purely by their osmotic action, thereby increasing the water content of the stool. If they are administered in hypotonic solution, water is quickly absorbed from the intestines until the administered solution becomes isotonic. If a hypertonic solution is administered, water is drawn from the body and retained in the bowel.

The same mechanism underlies the action of nonabsorbable sugars (mannose) and sugar alcohols (mannitol and sorbitol) of plant origin. With these compounds, however, a second mechanism is operative as well: the unabsorbed sugars enter the colon unchanged, where they are broken down into short-chain fatty acids. This process releases acetic, lactic, and butyric acids that stimulate peristalsis and promote osmotic water retention. The proliferation of normal intestinal flora probably also contributes to bowel regulation by increasing the fecal mass.

The prototype of this laxative group is lactulose, a partially synthetic transformation product of lactose that is not an herbal substance.

Mannitol is of plant origin, however, and occurs widely throughout the plant kingdom. Seaweed contains significant amounts of mannitol (up to 20 %), and manna, the dried sap of the manna ash (Fraxinus ornus), contains up to 13 %. Medicinal mannitol is a partially synthetic agent produced by the hydration of invertose.

Sorbitol is a sugar alcohol that also occurs in the plant kingdom. Relatively high concentrations are present in apples, pears, plums, apricots, cherries, and especially mountain ash berries (Sorbus aucuparia). Again, the commercial product is a partially synthetic agent produced by the reduction of glucose. Sorbitol acts as a mild laxative when taken in an oral dose of 20–30 g.

5.6.4
Anthranoid-Containing Herbs

While bulk-forming agents act mainly through physical effects within the bowel lumen, stimulant laxatives, particularly those containing anthranoids, act directly on the intestinal mucosa. The stimulant laxatives usually induce an unphysiologic bowel movement with loose stools and frequent griping (Gysling, 1976).

Several mechanisms are involved in this effect:

● Reflexes elicited by the stimulation of receptors in the mucosa and submucosa, leading to increased propulsive colonic motility, a shortened transit time, and a net decrease in the absorption of water and electrolytes.

- An increase of cyclic AMP (cAMP) in the enterocytes. As the intracellular calcium concentration changes, chloride enters the intestinal lumen; sodium and water follow for osmotic reasons and to maintain electroneutrality (= secretagogic action).
- Leakage of the junctional complexes (terminal bars) between the endothelial cells of the large intestine. Sodium and water that have already been absorbed can re-enter the lumen through the incompetent junctional complexes.
- Blockage of the sodium pump (sodium-potassium-ATPase) on the bowel epithelium facing away from the lumen. This inhibits the absorption of sodium and water (= antiabsorptive action).

The laxative effect of anthranoid-containing herbs is caused by the presence of chemically defined anthranoid compounds. Accordingly, commercial products are standardized on the basis of their anthranoid content. This group of phytomedicines should not be dosed according to their quantity of dried herb or raw extract, but only by the quantity of the key active constituents, i.e., anthranoids. The corresponding pharmaceutical dose equivalents are given in Table 5.8.

Our knowledge of the pharmacokinetics of anthranoid-containing herbs is fragmentary, sennosides being the only compounds for which studies are available. Anthranoids bound to sugars are pharmacologically inert and enter the colon unchanged. There they are metabolically altered by intestinal bacteria, yielding products that include free anthrones, which are considered the true active principles. Most of the metabolites are excreted in the stool; a quantitatively undetermined fraction is absorbed and appears as glucuronide or sulfate conjugates in the urine, turning the urine a dark yellow or even red if there is a positive alkaline reaction. In nursing mothers, anthranoid metabolites can enter the milk and give it a brownish tinge. There is debate as to whether the active ingredients become sufficiently concentrated in breast milk to cause diarrhea in nursing infants (Curry, 1982).

The principal adverse effect that can occur with occasional use is colicky abdominal pain, or griping. The susceptibility to this complaint varies greatly among different individuals. Anthranoids, particularly aloe, can cause a reflex engorgement of abdominal blood vessels throughout the pelvis, with a substantial augmentation of blood flow to the uterus and its appendages. This can increase the intensity of menstrual bleeding, and in pregnancy it can heighten the risk of fetal loss. Melanosis coli develops in about 5% of long-term anthranoid users over a period of 4–13 months, but this condition has no clinical importance and resolves in 6–12 months after the laxative is discontinued (Weber, 1988).

Table 5.8.
The dosage of an anthranoid-containing herb is based on its total anthranoid content, the daily dose of which should not exceed 20–30 mg of anthranoids.

Herb	Total anthranoids (%)	Daily dose (g)
Rhubarb	2–3	1
Senna leaf	2–3	1
Buckthorn berries	3–4	1
Senna pods	3–6	0.5–1
Fangula bark	6–9	0.5
Cascara	>8	0.5
Aloe	20–40	0.1

True adverse side effects result almost entirely from long-term abuse leading to severe electrolyte and water losses and eventual hyperaldosteronism (Ewe, 1988). The chronic hypokalemia worsens constipation and may cause damage to the renal tubules. These toxic side effects should not occur when anthranoid laxatives are taken intermittently and at low doses. Recent studies cast doubt on the notion that chronic laxative abuse causes irreversible damage to intramural ganglia and nerves of the intrinsic mucosal plexus (Dufour and Gendre, 1988).

Anthranoid preparations are contraindicated in partial or complete bowel obstruction, pregnancy, and lactation. Interactions with cardiac glycosides and other drugs may occur indirectly as a result of electrolyte imbalance (hypokalemia).

Chronic laxative use is undesirable by its very nature, but prolonged laxative use under the supervision and guidance of a physician (e. g., potassium replacement) is justified in severe forms of constipation (Ewe, 1988). The same applies to colonic inertia in the elderly. There is no apparent reason to discount the importance of laxatives more than any other symptom-relieving medication (Müller-Lissner, 1987). Recent epidemiologic studies have allayed fears that the melanosis coli caused by anthranoid laxatives represents a premalignant condition.

5.6.4.1
Rhubarb Root

Rhubarb root consists of the dried underground parts of medicinal rhubarb (*Rheum* spp.) (Fig. 5.11), native to the mountainous regions of western China and cultivated in Europe. The dried herb has a faint aromatic odor and a bitter, slightly astringent taste. Chewing the root produces a gritty sensation between the teeth caused by large calcium oxalate crystals, and it turns the saliva yellow. The crude drug contains about 2.5 % anthranoids (calculated as rhein), consisting mostly of anthraquinone glycosides (60–80 %) with lesser amounts of anthrone glycosides (10–25 %) and free anthraquinones (about 1 %). Rhubarb also contains about 5 % tannins of the gallotannin and catechin type along with flavonoids, pectins, and minerals.

Besides the anthranoids, which have a cathartic action, rhubarb also contains tannins and pectins, which produce an antidiarrheal effect. Both actions are superimposed during use. The overall effect is dose-dependent because emodins and tannins appear to have different dose-response characteristics. Rhubarb taken in smaller doses (0.1–0.3 g) has an astringent action in gastritis and dyspepsia and an antidiarrheal action in mild forms of diarrhea. Higher doses (1.0–4.0 g) produce a mild laxative effect. Since the relative contents of emodins and tannins are variable, the laxative action is somewhat uncertain. The German Pharmacopeia describes a rhubarb root extract that is made with 70 % alcohol. This extract is adjusted with lactose as needed to obtain a 4–6 % anthranoid content. Rhubarb extract is a brown, hygroscopic, powdered material with a distinctive odor and the bitter taste of rhubarb root.

5.6.4.2
Buckthorn Bark

This herb consists of the dried bark from the trunk and branches of the buckthorn (*Rhamnus frangula*). This deciduous shrub or small tree (family Rhamnaceae) is widely distributed in Europe and western Asia. The common German name for

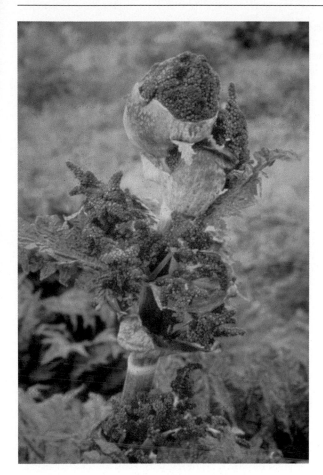

Fig. 5.11.
Flower head of medicinal rhubarb (*Rheum* sp.).

buckthorn, *Faulbaum*, means the "rotten tree," and refers to the offensive odor of the friable wood (frangere = "break").

Buckthorn bark contains 6–9 % anthraquinone glycosides, the most important of which are glucofrangulin A and B. The bark differs from other anthranoid-containing herbs in that its active constituents occur mainly as anthraquinones, which have less powerful antiabsorptive and hydragogic properties. This accounts for the relatively mild action of buckthorn bark.

The cut and dried herb is a frequent ingredient in commercially produced specialty teas. Additionally, powdered extracts are used for instant teas, and solid or powdered extracts are used as ingredients in combination products that are usually sold in capsule or tablet form.

The anthrones in the freshly dried herb are extremely potent, and the bark should be stored for at least 1 year before use or aged artificially by heating it while exposing it to the air. Use of the untreated fresh herb can cause severe vomiting and spasms.

Cascara bark, which is related to alder buckthorn bark, is obtained from *Rhamnus purshianus,* a tree resembling the buckthorn and native to Pacific North America. Cascara bark contains at least 8 % total anthranoids, approximately two-thirds of which are cascarosides. Preparations in the form of extracts and fluidextracts are used as ingredients in pharmaceutical products. Because of its disagreeable odor, the bark is not suitable for use in teas. Cascara bark is widely used in laxative products in the United States.

5.6.4.3
Senna Pods and Leaves

Senna pods and leaves are obtained from two different senna species: *Cassia senna* and *Cassia augustifolia.* The former species is a small shrub of the family Fabaceae that reaches a height of 60 cm. It grows along the Nile in Egypt and Sudan. The seed pods of Cassia senna (Alexandrian senna pods) have a bittersweet, mucilaginous taste. They contain 3.5–5.5 % anthranoids, principally sennosides A and B.

Cassia augustifolia is a shrub growing to 2 m that is native to the region about the Red Sea. Its seed pods (Tinnevelly senna pods) are cultivated in India and Indonesia. The anthranoid spectrum of *C. augustifolia* is mostly identical to that of *C. senna,* but its total anthranoid content, at 2–3 %, is considerably lower, so it must be given in a higher dose. Senna leaves can be harvested from both Cassia species. In fact, some modern taxonomists now place both species in a single taxon *Senna alexandrina.* However, in this volume, the classic nomenclature has been retained. The crude drug consists of the stripped leaflets rather than whole leaves and should contain at least 3 % total anthranoids including the key active constituents, sennosides A and B. Senna leaves are most commonly used in the form of teas, but extracts are frequently used in a wide variety of laxative products.

5.6.4.4
Aloe

Aloe refers to the dried juice or latex obtained from the pericyclic tubules of various *Aloe* species. If should not be confused with aloe gel, a mucilage from the inner parenchymal tissue of the leaf. Various techniques are used in eastern and southern Africa and the Antilles to collect and process the juice. Not an herb in the usual sense, aloe latex is an herbal preparation that is classified pharmaceutically as a juice. Due to the many varieties of aloe, commercial products are designated according to the country of origin. This section deals with cape aloe, the product obtained from *Aloe spicata* that is chiefly used in central Europe.

Cape aloe is obtained by cutting off the leaves and holding the cut surface down to drain the juice from the base of the leaf. The collected juice is thickened by heating over an open fire or by allowing the semisolid latex to harden in a canister. This yields a homogeneous, vitreous mass that is sold commercially under the brand name Lucida. Alternatively, the juice can be slowly evaporated (e. g., by letting it stand in the sun), causing the aloin (a mixture of anthraquinones) to crystallize out. This product has a flat, lusterless appearance and is sold under the brand name Hepatica. Powdered aloe is greenish-brown, has a pungent odor and a bitter, unpleasant taste. The main active constituents of the herb are aloin A and aloin B.

Aloe is the most powerful herbal anthranoid laxative and also the most widely used in Europe. Because of its drastic cathartic action it is not commonly employed in the United States. Research on the long-term toxicity and pharmacokinetics of aloe is still incomplete. In particular, it is not known what portions of the relatively lipophilic aloins undergo unwanted absorption. An accurate risk assessment cannot be made on the basis of available information.

5.6.5
Castor Oil

Castor oil is the oil that is mechanically pressed from the seeds of *Ricinus communis* (Fig. 5.12, family Euphorbiaceae) without heating. Cold pressing is carried out to keep the highly toxic protein ricin from entering the expressed oil. Castor oil has a very faint but characteristic odor; it has a mild initial taste and an acrid aftertaste.

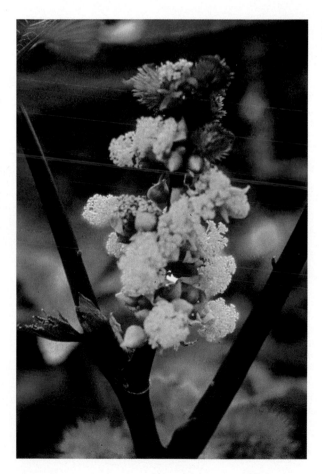

Fig. 5.12.
Raceme of castor *(Ricinus communis)*.

In contrast to most fatty oils, which are composed of mixed-acid triglycerides, up to 80 % of castor oil consists of triricinolein, which is broken down by saponification into glycerol and ricinoleic acid. Ricinoleic acid, or the sodium salt that forms from it, is the actual laxative agent. Because castor oil, like other triglycerides, is readily attacked by lipases and bile acids, its laxative action affects both the small and large intestine. The high polarity of the acid distinguishes it from other fatty acids and allows large portions of the acid to enter the colon.

A powerful cathartic, castor oil has a recommended dose of 5–10 g (1–2 teaspoons) for adults. It takes about 8 h to act. If more rapid catharsis is desired, the dose can be increased to a maximum of 30 g (6 teaspoons). Castor oil is most effective when taken on an empty stomach. Use in the form of gelatin capsules avoids the unpleasant taste, but a large number of capsules must be taken.

The contraindications and risks are similar to those of other laxatives. Because castor oil is a powerful stimulant of bile flow, it is also contraindicated by biliary tract obstructions and other biliary disorders. The laxative use of castor oil is contraindicated in poisonings with lipid-soluble agents because the oil can promote their absorption.

5.6.6
Suggested Formulations

Laxative tea I according to German Standard Registration

Rx	Senna leaves	60.0
	Fennelseed	10.0
	Chamomile	10.0
	Peppermint leaves	20.0
	Mix to make tea	

Directions: Prepare 1–2 teaspoons as an infusion, steep for 10 min. Drink 1 cup every evening.

Laxative tea according to R. F. Weiss (1982)

Rx	Senna leaves	25.0
	Buckthorn bark	25.0
	Chamomile	25.0
	Fennelseed, crushed	25.0
	Mix to make tea	

Directions: Prepare 1–2 teaspoons as an infusion, drink 1 cup every evening.

References

Cummings JH, Southgate DAT, Branch W, Houston H, Jenkins DJA, James WPT (1978) Colonic response to dietary fiber from carrot, cabbage, apple, bran, and guar gum. Lancet I: 5.

Curry CE (1982) Laxative products. In: Handbook of Nonprescription Drugs. Am Pharmac Assoc, Washington, pp 69–92.

Dufour P, Gendre P (1988) Long-term mucosal alterations by sennosides and related compounds. Pharmacology 36 (Suppl 1): 194–202.

Ewe K (1988) Schwer therapierbare Formen der Obstipation. Verhandl dtsch Ges Inn Med 94: 473–480.

Ewe K (1983) Obstipation – Pathophysiologie, Klinik, Therapie. Int Welt 6: 286–292.

Fingl E (1980) Laxatives and cathartics. In: Goodman AF, Goodman L, Gilman A (eds) The Pharmacological Basis of Therapeutics. 6th Ed. Macmillan, New York Toronto London, p 1004.

Gysling E (1976) Behandlung häufiger Symptome. Leitfaden zur Phamakotherapie. Huber, Basel Bern Stuttgart Vienna.

Huth K, Pötter C, Cremer CD (1980) Füll- und Quellstoffe als Zusatz industriell hergestellter Lebensmittel. In: Rottka H (ed) Pflanzenfasern-Ballaststoffe in der menschlichen Ernährung. Thieme, Stuttgart New York, pp 39–53.

Hutz J, Rösch W (eds) (1987) Funktionelle Störungen des Verdauungstrakts. Springer-Verlag, Berlin Heidelberg New York, pp 200, 222.

Kasper H (1980) Der Einfluß von Gallastoffen auf die Ausnutzung von Nährstoffen und Pharmaka. In: Rottka H (ed) Pflanzenfasern-Ballaststoffe in der menschlichen Ernährung. Thieme, Stuttgart New York, pp 93–112.

Kasper H (1985) Ernährungsmedizin und Diätetik. 5th Ed. Urban & Schwarzenberg, Munich Vienna.

Leng-Peschlow E, Mengs U (1990) No renal pigmentation by Plantago ovata seeds or husks. Med Sci Res 18: 37–38.

Müller-Lissner S (1987) Chronische Obstipation. Dtsch Med Wschr 112: 1223–1229.

Ruppin H, Bar-Meir S, Soergel KH, Wood CM, Schmitt MG (1980) Absorption of short-chain fatty acids by the colon. Gastroenterol 78: 1500–1507.

Schulz V, Löffler A, Gheeorghiu T (1983) Resorption von Blausäure aus Leinsamen. Leber Magen Darm 13: 10–14.

Schulz V (1984) Clinical pharmacokinetics of nitroprusside, cyanide, thiosulphate, and thiocyanate. Clinical Pharmacokinetics 9: 239–251.

Sewing KFR (1986) Obstipation. In: Fülgraff G, Palm D (eds) Pharmakotherapie, Klinische Pharmakologie. 6th Ed. Fischer, Stuttgart, pp 162–168.

Smith AN, Drummond E, Eastwood MA (1981) The effect of coarse and fine wheat bran on colonic motility in patients with diverticular disease. Am J Clin Nutr 34: 2460–2464.

Stephen AM, Cummings JH (1980) The microbial contribution to human fecal mass. J Med Microbiol 13: 45–66.

USD (1967) The United States Dispensatory and Physicians' Pharmacology. In: Osol R, Pratt R, Altschule MD (eds) Lippincott, Philadelphia Toronto, p 917.

Weber E (1988) Taschenbuch der unerwünschten Arzneiwirkungen. Fischer, Stuttgart New York.

Weinrich J (1980) Therapy of colon disease with a fiber-rich diet. In: Rottka H (ed) Pflanzenfasern-Ballaststoffe in der menschlichen Ernährung. Thieme, Stuttgart New York, pp 154–157.

Weiss RF (1982) Lehrbuch der Phytotherapie. 5th Ed. Hippokrates, Stuttgart, p 132.

Yajima T (1985) Contractile effect of short-chain fatty acids on the isolated colon of the rat. J Physiol 368: 667–678.

5.7
Liver Diseases

Most liver remedies were introduced into therapeutic use because they were found to have protective properties in certain animal species. The experimental agent (drug substance) was administered to the laboratory animal for a specified period of time, then a hepatotoxic agent was administered. In some models, the protective and toxic agents were administered concurrently. There have been studies in which liver damage was induced first and the experimental agent was administered afterward to test its curative properties, but in most cases the agent did not favorably affect the course of the hepatotoxicity. Even when curative effects were seen, experimental designs based on the administration of a hepatotoxic substance (carbon tetrachloride, galactosamine, thioacetamide, phalloidin) are not a valid model for studying liver diseases in humans. The main problem is that the alcohol-related liver damage so common in humans cannot be adequately reproduced in experimental animals except for certain species of higher apes (Bode, 1981). Thus, the antihepatotoxic and hepatoprotective effects seen in animal studies do not allow us to predict therapeutic efficacy in human patients with liver disease (alcoholic liver disease, hepatitis, fatty degeneration). A far more useful indicator is the finding that certain agents promote hepatic regeneration, as in the case of silymarin, which is described below (Sect. 5.7.1.4).

The following therapeutic goals have been defined as criteria for the clinical testing of hepatic remedies (Bode, 1986):

- improving the patient's subjective symptoms,
- shortening the duration of the disease, and
- reducing the number of fatal outcomes.

A very important criterion for the patient is the relief or improvement of complaints: anorexia, nausea, vomiting, epigastric pain and pressure, flatulence, and itching. This is a critical point in the objective assessment of drug actions, for an improvement in complaints is not necessarily linked to an objective amelioration of the disease process. The problem of assessment is made even more difficult by the extreme fluctuations that can occur in the spontaneous course of liver diseases.

The best criteria to use in the objective assessment of therapeutic response are (Bode, 1986): the regression of clinical symptoms of functional decompensation and laboratory findings.

It is commonly argued that the course of liver diseases cannot be significantly influenced by therapy (Dölle and Schwabe, 1988; Martini, 1988). However, molecular biochemical studies on the regeneration-promoting action of silybinin (Sonnenbichler et al., 1984, 1987, 1988) and supporting clinical reports (survey in Reuter, 1992) suggest that adequate doses of silymarin preparations can inhibit the progression of liver diseases when combined with appropriate general measures.

5.7.1
Milk Thistle Fruits, Silymarin

The majority of all biochemical, pharmacologic, and clinical tests of herbal liver remedies have employed a fraction extracted from the fruits ("seeds") of the milk thistle. Seventy percent of this fraction consists of silymarin, a mixture of four isomers including the main active constituent silybinin.

5.7.1.1
Medicinal Plant and Crude Drug

Milk thistle (*Silybum marianum*, Fig. 5.13) is an annual to biennial plant of the Asteraceae family growing to 2 m. It is native principally to southern Europe and northern Africa and grows in warm, dry locales. The milk thistle is a protected plant in Germany and is cultivated for medicinal purposes mainly in northern Africa and South America. It blooms in July and August at Central European latitudes.

The crude drug consists of the ripe fruits from which the pappus has been removed. Each fruit is about 6–7 mm long and 3 mm wide with a glossy, brownish black to grayish brown husk. The freshly milled fruits have a cocoa-like odor and an oily taste.

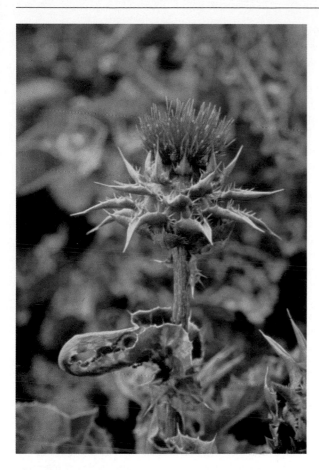

Fig. 5.13.
Milk thistle *(Silybum maria-num).*

5.7.1.2
Components and Active Constituents

Milk thistle fruits contain 15-30% fatty oil and about 20-30% proteins. The true active constituents constitute only about 2-3% of the dried herb. The mixture of active principles, called silymarin, consists of four isomers: silybinin (about 50%) and lesser amounts of isosilybinin, silydianin, and silychristin (Arnone et al., 1979; Wagner, 1976). Silymarin is most concentrated in the protein layer of the seed husk.

5.7.1.3
Pharmacokinetics

About 20-50% of silymarin is absorbed following oral administration in humans. About 80% of the dose, whether administered orally or by intravenous injection, is excreted in the bile (Mennicke, 1975); about 10% enters the enterohepatic circulation. With repetitive use, the circulating levels of silybinin reach an equilibrium state after just one day (Lorenz et al., 1982). The absorption rate depends on the galenic form of the preparation and can vary by a factor of at least two among different commercial products (Schulz et al., 1995).

5.7.1.4
Pharmacology and Toxicology

Pharmacologic studies have been performed on silymarin and its main component silybinin. It was found that silymarin mainly exerts antitoxic effects and promotes the regeneration of liver tissue. The antitoxic effects are based in part on membrane-stabilizing and radical-antagonizing actions. The regeneration-promoting effects are attributed to the stimulation of protein biosynthesis (survey in Reuter, 1992).

Antitoxic effects: Silymarin premedication in rats was found to prevent the injurious effects of various liver toxins such as carbon tetrachloride, galactosamine, thioacetamide, and praseodymium (Hahn et al., 1968; Rauen and Schriewer, 1971). Silymarin also protects the liver from drug toxicity (Martines et al., 1980; Leng-Perschlow et al., 1991). Particularly impressive are experimental reports of protective effects against the toxins of the mushroom Amanita phalloides, phalloidin and α-amanitin which attack the liver at various sites. Silymarin forms the basis for the only antidote to amanita poisoning (Sect. 5.7.1.6).

It is believed that the antidotal efficacy of silymarin against phalloidin, hepatotoxic chemicals, and alcohol is based on its tendency to bind to proteins and receptors on cell membranes, displacing toxic substances and preventing their entry into the cells.

Regeneration-promoting action: Silymarin may derive its curative properties from the capacity, especially of its silybinin component, to stimulate the regeneration of liver cells (Sonnenbichler and Zetl, 1988). In biochemical terms, the regenerative capacity of a tissue is based on stimulation of the cell metabolism and of macromolecular synthesis. Silybinin induces a global increase in cellular protein synthesis (Sonnenbichler and Zetl, 1986, 1987). The mechanism for stimulating protein synthesis is based on the ability of silybinin to bind to a subunit of the RNA polymerase of the cell nucleus, taking the place of an intrinsic cell regulator. The presence of the silybinin stimulates the polymerase to synthesize more ribosomal RNA, whose rate of transcription is increased. This leads to an increase in ribosome formation and, as a secondary effect, to an augmentation of cellular protein synthesis (Sonnenbichler and Zetl, 1988).

In evaluating silybinin-containing drugs, it is important to consider that silybinin not only protects the liver when administered prophylactically but also acts curatively to promote the regeneration of cells that are already damaged. It is also noteworthy that silybinin exerts its regeneration-promoting action at a 10 times lower concentration than is needed for antihepatotoxic membrane effects, and that the regenerative action is less structure specific. The regeneration-promoting action of silybinin may well account for the clinically observed acceleration of liver cell regeneration in response to silymarin preparations (Fintelmann and Albert, 1980).

5.7.1.5
Therapeutic Efficacy in Chronic Liver Diseases

By far the most frequent cause of chronic liver disease is alcohol abuse. The regular consumption of more than 50 g of ethanol per day is sufficient to pose an excess risk. The most effective therapeutic measure is abstinence from alcohol. Alcohol-re-

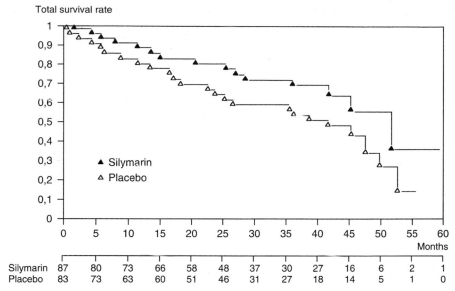

Total survival rate												
Silymarin	87	80	73	66	58	48	37	30	27	16	6	2	1
Placebo	83	73	63	60	51	46	31	27	18	14	5	1	0

Fig. 5.14. Survival rates of 170 patients with hepatic cirrhosis treated with silymarin or a placebo. The Kaplan-Meier method was used for statistical analysis. Significantly better survival rates (p < 0.05) were observed in the group treated with silymarin (Ferenci et al., 1989).

lated fatty liver changes, for example, will regress in most patients within a few months after alcohol is withdrawn.

Seven controlled clinical studies have been performed in patients with alcohol-related toxic liver damage using a standardized product with the brand name Legalon (Varis et al., 1978; Fintelmann and Albert, 1980; Benda et al., 1980; Salmi and Sarna, 1982; Feher et al., 1988, 1989; Ferenci et al., 1989). Most of the studies involved about 50–100 patients, and one study included 170 patients (Ferenci et al., 1989). Two studies (Benda et al., 1980; Ferenci et al., 1989) involved treatment periods of up to 4 years and used survival rate as their confirmatory parameter. Both of these studies showed a significant (p < 0.05) improvement in survival rate in the silymarin-treated group versus a placebo (Fig. 5.14). Most of the other studies also showed statistically significant gains in patients treated with the milk thistle preparation.

The tolerance toward silymarin preparations was very good. One observational study in 2169 patients revealed 21 cases (1%) of reported side effects, consisting mainly of transient gastrointestinal complaints.

5.7.1.6
Use in Mushroom Poisoning
More than 90% of all fatal mushroom poisonings are caused by ingestion of the death cup mushroom *Amanita phalloides*. A death cup of moderate size contains about 10 mg of amanitin – a potentially lethal quantity for an adult. The toxins in amanita mushrooms block the RNA polymerase in liver cells, culminating in cell death after a typical latent period of about 12–24 h. It is believed that silybinin com-

petitively displaces the amanitin from the enzyme, thereby reactivating the process of protein biosynthesis (Sonnenbichler, 1988).

Placebo-controlled double-blind studies in humans are prohibited for this indication. To date, some 150 case reports have been published on the therapeutic use of silybinin in patients with amanita poisoning. While older publications cited mortality rates of 30–50 % from this type of poisoning, studies using silybinin infusion therapy reported dramatically lower death rates: 1 death in 18 patients (Hruby et al., 1983) and 1 death in 13 patients (Marugg and Reutter, 1985).

5.7.1.7
Indications, Dosages, Risks, and Contraindications

The Commission E monograph of March, 1986, states that milk thistle is used for "dyspeptic complaints." It cites the following indications for silymarin preparations: "toxic liver damage; also the supportive treatment of chronic inflammatory liver diseases and hepatic cirrhosis."

There are no known contraindications, side effects, or interactions with other drugs. The recommended average daily dose is 12–15 g of the dried herb or 200–400 mg silymarin, calculated as silybinin.

The recommended regimen for amanita poisoning is infusion therapy with a silybinin derivative (brand name Legalon SIL). The manufacturer recommends a total dose of 20 mg silybinin per kg body weight over a 24-h period, divided into 4 infusions, each administered over a 2-h period.

5.7.2
Soybean Phospholipids

The term essential phospholipids (EPLs) denotes a soybean lecithin fraction that the manufacturer describes as a "choline phosphoric acid glyceride ester of natural origin containing predominantly unsaturated fatty acids, specifically linoleic acid (about 70 %), linolenic acid, and oleic acid." Phospholipids are an integral component of biomembranes and are involved in numerous membrane-dependent metabolic processes. It is postulated that phospholipids with polyunsaturated fatty acids prevent the hydrocarbon chains of the membrane phospholipids from assuming a parallel alignment owing to the cis double bonds of their polyunsaturated fatty acids. This would reduce the packing density of the micellar phospholipid structure, thereby increasing the rate of transmembrane exchange processes. This hypothesis underlies the presumed ability of soybean phospholipids to enhance the biochemical functioning of the liver parenchyma (Vogel and Görler, 1981; Peeters, 1976).

EPLs reportedly are absorbed unchanged after oral administration (Koch, 1980). Pharmacologic studies in rats showed a 100 % absorption of orally administered EPLs within 24 h, which reached the liver almost entirely by the lymphatic pathway. The liver absorbs 10–25 % of administered EPLs, which are gradually excreted via the urine and bile.

A total of 10 controlled therapeutic studies have been performed in patients with chronic liver disease. A review of these studies by Commission E in May of 1994 stated that 4 of the 10 studies demonstrated statistically significant benefits from EPL therapy. The Commission concluded that EPL preparations are indicated "for the improvement of subjective complaints such as anorexia and pressure in the right upper abdomen due to toxic-nutritional liver damage or chronic hepatitis." The recommended dose is 1.5–2.7 g of soybean phospholipids containing 73–79 % phosphatidylcholine. There have been rare reports of gastrointestinal complaints; there are no known contraindications or drug-drug interactions.

5.7.3
Drug Products

The *Rote Liste 1995* includes 28 single-herb products under the heading "Liver Remedies," consisting of 27 standardized silymarin preparations and one soybean phospholipid preparation, in addition to numerous combinations. None of the combination products are included among the 100 most commonly prescribed herbal medications (see Appendix).

References

Arnone A, Merlini L, Zanarotti A (1979) Constituents of Silybum marianum. Structure of isosilybin and stereochemistry of isosilybin. J Chem Soc (Chem Commun): 696–697.

Benda L, Dittrich H, Ferenzi P, Frank H, Wewalka F (1980) The influence of therapy with silymarin on the survival rate of patients with liver cirrhosis. Wien Klin Wschr 92 (19): 678–683.

Bode JC (1986) Arzneimittel für die Indikation "Lebererkrankungen". In: Dölle W, Müller-Oerlingshausen B, Schwabe U (eds) Grundlagen der Arzneimitteltherapie. Entwicklung, Beurteilung und Anwendung von Arzneimitteln. B.I.-Wissenschaftsverlag, Mannheim Vienna Zurich, pp 202–211.

Bode JC (1981) Die alkoholische Hepatitis, ein Krankheitsspektrum. Internist 220: 536–545.

Dölle W, Schwabe U (1988) Leber- und Gallenwegstherapeutika. In: Schwabe U, Paffrath D (eds) Arzneiverordnungsreport 88. Gustav Fischer, Stuttgart New York, pp 242–253.

Feher J, Deak G, Muezes G, Lang I, Niederland V, Nekam K, Karteszi M (1989) Hepatoprotective activity of silymarin Legalon therapy in patients with chronic alcoholic liver disease. Orv Hetil 130 (51): 2723–2727.

Ferenci P, Dragosics B, Dittrich H, Frank H, Benda L, Lochs H, Meryn S, Base W, Schneider B (1989) Randomized controlled trial of silymarin treatment in patient swith cirrhosis of the liver. J Hepatol 9 (1): 105–113.

Fintelmann V, Albert A (1980) Nachweis der therapeutischen Wirksamkeit von Legalon bei toxischen Lebererkrankungen im Doppelblindversuch. Therapiewoche 30 (35): 5589–5594.

Hahn G, Lehmann HD, Kürten M et al. (1968) Zur Pharmakologie und Toxikologie von Silymarin, des antihepatotoxischen Wirkprinzips aus Silybum marianum (L.) Gaertn. Arzneim Forsch/Drug Res 18: 696–704.

Hruby K, Fuhrmann M, Csomos G, Thaler H (1983) Pharmakotherapie der Knollenblätterpilzvergiftung mit Silibinin. Wien Klin Wschr 95 (7): 225–231.

Koch H (1980) Leberschutz-Therapeutika. Pharmazie in unserer Zeit 9; 33–44, 65–74.

Leng-Peschlow E, Strenge-Hesse A (1991) Die Mariendistel (Silybum marianum) und Silymarin als Lebertherapeutikum. Z Phytother 12: 162–174.

Lorenz D, Mennicke WH, Behrendt W (1982) Untersuchungen zur Elimination von Silymarin bei cholecystektomierten Patienten. Planta Med 45: 216–233.

Martines G, Copponi V, Cagnetta G (1980) Aspetti del danno epatico dopo somministrazione sperimentale diarrhea alcuni farmaci. Arch Sci Med 137: 367–386.

Martini GA (1988) Hepatocelluläre Erkrankungen, Leberkrankheiten. In: Riecker G (ed) Therapie innerer Krankheiten. Springer, Berlin Heidelberg New York, pp 638–652.

Marugg D, Reutter FW (1985) Die Amanita-phalloides-Intoxikation. Moderne therapeutische Maßnahmen und klinischer Verlauf. Schweiz Rundschau Med (Praxis) 14 (37): 972–982.

Mennicke WH (1975) Zur biologischen Verfügbarkeit und Verstoffwechselung von Silybin. Dtsch Apoth Z 115 (33): 1205–1206.

Peeters H (ed) (1976) Phosphatidylcholine. Biochemical and Clinical Aspects of Essential Phospholi-
pids. Springer-Verlag, Berlin Heidelberg New York.
Rauen HM, Schriewer H (1971) Die antihepatotoxische Wirkung von Silymarin bei experimentellen
Leberschäden der Ratte durch Tetrachlorkohlenstoff, D-Galaktosamin und Allylalkohol. Arzneim
Forsch/Drug Res 21: 1194–1201.
Reuter HD (1992) Spektrum Mariendistel und andere leber- und gallewirksame Phytopharmaka. In:
Bundesverband Deutscher Ärzte für Naturheilverfahren (ed). Arzneimitteltherapie heute. Aesopus
Verlag, Basel.
Salmi HA, Sarna S (1982) Effect of silymarin on chemical, functional and morphological alterations
of the liver. A double-blind controlled study. Scand J Gastroenterol 17 (4): 517–521.
Schulz HU, Schürer M, Krumbiegel G, Wächter W, Weyhenmeyer R, Seidel G (1995). Untersuchungen
zum Freisetzungsverhalten und zur Bioäquivalenz von Silymarin-Präparaten. Arzneim Forsch/
Drug Res 45: 61–64.
Sonnenbichler J, Zetl I (1984) Untersuchungen zum Wirkungsmechanismus von Silibinin, Einfluß
von Silibinin auf die Synthese ribosomaler RNA, mRNA und tRNA in Rattenlebern in vivo. Hop-
pe-Syler's Physiol Chem 365: 555–566.
Sonnenbichler J, Zetl I (1986) Biochemical effects of the flavonolignane silibinin in RNA, protein and
DNA synthesis in rat livers. Prog Clin Biol Res 213: 319–331.
Sonnenbichler J, Zetl I (1987) Stimulating influence of a flavonolignane on proliferation, RNA syn-
thesis and protein synthesis in liver cells. In: Okoliczányi L, Csomós G, Crepaldi G (eds) Assess-
ment and Management of Hepatobiliary Disease. Springer, Berlin Heidelberg New York, pp 265–
272.
Sonnenbichler J, Zetl I (1988) Specific binding of a flavonolignane to an estradiol receptor. In: Plant
Flavonoids in Biology and Medicine II: Biochemical, Cellular, and Medicinal Properties. Alan R
Liss, New York, pp 369–374.
Varis K, Salmi HA, Siurala M (1978) Die Therapie der Lebererkrankung mit legalon; eine kontrollier-
te Doppelblindstudie. In: Aktuelle Hepatologie, Third International Symposium, Cologne, Nov. 15–
17, 1978. Hanseatisches Verlagskontor. Lubeck, pp 42–43.
Vogel G, Görler K (1981) Lebertherapeutika. In: Ullmanns Enzyklopädie der technischen Chemie.
Vol. 18, 4th Ed. Verlag Chemie, Weinheim New York, pp 132–136.
Vogel G (1980) The anti-amanita effect of silymarin. In: Faulstich et al. (eds) Amanita toxins and poisoning. Witzstrock, Baden-Baden Cologne New York, pp 180–187.
Wagner H, Seligmann O, Seilz M, Abraham D, Sonnenbichler J (1976) Silydianin und Silychristin,
zwei isomere Silymarine aus Silybum marianum L. Gaertn. (Mariendistel). Z Naturforsch 31 b:
876–884.

6 Urinary Tract

The two main urologic indications for plant drugs are inflammatory urinary tract diseases and benign prostatic hyperplasia (BPH). The first of these indications includes renal gravel and more severe types of lithiasis. Herbal remedies for these conditions consist mainly of kidney and bladder teas, most of which are relatively heterogeneous mixtures of various herbs. Only three herbs are commonly used in the treatment of BPH: saw palmetto berries, nettle root, and pumpkin seeds. The compound β-sitosterol, a plant sterol derived from *Hypoxis rooperi,* is also used. In Germany, the nonsurgical treatment of BPH relies predominantly on herbal medications (Schmitz, 1995).

6.1
Inflammatory Diseases of the Urinary Tract

Inflammatory urinary tract disorders are treated mainly with medicinal teas. The designation kidney and bladder teas is somewhat misleading, for while the herbal ingredients of these teas are often purported to have a diuretic action, this has never been proven conclusively. Juniper berries are the only herb deemed likely to have a direct action on the renal parenchyma. As for the other herbs used in urologic teas (Table 6.1), it is probable that they derive most or all of their aquaretic effect (Schil-

Table 6.1. Twelve tea herbs recognized by Commission E as having value in the treatment of inflammatory urinary tract disorders and mild renal stone disease.

Herb	Latin name	Daily dose (g)
Birch leaf	Betulae folium	12
Dandelion herb and root	Taraxaci herba cum radice	3
Field Horsetail	Equiseti herba	6
Goldenrod and Early Goldenrod	Virgaureae herba and Virgaureae giganteae herba	6–12
Lovage root	Levistici radix	4–8
Nettle leaf	Urticae herba	8–12
Orthosiphon leaf	Orthosiphonis folium	6–12
Parsley herb and root	Petroselini herba cum radice	6
Petasite rhizome	Petasitidis rhizoma	5–7
Red Sandalwood	Santali lignum rubri	10
Restharrow root	Ononidis radix	12
Triticum rhizome	Graminis rhizoma	6–9
Uva Ursi leaf	Uvae ursi folium	3

cher, 1987, 1992) from the fluid that is ingested with the tea. Although various plant constituents were described as diuretic in the older literature (flavonoids, phenols, volatile oils, silicic acid), their low concentrations alone make it unlikely that they could produce a significant diuretic action (Nahrstedt, 1993; Veit, 1994).

Commission E, after reviewing mostly traditional reports, has declared the herbs listed in Table 6.1 to be effective in the treatment of inflammatory urinary tract diseases. Most of these herbs have also been declared useful in the treatment of mild renal stone disease (gravel). It appears that positive experience with the use of these herbal teas, especially in relieving dysuric complaints associated with inflammatory urinary tract diseases and infections, is reflected in current medical practice as significant numbers of these preparations are still being recommended and prescribed by German doctors (see Appendix, p. 287).

In patients with urinary tract infections or with stone-related and other inflammatory irritations of the urinary tract, increasing the output of a hypo-osmolar urine appears to be an effective way to clear ascending bacteria, crystallization nuclei, and other inflammatory agents from the urinary tract, thus protecting the damaged epithelium. While this pharmacodynamic principle has been challenged with respect to the prevention of urolithiasis (Ljunghall, 1988), we cannot question the plausibility of flushing out the urinary tract as a general treatment strategy in inflammatory urinary tract diseases. A related question is whether urologic teas owe their therapeutic effect to the fluid intake or to specific aquaretic actions of the administered herbs, provided the latter have a reasonable cost and can be used with an acceptable risk.

In 1992, Commission E reversed its position on madder root *(Rubia tinctorium)*, which it formerly recommended for the prevention of stone disease, and condemned the herb due to suspicion of excessive therapeutic risk. Madder root contains lucidin. A number of experimental studies, including the Ames test, strongly suggest that lucidin has mutagenic and carcinogenic properties.

Two herbs from this group (Table 6.1) have more specific actions: uva ursi (bearberry) leaves, whose hydroquinone constituents give it demonstrable antibacterial properties, and petasite rhizome, whose antispasmodic actions are beneficial in relieving spasmodic flank pain, especially when caused by urinary stones. Both herbs are discussed below in greater detail.

6.1.1
Uva Ursi Leaves

This herb consists of the dried leaves of the uva ursi or bearberry shrub (*Arctostaphylos uva-ursi,* family Ericaceae, Fig. 6.1). The trailing, perennial ground cover is similar to the cranberry in appearance and is widely distributed in the cool, temperate, forested zones of the northern hemisphere. Uva ursi leaves are odorless and have a bitter, astringent taste.

The key constituents of the herb are phenolic heterosides such as arbutin (5–12%), small amounts of the free aglycone hydroquinone (0.2–0.5%), tannins (10–20%), and flavonoids. The relatively high tannin content of the herb limits the duration of its use to about 2–3 weeks. The antibacterial principle is arbutin or its hydrol-

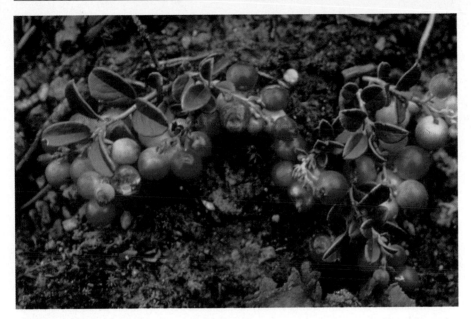

Fig. 6.1. Fruits of *Arctostaphylos uva-ursi* (bearberry).

ysis product hydroquinone. Relatively little is known about the pharmacokinetics of arbutin; all data are based essentially on studies by Frohne (1986). Arbutin itself is poorly absorbed from the gastrointestinal tract. The aglycone hydroquinone is well absorbed following hydrolytic cleavage of the glycosidic bond by intestinal flora. Hydroquinone is probably conjugated in the intestinal mucosa or liver and excreted as a conjugate via the renal pathway. If the urine is alkaline, it is believed that hydroquinone reforms from the conjugates and, when present in sufficient quantities, acts as a urinary antiseptic. Thus, the urine should be adjusted to a slightly alkaline pH (about 8) through dietary measures. These concepts, though plausible, are supported only by scant experimental data. Meanwhile, phenols normally are antimicrobial in an undissociated state, which requires an acidic urinary pH. An urgent need exists for new studies on the antibacterial properties of uva ursi (Nahrstedt, 1993).

So far, there have been no statistically and medically valid studies on the clinical use of uva ursi leaves administered as a single-herb preparation. There is a pressing need for up-to-date, controlled clinical studies using a high-dose, single-herb product. Nevertheless, documented experience, several clinical reports, and a number of experimental studies attest to the efficacy of the herb in bacterial inflammatory diseases.

No studies have yet been conducted on the acute and chronic toxicity, mutagenicity, or carcinogenicity of uva ursi leaves or their preparations. There is reason to suspect, however, that hydroquinone, which is partially derived from arbutin, does have mutagenic and carcinogenic effects. This prompted Commission E in 1993 to reevaluate uva ursi leaves as part of a general review of hydroquinone-containing drugs. While the Commission affirmed the value of uva ursi leaves for "inflammatory diseases of the urinary tract," it cautioned against use of the herb in pregnancy, lactation, or in children under 12 years of age. The recommended dosage is 3 g of the dried herb, or 400–800 mg of hydroquinone derivatives, taken up to 4 times daily. Due to the risk potential, uva ursi leaves and their preparations should not be taken for more than one week without the advice of a physician, and they should be used no more than five times in one year.

6.1.2
Petasite Rhizome

Petasite rhizome consists of the dried underground parts of *Petasites hybridus,* a native European perennial that flourishes along the banks of streams and other moist areas. The active principles are a group of sesquiterpene compounds, the petasins, which are reputed to have antispasmodic and analgesic actions based on earlier studies (Bucher, 1951). The herb also contains pyrrolizidine alkaloids.

Based on medical experience with petasite rhizome and the results of several experimental studies, Commission E in 1990 recognized the herb as being useful for the "supportive treatment of acute colicky urinary tract pain, especially when due to stone disease," recommending a daily dose of about 5–7 g of the dried herb. Given the possible therapeutic risk, however, the daily dose should not exceed 1 µg pyrrolizidine alkaloids, and the duration of use should not exceed 4–6 weeks per year.

Another herb traditionally used to relieve the pain of renal colic and spastic urinary tract disorders, ammi fruit *(Ammi visnaga),* was condemned by Commission E in 1994 because of its excessive therapeutic risk and unproven efficacy. Consequently, preparations made from ammi fruits may no longer be prescribed in Germany for this or any other indication.

6.2
Benign Prostatic Hyperplasia

Benign prostatic hyperplasia (BPH) is the most important urologic disorder affecting males. It generally affects men over 40 years of age and is present in more than 90% of men over age 65. Only about 50% of patients develop symptoms and complaints, however. The main obstructive signs of BPH are hesitancy in initiating the urinary stream, a weak and/or intermittent stream, and the terminal dribbling of urine. Up to 80% of patients also have irritative symptoms such as pollakiuria, urgency, nocturia, pressure over the bladder, and a feeling of incomplete bladder emptying (Dreikorn et al., 1990). The anatomic cause is an enlargement of the prostate due to hyperplastic changes in the periurethral glands, causing narrowing of the urethra and voiding difficulties. The Vahlensieck classification (Table 6.2) is one of several staging systems that have been developed for diagnostic and therapeutic purposes.

The etiology and pathogenesis of BPH are not fully understood, so a causal medical treatment is not yet available. BPH is generally regarded as an endocrine disorder of older males caused by changes in the hormone balance associated with aging

Table 6.2. Stages of benign prostatic hyperplasia (Vahlensiek, 1985)

Stage I	Stage II
▶ No voiding difficulties ▶ Urine flow > 15 mL/s ▶ No residual urine ▶ No trabeculation of the bladder	▶ Transient voiding difficulties ▶ Urine flow > 10–15 mL/s ▶ Little or no trabeculation of the bladder
Stage III	Stage IV
▶ Permanent voiding dysfunction ▶ Urine flow < 10 mL/s ▶ Residual urine > 50 mL ▶ Trabeculated bladder	▶ Permanent voiding dysfunction ▶ Urine flow < 10 mL/s ▶ Residual urine > 100 mL ▶ Bladder dilatation ▶ Urinary retention

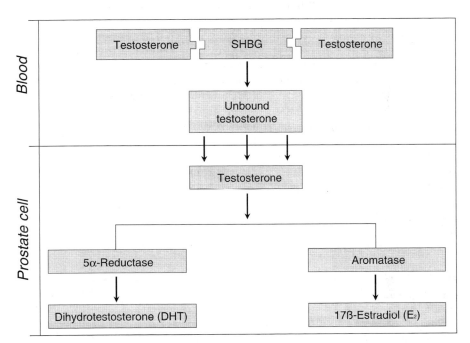

Fig. 6.2. Metabolism of testosterone. The hormonal hypothesis for prostatic hyperplasia is based on the assumption of increased DHT synthesis in the prostate and a shift in the androgen/estrogen ratio in favor of estrogens. This implies that the inhibition of a α-reductase and aromatase would be of therapeutic benefit. SHBG = Sex-hormone-binding globuline.

(Ekman, 1989). Three specific hypotheses on the pathogenesis of BPH will be reviewed below to help clarify the mechanisms of actions of herbal remedies.

The most widely favored hypothesis is based on an increase in the prostatic synthesis of dihydrotestosterone accompanied by an increase in the estrogen : androgen ratio (Fig. 6.2). The best known therapeutic approach based on this hypothesis is to inhibit the two prostatic enzymes 5 α-reductase (which converts testosterone to dihydrotestosterone) and aromatase (which converts testosterone to estrogens). In close association with the hormonal transformations in the prostatic tissue, changes in the binding capacity of sex-hormone-binding globulin (SHBG) also have been implicated in the pathogenesis of BPH (Schmidt, 1983). But an elevation of SHBG with aging is seen even in men without BPH symptoms, so it is difficult to draw therapeutic implications (Dreikorn et al., 1990). A third hypothesis holds that elevated levels of inflammatory mediators (prostaglandins and leukotrienes) are partly responsible for the development of BPH. This multifactorial pathogenesis suggests that plant constituents with anti-inflammatory and antiedematous actions would be of therapeutic benefit in BPH patients.

Koch (1995) may be consulted for an up-to-date review of the pharmacologic actions of extracts from saw palmetto berries, nettle roots, and pumpkin seeds.

There is controversy regarding the indications and efficacy of the various treatment options for BPH (Dreikorn et al., 1990). While prostatic hyperplasia in the U.S. is usually managed by surgical resection, conservative treatment is considered an acceptable option in Europe and especially in Germany. The conservative regimen starts with a change in living habits. To reduce congestion and bladder irritation, the patient should urinate promptly when the urge is felt, avoid overdistending the bladder by rapidly drinking large amounts of fluid, and avoid prolonged sitting or excessive cold. Emphasis is also placed on regular bowel habits and ample physical exercise; excessive alcohol intake, cold carbonated beverages, and pungent spices should be avoided (Sökeland, 1987). It should be noted that adrenomimetic drugs such as ephedrine in cough syrups and phenylephrine in nosedrops can exacerbate voiding difficulties, as can anticholinergics and antihistamines.

Synthetic preparations are also available for the pharmacotherapy of BPH; their role is discussed in Sect. 6.3.

6.2.1
Saw Palmetto Berries

The use of preparations made from the ripe fruits (berries) of a small fan palm known as saw palmetto or sabal (*Serenoa repens,* Fig. 6.3) for the treatment of BPH can be traced back to the early 1900's (Harnischfeger and Stolze, 1989). Saw palmetto berries are about 1–2 cm long and are usually gathered in the wild. The main supplier is the United States. Commercial preparations contain only lipophilic (fat-soluble) extracts, which are obtained from the powdered herb by extraction with hexane or liquid carbon dioxide. The principal ingredients in these extracts are saturated and unsaturated fatty acids, which occur mostly in free form. Free and conjugated plant sterols are also key constituents.

The results of animal studies and in vitro experiments with saw palmetto extracts have been published in about 20 original papers (surveys in Hänsel et al., 1994, and Koch, 1995). Studies in mice and rats demonstrated antiandrogenic actions in various models. Several in vitro studies confirmed inhibitory effects of saw palmetto extracts on 5 α-reductase. A comparison of relative efficacies showed that saw palmetto extract was some 6000 times less potent than an equal weight of the synthetic inhi-

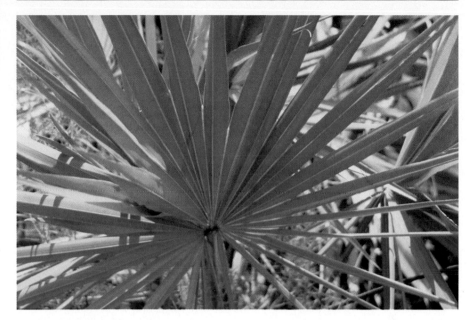

Fig. 6.3. Saw palmetto (Serenoa repens).

bitory agent finasteride (Rhodes et al., 1993), but allowance for the therapeutic dosage of both agents narrowed the potency difference by a factor of 100 (Koch, 1995). The inhibition of 5 α-reductase by saw palmetto extract is partly due to its content of free fatty acids. A recently published study compared the effect of saw palmetto extract with that of free fatty acids of various chain lengths. It was found that several common dietary fatty acids (e. g., linoleic acid) exerted stronger inhibitory effects on 5 α-reductase than equivalent concentrations of saw palmetto extract (Niederprüm et al., 1994), raising some unanswered questions regarding this mechanism of action. Saw palmetto extracts have other effects as well. For example, fractions from saw palmetto berries as well as commercial saw palmetto extracts demonstrated anti-inflammatory and antioxidant actions in typical experimental models of inflammation (carrageenan-induced rat's paw edema) (Koch, 1995).

The results of 15 therapeutic studies were published from 1983 to 1993 (surveys in Dreikorn et al., 1990, and Hänsel et al., 1994). Eight of these studies did not use control groups. The remaining seven had a double-blind, placebo-controlled design and involved a total of 490 patients. All the studies used lipophilic saw palmetto extracts administered in doses of 320 mg/day. The duration of treatment was 1–3 months in most studies and up to 6 months in 2 studies. A long-term study covering a treatment period of 3 years was published in 1995 (Bach, 1995), but it did not utilize a control group.

Most of the patients in the studies had Vahlensieck stage II BPH; smaller numbers had stage I or stage III disease. Therapeutic response was assessed on the basis of symptom scores, frequency of nocturia, ultrasound-determined residual urine volumes, and in some studies by measurements of urine flow. Plasma hormone levels (testosterone, dihydrotestosterone, estradiol, FSH, and LH) were measured during

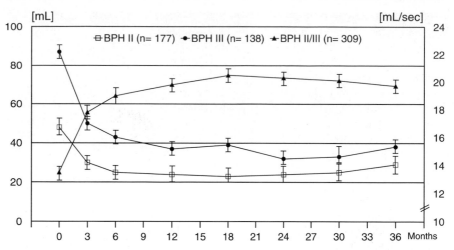

Fig. 6.4. Results of a therapeutic study with 320 mg saw palmetto extract per day taken over a 3-year period. Lower curves: residual urine volume; upper curve: maximum urine flow rate (Bach, 1995).

the course of treatment in two studies, but no treatment-associated changes were observed (Casarosa et al., 1988).

By contrast, nearly all the studies found statistically significant improvements in typical symptoms or symptom scores during the course of therapy in comparison to patients taking a placebo. The improvement rates were comparable to those achieved with other prostate remedies (see Sect. 6.3). Most of the studies that measured urine flow demonstrated increases of approximately 2–6 mL/s during the treatment period. Most of the studies also showed a marked decrease in residual urine volumes. These effects remained stable over a 3-year treatment period (Fig. 6.4).

The Commission E monograph on saw palmetto in its January, 1991, revision states that certain preparations made from saw palmetto berries are indicated for "micturition difficulties associated with stage I–II benign prostatic hyperplasia," recommending a daily dose of 1–2 g of the crude drug or 320 mg of an extract made with lipophilic solvents. As for side effects, there have been rare reports of gastric upset. Thirty-four of 435 patients who completed a 3-year study reported a total of 46 adverse effects, consisting mostly of gastrointestinal disturbances. The dropout rate due to adverse effects in this population was 1.8%. There are no known contraindications to saw palmetto preparations.

6.2.2
Nettle Root

Familiar to everyone, nettle *(Urtica dioica)* is a traditional medicinal plant cited in medieval herbals for its usefulness as a diuretic and a remedy for joint ailments. It is only in the past 15 years or so that nettle root and its preparations have been applied to the treatment of benign prostatic hyperplasia (Nöske, 1994).

All experimental pharmacologic studies and several clinical studies of nettle root have used hydroalcoholic extracts prepared with relatively hydrophilic solvents, i.e., methanol or ethanol in concentrations of 20–60%. The main components of these extracts include phytosterols, triterpene acids, lignans, polysaccharides, and simple phenol compounds.

Numerous experimental pharmacologic studies (survey in Koch, 1995) have shown that nettle root extract inhibits prostatic aromatase, interacts with sex-hormone-binding globulin (Hryb et al., 1995), and exerts multiple inhibitory effects on inflammatory mediators. An aqueous extract of nettle root showed weak anti-inflammatory activity when tested in the model of carrageenan-induced rat's paw edema. The authors attributed the anti-inflammatory action to an acid polysaccharide fraction in the extract (Wagner et al., 1994).

The positive effects of nettle root extract in patients with BPH have been attributed in part to the competitive displacement of sex-hormone-binding globulin (SHBG). However, such an effect requires extract concentrations on the order of 1–10 mg/mL (Hryb, 1995), which probably are too high for to be attained by therapeutic doses.

In addition to eight open and observational studies, only two groups of authors (Vontobel et al., 1985; Dathe and Schmid, 1987) have performed placebo-controlled double-blind studies on the therapeutic efficacy of nettle root extract.

Vontobel et al. found a statistically significant reduction of SHBG and a significant increase in urinary output compared with a placebo. A comparison of extract versus placebo showed no significant change in subjective symptoms, urine flow, residual urine volume, or serum levels of acid phosphatase.

Dathe and Schmid (1987) conducted a double-blind study in a total of 79 patients over a period of 4–6 weeks. The patients received the same preparation at the same dosage (600 mg extract daily) as in the study of Vontobel et al. The patients had BPH, but the stage was not specified. Response was assessed by the measurement of urine flow, which increased significantly by 2 mL/s (14%) relative to the placebo group.

The tolerance to nettle root extract is demonstrated by an observational study in 4087 patients with BPH who took 600–1200 mg of the extract daily for 6 months. Only 35 of the patients reported side effects, with 33 citing gastrointestinal complaints (0.65%), 9 noting skin allergies (0.19%), and 2 reporting hyperhidrosis (Sonnenschein, 1987).

The Commission E monograph on the nettle root in its January, 1991, revision states that the herb is indicated for "micturition difficulties associated with stage I–II prostatic adenoma," recommending a daily dose equivalent to 4–6 g of the crude drug. No contraindications are stated. Occasional, mild gastrointestinal complaints are mentioned as possible side effects.

6.2.3
Pumpkin Seeds

Seeds of the pumpkin, *Cucurbita pepo* (family Cucurbitaceae) have long been used in folk medicine, especially in southeastern Europe, as a remedy for irritable bladder and benign prostatic hyperplasia. The soft-shell varieties are particularly recommended and are the only ones for which scientific data have been acquired.

The seeds, which have a sweet, oily taste, contain fatty oil consisting mainly of linoleic acid (64%) in addition to plant sterols, tocopherols, carotinoids, and minerals. The identify of the constituents responsible for the therapeutic efficacy of pumpkin seeds remains to be established (Schilcher, 1987, 1992).

Pumpkin seeds are used medicinally in various forms. The most common practice is to use the whole or ground seeds. Expressed oils and dry extracts are also used. An isolated protein known as pumpkin globulin is employed mainly in combination products. How the different preparations may differ in their pharmacologic actions is unknown (Koch, 1995).

The use of pumpkin seeds and their preparations in the treatment of benign prostatic hyperplasia is based almost entirely on empirical knowledge. One experimental study showed that the Δ-7 sterols contained in pumpkin seeds have the ability to displace dihydrotestosterone from androgen receptors on human fibroplasts. In an open clinical study, 6 patients with BPH each received 90 mg of an isolated pumpkin sterol mixture 3 and 4 days before undergoing a radical prostatectomy. Examination of the excised tissue showed a highly significant decline in the dihydrotestosterone levels of the prostatic tissue compared with an untreated control group (Schilcher, 1987, 1992).

Further experimental and clinical studies on pumpkin seed preparations, especially placebo-controlled double-blind studies, are urgently needed in this area.

The 1985 Commission E monograph states that pumpkin seeds are indicated for "micturition difficulties associated with stage I–II prostatic adenoma," recommending a daily dose of 10 g of ground seeds or corresponding preparations. There are no known side effects or drug-drug interactions.

6.2.4
Grass Pollens

In 1994, Commission E recommended a preparation for the treatment of BPH whose active ingredient is a complex extract of 92% rye pollen (Secale cereale), 5% timothy pollen (Phleum pratense), and 3% corn pollen (Zea mays). The herbs are extracted with a water and acetone mixture, yielding a product with an herb-to-extract ratio of 2.5:1.

This extract has been the subject of numerous pharmacologic studies. One in vitro study showed a dose-dependent inhibition of inflammatory mediators (Loschen and Ebeling, 1991); another demonstrated growth-inhibiting effects in cultured prostatic epithelial cells and fibroblasts (Habib et al., 1992). Toxicologic studies showed no evidence of increased therapeutic risks or mutagenic effects.

The therapeutic efficacy of the pollen extract in benign prostatic hyperplasia was tested in two placebo-controlled double-blind studies in patients with Vahlensieck stage II or stage III disease. The first was a multicenter study involving a total of 103 patients from 6 urologic practices. The extract was administered in a dose of 138 mg/day for 12 weeks. Response was assessed on the basis of FDA-recommended criteria for voiding difficulties (residual urine volume, urine flow, palpable findings, and overall rating by the physician and patient). Comparison of the extract-treated and placebo-treated groups showed a statistically significant improvement in nocturia (in 69% vs. 37% of cases, respectively, $p < 0.005$) and in residual urine volumes (reduced by 24 mL vs. 4 mL in the placebo group). There was no significant difference in urine flow (Becker and Ebeling, 1988, 1991).

In the second placebo-controlled double-blind study, 60 patients with BPH received a daily dose equivalent to 92 mg of the pollen extract for 6 months. The parameters of interest were urine flow, urinary output, ultrasound-determined residual urine volume, transrectal palpation of prostate size, and clinical symptoms. Fifty-three of the patient protocols were deemed satisfactory for analysis. The extract showed statistically significant advantages over the placebo in the total complaint score (69% vs. 29% with a placebo, $p < 0.01$), residual urine, and prostate volume. Neither group showed significant changes in urine flow (Buck et al., 1990).

Based largely on the results of the two placebo-controlled double-blind studies, which meet current minimum standards for such research, Commission E declared the pollen extract to be useful in the treatment of "micturition difficulties associated with Alken stage I–II benign prostatic enlargement (BPH)." The recommended daily dose is 80–120 mg of the extract taken in 2 or 3 divided doses. As for side effects, rare instances of gastrointestinal complaints or allergic skin reactions have been reported. There are no contraindications. At least a 3-month course of treatment is advised.

6.2.5
Phytosterols from *Hypoxis rooperi*

The tuber of the South African plant *Hypoxis rooperi* (botanically related to asparagus) was used by the natives and later by European immigrants as a natural remedy for ailments of the bladder and prostate. Extraction of the herb with lipophilic solvents yields a β-sitosterol fraction that contains 10% β-sitosterolin (a glycoside of sitosterol).

β-Sitosterol resembles cholesterol in its chemical structure and interferes with the intestinal absorption of cholesterol, so it is also useful in the treatment of hypercholesterolemia. Pharmacologic studies have shown that prostatic tissue tends to bind sitosterol, which then acts on prostaglandin metabolism (Pegel and Walker, 1984). Besides β-sitosterol, β-sitosterolin is also considered a key active ingredient of *Hypoxis rooperi* preparations.

One placebo-controlled double-blind study showed a beneficial effect of β-sitosterol on residual urine volume and urine flow (Ebbinghaus and Baur, 1977). Another double-blind study using ultrasonography showed a significant improvement in the internal echo pattern of prostatic adenoma, which was interpreted as a reduction of interstitial edema by β-sitosterol (Szutrely, 1982).

Another placebo-controlled double-blind study applied the test criteria of the International Consensus Conference on Benign Prostatic Hyperplasia (Aso et al., 1993) to 200 patients with BPH. When the treatment period was concluded at 6 months, 96 of the patients receiving sitosterol (60 mg/day β-sitosterol) and 91 of those given the placebo were deemed satisfactory for evaluation. Efficacy was judged using a modification of the Boyarsky symptom score (Boyarsky, 1977) in addition to urine flow and prostate volume. On average, the symptom score improved by 6.7 points in the sitosterol-treated group vs. 2.1 points in the placebo group (Fig. 6.5). The difference

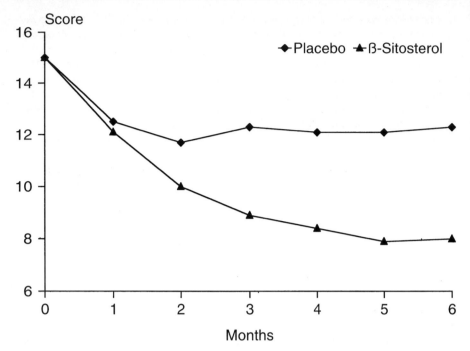

Fig. 6.5. Results of a therapeutic study with β-sitosterol from *Hypoxis rooperi*. The graph shows the progression of total symptom scores according to the Boyarsky scale (after Berges et al., 1995).

between the groups was statistically significant ($p < 0.01$). Significant intergroup differences were also seen in maximum urine flow and residual urine volume, but not in prostate volume. No significant side effects were noted during the 6-month course of treatment (Berges et al., 1995).

6.2.6
Pygeum

The powered bark of pygeum *(Prunus africana),* an evergreen tree native to southern and central Africa, was long used in Natal in the form of a milk suspension for micturition problems. Pharmacological studies subsequently verified the utility of the botanical in treating benign prostatic hyperplasia.

Lipophilic extracts of pygeum have been shown to contain at least three classes of active constituents that exert a beneficial influence on this condition. Phytosterols, present in both free and conjugated form, compete with androgen precursors and also inhibit prostaglandin biosynthesis. Pentacyclic terpenes, including oleanolic, crataegolic, and ursolic acids, exhibit anti-inflammatory activity by inhibiting the glucosyl transferase and β-glucuronidase enzymes involved in the depolymerization of proteoglycans in the connective tissue. Ferulic acid esters of fatty alcohols reduce the level of cholesterol in the prostate, thereby limiting androgen synthesis.

During the past 20 years, 26 clinical trials were concluded with pygeum extract involving a total of some 600 patients. Twelve of the trials were double blind versus placebo. Results indicated that administration of 100–200 mg per day of the lipophilic botanical extract resulted in a significant improvement of the various symptoms of benign prostatic hyperplasia, including dysuria, nocturia, pollakiuria, and volume of residual urine (Anon, 1991).

Acute and chronic toxicity tests in small animals showed pygeum to be devoid of severe side effects. Likewise, tests for mutagenesis and teratogenesis were negative. The extract appears to be well tolerated in humans following long-term administration.

The use of pygeum is far more widespread in Italy and, especially, in France than in Germany, so the botanical was never monographed by Commission E. In the United States, products containing pygeum, often in combination with other botanicals such as saw palmetto, are now widely marketed.

6.3
Therapeutic Significance

Herbal medications are frequently prescribed urinary remedies in Germany, and plant drugs are used almost exclusively in patients treated for benign prostatic disorders (Schmitz, 1995).

Tea preparations, whether by virtue of their fluid content or specific pharmacodynamic actions, are considered beneficial adjuncts in the symptomatic treatment of mild forms of inflammatory urinary tract disease. Of course, there are far more potent synthetic drugs available for the treatment of pain, spasms, and bacterial infections, and the prescribing physician must decide on an individual basis whether such products are preferred. Moreover, there is no rigorous scientific proof that any of the tea herbs listed in Sect. 6.5 are effective in treating urologic disorders. Thus, the supportive use of these teas in inflammatory urinary tract diseases can be justified only if their use does not pose any additional risk. This policy would contraindicate the use of tea therapy in patients with advanced cardiac or renal failure. It also justifies the actions of Commission E in withdrawing its approval of two herbs (madder root and ammi fruit) for urologic indications because of their unacceptable risks.

In Germany, phytomedicines have come to be preferred over synthetic drugs in the treatment of benign prostatic hyperplasia (BPH). In assessing the efficacy of the medical or surgical treatment of BPH, and in selecting patients for a specific type of therapy, our task is made difficult by the fact that purely obstructive symptoms, which today can be verified by urodynamic studies, are generally associated with marked subjective complaints that are very difficult to evaluate and confirm objectively. As a way out of this dilemma, many studies make use of scoring systems and rating scales (Boyarsky, 1977; Aso et al., 1993). But even when studies are properly designed and conducted, it is likely that 30–60 % of the results will be referable to placebo effects. To produce a significant, demonstrable therapeutic change, the tested drug must achieve an improvement rate on the order of at least 70–80 % (Dreikorn et al., 1990). Moreover, evaluations of subjective symptoms are subject to considerable spontaneous variation during the initial months of therapy, and a valid assessment requires treatment periods of at least 6 months' and preferably 12 months' duration (Aso et al., 1993).

An obvious alternative to phytotherapy in stage I–III BPH is synthetic drugs, specifically α-receptor blocking drugs and 5 α-reductase inhibitors (e.g., finasteride). On comparing the results of studies with a typical synthetic drug (Rhodes et al., 1993) and a typical herbal prostate remedy (Berges et al., 1995), we observe no fundamental differences in terms of therapeutic efficacy. Given the far better tolerance of herbal remedies, a strong rationale exists for favoring these medications over synthetic agents. At present, neither phytomedicines nor synthetic drugs can provide a causal treatment for benign prostatic hyperplasia.

6.4
Drug Products Other than Teas

The *Rote Liste 1995* includes herbal medications for inflammatory urinary tract diseases under the headings "Therapeutic agents for urinary tract infection" and "Urolithiasis remedies." A total of 15 single-herb products are listed for these indications, 9 of them containing goldenrod extract, 3 containing uva-ursi leaf extract, and 3 containing orthosiphon leaf extract. Due to the uncertain intrinsic actions of these three herbs and the likelihood that most of their effect derives from the fluid intake itself (see Sect. 6.1), their tea preparations (Sect. 6.5) are recommended in preference to the extract-based products. For the treatment of benign prostatic hyperplasia, *the Rote Liste 1995* includes a total of 35 single-herb preparations under the headings "Micturition remedies" and "Prostate remedies." Thirteen of these preparations are based on saw palmetto berries, 11 on nettle root, 10 on pumpkin seeds, and 1 on grass pollens. Also, the list of the 100 most commonly prescribed herbal medications in Germany (see Appendix) includes two combination products for inflammatory diseases of the urinary tract and two for benign prostatic hyperplasia.

6.5
Bladder and Kidney Teas

More than 100 medicinal herbs, including those listed in Table 6.1, are said to promote the flow of urine when administered in the form of an infusion or decoction. The patient should be taken off the medicinal tea at periodic intervals to ensure that the tea remains palatable. Alternatively, the daily dose can be reduced and supplemented by other forms of fluid intake. Infusions can be prepared from black or green tea, maté, or hibiscus flowers, or mineral water can be taken to provide fluid supplementation.

Patients with a sensitive stomach may find it difficult to tolerate teas with a high tannin content, including tea made from uva ursi leaves.

Suggested tea formulations. These teas are based on herbs that are reputed to have antibacterial and/or diuretic actions. To make the appearance of the tea mixtures more appealing or to improve the taste of the infusion, bladder and urine teas also contain one or more of the following herbs as correctives: calendula flowers, rose hips, fennelseed, peppermint leaves, and licorice root.

Suggested Formulations
Note: The provisions of the German Standard Registration specify the quantitative proportions of key active ingredients and correctives in urologic teas. The total content of correctives may not exceed 30 %, and the content of any one corrective may not exceed 5 %.

General Information
Preparation and use: Pour boiling water (about 150 mL) over 2–3 teaspoons of the tea mixture, cover and steep for about 10 min, and pour through a strainer. Prepare the tea fresh for each use.
Directions to patient: Drink 1 cup 3 or 4 times daily between meals.

Urologic tea according to German Prescription Formula Index

Rx	Maté leaves	10.0
	Orthosiphon leaves	10.0
	Uva ursi leaves	20.0
	Kidney bean pods	20.0
	Horsetail tops	20.0
	Birch leaves	20.0
	Directions (see above).	

Bladder tea according to Swiss Pharmacopeia 6

Rx	Uva ursi leaves	40.0
	Birch leaves	20.0
	Licorice root	25.0
	Couch grass rhizome	15.0
	Directions (see above).	

Urologic tea according to Austrian Pharmacopeia

Rx	Uva ursi leaves	35.0
	Birch leaves	30.0
	Rupturewort	35.0

Bladder and kidney tea I according to German Standard Registration

Rx	Birch leaves	
	Couch grass rhizome	
	Early goldenrod	
	Restharrow root	
	Licorice root	aa to make 100.0

Bladder and kidney tea II according to German Standard Registration

Rx	Uva ursi leaves	35.0
	Birch leaves	20.0
	Kidney bean pods	20.0
	Horsetail	15.0
	Nettle herb	5.0
	Licorice root	5.0
	Directions (see above).	

Bladder and kidney tea III according to German Standard Registration

Rx	Birch leaves	20.0
	Early goldenrod	20.0
	Restharrow root	20.0
	Horsetail	20.0
	Fennelseed	5.0
	Licorice root	5.0
	Rose hips	5.0
	Calendula flowers	5.0
	Directions (see above).	

Bladder and kidney tea III according to German Standard Registration

Rx	Birch leaves	20.0
	Early goldenrod	20.0
	Restharrow root	20.0
	Orthosiphon leaves	30.0
	Peppermint leaves	5.0
	Red sandalwood	5.0
	Directions (see above).	

Bladder and kidney tea IV according to German Standard Registration

Rx	Uva ursi leaves	35.0
	Kidney bean pods	20.0
	Early goldenrod	25.0
	Orthosiphon leaves	20.0
	Directions (see above).	

Bladder and kidney tea according to Pahlow

Rx	Dandelion root and herb	30.0
	Horsetail	20.0
	Restharrow root	20.0
	Birch leaves	20.0
	Goldenrod	20.0
	Directions (see above).	

Bladder tea according to W. Zimmermann

Rx	Marshmallow leaves	10.0
	Uva ursi leaves	20.0
	Speedwell	20.0
	Sage leaves	20.0
	Horsetail	30.0
	Directions (see above).	

Diuretic tea according to W. Zimmermann

Rx	Heather	20.0
	Kidney bean pods	10.0
	Lovage root	10.0
	Parsley fruit	20.0
	Horsetail	20.0
	Early goldenrod	10.0
	Hops	10.0
	Directions (see above).	

References

Anon (1991) Prunus africana. Indena SpA Milan Italy Technical documentation, pp 1–11.

Aso Y, Boccon-Gibob L, Brendler CB, et al. (1993) Clinical research criteria. In: Cockett AT, Aso Y, Chatelain C, Denis L, Griffith K, Murphy G (eds) Proceedings of the second international consultation on benign prostatic hyperplasia (BPH). Paris, SCI, pp 345–355.

Bach D (1995) Medikamentöse Langheitbehandlung der BPH. Ergebnisse einer prospektiven 3-Jahres Studie mit dem Sabalextrakt IDS 89. Urologe [B] 35: 178–183.

Becker H, Ebeling L (1988) Konservative Therapie der benignen Prostata-Hyperplasie (BPH) mit Cernilton®N – Ergebnisse einer placebokontrollierten Doppelblindstudie. Urologe [B] 28: 301.

Becker H, Ebeling L (1991): Phytotherapie der BPH mit Cernilton®N – Ergebnisse einer kontrollierten Verlaufsstudie. Urologe [B] 31: 113.

Berges RR, Windeler J, Trampisch HJ, Senge Th (1995) Randomised, placebo-controlled, double-blind clinical trial of β-sitosterol in patients with benign prostatic hyperplasia. Lancet 345: 1529–1532.

Boyarsky S (1977) Guidelines for investigation of benign prostatic hypertrophy. Trans Am Assoc Gen Urin Surg 68: 29–32.

Bucher K (1951) Über ein antispastisches Prinzip in Petasites officinalis Moendi. Arch Exp Path Pharmacol 213: 69.

Buck AC, Cox R, Rees RWM, Ebeling L, John A (1990) Treatment of outflow tract obstruction due to benign prostatic hyperplasia with the pollen extract Cernilton®. A double-blind, placebo-controlled study. Br J Urol 66: 398.

Casarosa C, Cosci M, o di Coscio, Fratta M (1988) Lack of effects of a Iyposterolic extract of Serenoa repens on plasma levels of testosterone, follicle-stimulating hormone and luteinizing hormone. Clin Ther 10: 5.

Dathe G, Schmid H (1987) Phytotherapie der benignen Prostatahyperplasie (BPH). Doppelblindstudie mit Extraktum Radicis Uricae (ERU). Urologe [B] 27: 223–226.

Dreikorn K, Richter R, Schönhöfer PS (1990) Konservative, nicht-hormonelle Behandlung der benignen Prostatahyperplasie. Urologe [A] 29: 8–16.

Ebbinghaus KD, Baur MP (1977) Ergebnisse einer Doppelblindstudie über die Wirksamkeit eines Medikaments zur konservativen Behandlung des Prostata-Adenoms. Z Allg Med 53: 1054–1058.

Ekman P (1989) BPH epidemiology and risk factors. Prostate (Suppl 2): 3–31.

Frohne D (1986) Arctostaphylos uva-ursi: Die Bärentraube. Z Phytother 7: 45–47.

Habib FK (1992) Die Regulierung des Prostatawachstums in Kultur mit dem Pollenextrakt Cernitin T60 und die Wirkung der Substanz auf die Verteilung von EGF im Gewebe. In: Vahlensieck W, Rutishauser G (eds) Benigne Prostatopathien. Thieme, Stuttgart, p 120.

Hänsel R, Keller K, Rimpler H, Schneider G (eds) (1994) Hagers Handbuch der Pharmazeutischen Praxis. 5th Ed, Vol 6, Drogen P–Z. Springer Verlag, Berlin Heidelberg New York, pp 680–687.

Harnischfeger G, Stolze H (1989) Serenoa repens – Die Sägezahnpalme. Z Phytother 10: 71–76.

Hryb DJ, Khan MS, Romas NA, Rosner W (1995) The effect of extracts of the roots of the stinging nettle (Urtica dioica) on the interaction of SHBG with its receptor on human prostatic membranes. Planta Med 61: 31–32.

Koch E (1995) Pharmakologie und Wirkmechanismen von Extrakten aus Sabalfrüchten (Sabal fructus), Brennesselwurzeln (Urticae radix) und Kürbissamen (Cucurbitae peponis semen) bei der Behandlung der benignen Prostatahyperplasie. In: Loew D, Rietbrock N (eds) Phytopharmaka in Forschung und klinischer Anwendung. Steinkopff Verlag, Darmstadt, pp 57–79.

Ljunghall S, Fellström B, Johansson G (1988) Prevention of renal stones by a high fluid intake? Eur Urol 14: 381–385.

Loschen G, Ebeling L (1991) Hemmung der Arachidonsäure-Kaskade durch einen Extrakt aus Roggenpollen. Arzneim Forsch/Drug Res. 41 (1) 2:162.

Nahrstedt A (1993) Pflanzliche Urologica – eine kritische Übersicht. Pharm Z 138:1439–1450.

Niederprüm HJ, Schweikert HU, Zänker KS (1994) Testosterone 5 α-reductase inhibition by free fatty acids from Sabal serrulata fruits. Phytomedicine 1: 127–133.

Nöske HD (1994) Die Effektivität pflanzlicher Prostatamittel am Beispiel von Brennesselwurzelextrakt. ÄrzteZ Naturheilverfahren 35 (1):18–27.

Pegel KH, Walker H (1984) Neue Aspekte zur benignen Prostatahyperplasie (BHP). Die Rolle der Leukotriene und Prostaglandine bei der Entstehung sowie bei der konservativen Therapie der durch sie verursachten Symptome. Extr Urologica 7 (Suppl 1): 91–104.

Rhodes L, Primka RL, Berman Ch, Vergult F, Gabriel M, Pierre-Malice M, Gibelin B (1993) Comparison of finasteride (Proscar®), a 5 α-reductase inhibitor, and various commercial plant extracts in in vitro and in vivo 5 α-reductase inhibition. Prostate 22: 43–51.

Schilcher H (1987a) Pflanzliche Diuretika. Urologe [B] 27: 215–222; (1987b) Möglichkeiten und Grenzen der Phytotherapie am Beispiel pflanzlicher Urologika. Urologe [B] 27: 316–319.

Schilcher H (ed) (1992) Phytotherapie in der Urologie. Hippokrates Verlag Stuttgart.

Schmidt K (1983) Die Wirkung eines Radix Urticae-Extrakts und einzelner Nebenextrakte auf das SHBG des Blutplasmas bei der benignen Prostatahyperplasie. Fortschr Med 101: 713–716.

Schmitz W (1995) Urologika. In: Schwabe U, Paffrath D (eds) Arzneiverordnungs-Report '95. Gustav-Fischer Verlag, Stuttgart Jena, pp 410–420.

Sökeland J (1987) Urologie. Thieme, Stuttgart, pp 258, 260.

Sonnenschein R (1987) Untersuchung der Wirksamkeit eines prostatotropen Phytotherapeutikums (Urtica plus) bei benigner Prostatahyperplasie und Prostatitis – eine prospektive multizentrische Studie. Urologe [B] 27: 232–237.

Szutrely HP (1982) Änderung der Echostruktur des Prostataadenoms unter medikamentöser Therapie. Med Klin 77: 42–46.

Vahlensiek W (1985) Konservative Behandlung der benignen Prostatahyperplasie (BPH). Therapiewoche 35: 4031–4040.

Veit M (1994) Probleme bei der Bewertung pflanzlicher Diuretika. Z Phytother 16: 331–341.

Vontobel HP, Herzog R, Rutishauser G, Kres H (1985) Ergebnisse einer Doppelblindstudie über die Wirksamkeit von ERU-Kapseln in der konservativen Behandlung der benignen Prostatahyperplasie. Urologe [A] 24: 49–51.

Wagner H, Willer F, Samtleben R, Boos G (1994) Search for the antiprostatic principle of stinging nettle (Urtica dioica) roots. Phytomedicine 1: 213–224.

Zimmermann W (1994) Praktische Phytotherapie. Sonntag Verlag, Stuttgart, pp 185–187.

7 Gynecologic Indications for Herbal Remedies

Herbal remedies cover a small but very important range of indications in the treatment of gynecologic diseases and functional disorders. They are used principally in the treatment of premenstrual syndrome (PMS), dysmenorrhea, and menopausal complaints in cases where stronger-acting drugs are not indicated or are declined by the patient. Two medicinal plants stand out in the frequency with which they are prescribed for gynecologic complaints: chasteberries (used chiefly for PMS) and black cohosh rhizome (used principally for menopausal complaints) (Schwabe and Rabe, 1995). Table 7.1 also lists four other herbs recommended by Commission E as having gynecologic indications. It can be seen that the range of recommended dosages (column 3 in Table 7.1) is greater for gynecologic herbal remedies than for any other class of phytomedicines. Some of the dosages are many times lower than the traditional single dose of about 1–4 g of crude drug taken in a cup of medicinal tea. There is an urgent need for pharmacologic and clinical studies to investigate the dose-dependency of the actions and efficacy of these drugs.

Historically, most herbal remedies for gynecologic problems were classified as emmenagogues. Hippocrates mentioned a number of herbs that were reputed to induce menstruation or increase menstrual flow. It was recognized in ancient times that regular menstruation was important in the preservation of health, and con-

Table 7.1. Herbal drugs used for gynecologic indications.

Herbs	Indications*	Daily dose*
Black cohosh (Cimicifugae racemosae rhizoma)	Premenstrual, dysmenorrheic, and menopause related neuroautonomic complaints	40 mg
Bugle weed (Lycopi herba)	Breast pain and tension; mild hyperthyroidism with neuroautonomic disturbances	0.02–2 g
Chasteberry (Agni casti fructus)	Abnormal frequency of menstrual bleeding, premenstrual complaints, mastodynia	30–40 mg
Shepherd's purse (Bursae pastoris herba)	Symptomatic treatment of mild menorrhagia and metrorrhagia	5–15 g
Silverweed (Potentillae anserinae herba)	Mild dysmenorrheic complaints	4 g
Yarrow (Achilleae millefolii herba)	In sitz baths: painful spastic conditions of psychoautonomic origin involving the lesser pelvis	100 g per 20 L water

* according to the monograph of Commission E

versely a variety of ailments were attributed to the absence or irregularity of menstrual bleeding. Classic emmenagogic herbs included locally irritating essential oils and a number of cathartics. With the estrogens and progestins available today, there is no longer a need to use plant drugs for this indication, and indeed the risks of many herbal drugs (abortion in undetected pregnancy) would contraindicate their use.

Herbal remedies continue to be of benefit in PMS, a symptom complex that commonly appears several days before the onset of menstrual bleeding. Many women experience an array of physical and behavioral symptoms that usually subside with the start of menstruation. The physical symptoms are mostly congestive in nature and consist of painful breast swelling and tension (mastodynia); abdominal discomfort with fullness, bloating, and constipation; and edema that typically involves the ankles, the area around the eyes, and the hands. Behavioral symptoms are also a common feature of PMS.

The breast discomfort in PMS is believed to relate causally to a latent hyperprolactinemia (Halbreich et al., 1976; Schneider and Bohnet, 1981). Falling estradiol and progesterone levels combined with stress can lead to an increased pituitary secretion of prolactin in these women. Dopaminergic agents inhibit prolactin secretion, thus providing an experimental approach to confirming the efficacy of chasteberry and other herbal preparations (Wuttke et al., 1995).

The waning of ovarian function that occurs at about age 50 is marked by a number of physical and psychologic complaints collectively referred to as menopausal syndrome. The most frequent and characteristic symptom is hot flashes, which occur in about three-fourths of affected women. Some 50 % of women also experience psychologic complaints such as nervousness, irritability, sleeplessness, or depression (Bates, 1981). Since menopausal discomforts are the result of declining hormone production, hormone replacement can be an effective therapy but is associated with various risks and side effects that many women find objectionable. The need for an alternative therapy with gentle-acting agents forms the basis for the second major indication for gynecologic herbal remedies: menopausal complaints.

7.1
Chasteberry

This herb consists of the dried, ripe fruits of the Chaste tree, *Vitex agnus-castus* (Fig. 7.1), a shrub of the family Verbenaceae that is native to the Mediterranean region. The hard, black, round berries are about 0.5 cm in size and contain 4 seeds. They have an aromatic odor and an acrid, slightly peppery taste. Chasteberry contains about 0.5 % volatile oil along with the iridoid glycosides agnoside and aucubin. The constituents responsible for the actions and efficacy of the herb have not been identified.

The Greek physician Dioscorides mentioned chasteberry as a medicinal plant some 2000 years ago, noting that its Latin name *agnus castus,* meaning chaste lamb, referred to the property of its seeds, when taken as a drink, to reduce sexual desire. Reportedly, the herb aided medieval monks in keeping their vow of chastity; hence, the common name Monk's pepper.

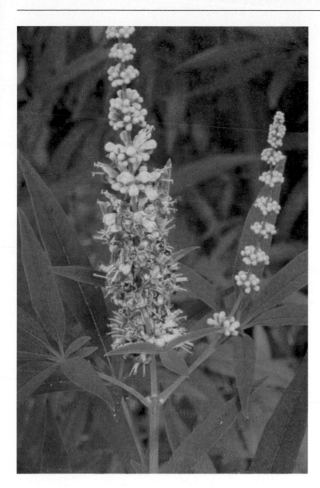

Fig. 7.1.
Chasteberry plant *(Vitex agnus-castus).*

Experimental studies in vitro and in live animals have shown that chasteberries have a prolactin-inhibiting action. This effect is described more specifically as a dopaminergic action based on the selective stimulation of D_2-type dopamine receptors (Jarry et al., 1991, 1994; Winterhoff, 1993). Regarding the dosage used in human beings (see Table 7.1), it is noteworthy that experimental studies had to use extract concentrations of 3.3 mg/mL in vitro (Fig. 7.2) and single doses of 60 mg injected intravenously in experimental rats (Fig. 7.3) in order to achieve significant effects (Wuttke et al., 1995).

A placebo-controlled double-blind study was performed in 20 healthy male subjects to test the effect of chasteberry on prolactin levels in humans. A cross-over design was used in which the subjects took an extract in doses equivalent to 120 mg, 240 mg, or 480 mg of the crude drug. The study did not show any definite dose-dependent changes in the 24-h serum prolactin profile. The changes that occurred during the treatment period depended strongly on the baseline values of the individual subjects (Merz et al., 1995). A pilot study in 56 women with mastodynia showed that

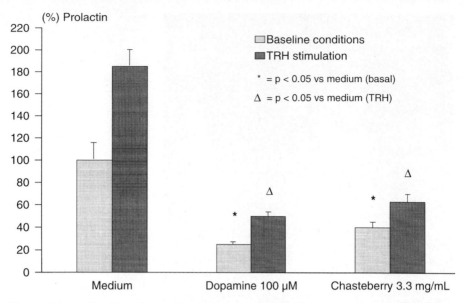

Fig. 7.2. Release of prolactin from cultured pituitary cells under baseline conditions, after stimulation with thyrotropin-releasing hormone (TRH), and after incubation with dopamine and chasteberry extract (Wuttke et al., 1995).

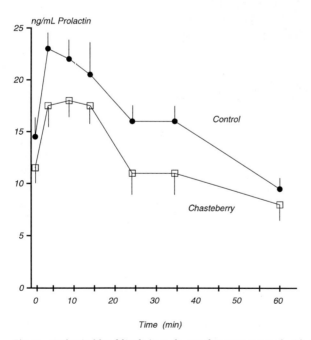

Fig. 7.3. Prolactin blood levels in male rats that were stressed with and without prior treatment with 60 mg chasteberry extract per animal (Wuttke et al., 1995).

a chasteberry combination product taken for three menstrual cycles significantly reduced serum prolactin levels in comparison to a placebo (Wuttke et al., 1995). In a multicenter controlled double-blind study, a 3-month regimen of 175 mg/day of a chasteberry tincture (1:5) was compared with the vitamin preparation pyridoxine (200 mg/day). The women in the study ranged from 18 to 45 years of age, and all were diagnosed with premenstrual syndrome. The main confirmatory parameter was the change in a total symptom score (PMTS scale). In patients treated with the botanical preparation, the total score decreased from 15 to 5 points; the score in patients treated with the vitamin preparation decreased from 12 to 5 (Reuter et al., 1995).

No studies have yet been published on the pharmacokinetics or toxicology of chasteberry preparations. Previous use of the herb has not been associated with any serious side effects. A clinical pharmacologic study using higher dosages did find a number of non-dose-dependent side effects, but they were so mild that the authors did not believe that chasteberry extract would cause tolerance problems even at higher doses (Merz et al., 1995).

7.2
Black Cohosh

Black cohosh (Fig. 7.4), known also as black snakeroot or cimicifuga, is a native North American herbaceous plant *(Cimicifuga racemosa)* of the family Ranunculaceae. The crude drug, consisting of the dried rhizome and roots, is nearly odorless and has a bitter, acrid taste. The drug contains triterpene glycosides, including actein and cimicifugoside, which are considered the key constituents. Researchers have also isolated from the botanical very small amounts of the isoflavonoid compound formononetin, an active principle that possesses hormonal activity (Jarry et al., 1995).

The endocrine effects of *Cimicifuga racemosa* extracts, which presumably are exerted on the pituitary, have been investigated in vitro, in ovariectomized rats, and in patients with menopausal complaints. Unlike synthetic estrogens, which affect follicle stimulating hormone (FSH), luteinizing hormone (LH), and prolactin release, the investigated black cohosh extract only reduced the serum levels of LH. Estrogen-binding studies in vitro and evidence of antiproliferative effects on the growth of breast carcinoma cells suggest that black cohosh acts on hormonal regulation. Studies of various extracts indicate that the lipophilic fraction contains the hormonally active principle (Jarry et al., 1985; Düker et al., 1991; Winterhoff, 1993; Jarry et al., 1995). The toxicology of cimicifuga extracts has not been adequately studied. More data are needed on acute toxicity, genotoxicity, mutagenicity, and carcinogenicity. There are no case reports of toxic effects from the herb, and there appears to be no specific toxicity associated with any of its known constituents.

The clinical efficacy of black cohosh extracts is based not just on older studies and anecdotal reports but on five controlled studies comparing the extract with a placebo or with estrogen therapy in women with physical, psychologic, and neuroautonomic complaints relating to menopause (Vorberg, 1984; Warnecke, 1985; Lehmann-Willenbrock, 1988; Daiber, 1983; Düker, 1991). Unfortunately, none of these studies employed a double-blind design. But significant changes in the Kupperman

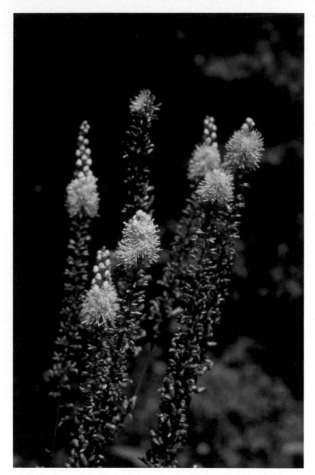

Fig. 7.4. Black cohosh *(Cimicifuga racemosa).*

index and a series of standard psychometric scales (CGI, POMS, HAMA, STS) do support the therapeutic efficacy of black cohosh extract in menopausal women. All the studies used doses equivalent to 40 mg/day of the crude drug. Mild side effects (gastrointestinal complaints, headache, dizziness, weight gain) were noted in two of the studies. Because of insufficient data, use during pregnancy and lactation is not advised. No other contraindications are known. The duration of use should not exceed three months.

7.3
Other Herbs

Several other herbs used for gynecologic indications are listed in Table 7.1. Only some are available as proprietary products (Sect. 7.5).

The aerial parts of the **bugle weed** (*Lycopus* spp., family Lamiaceae) are harvested just before the plant blooms. Tinctures and infusions of it were used in nineteenth-century America as a remedy for bleeding, especially nosebleeds and menorrhagia. Experimental pharmacologic studies have demonstrated antigonadotropic actions (Gumbinger et al., 1981; Winterhoff et al., 1983), antithyrotropic actions (Frömbling-Borges, 1987), and a lowering of serum prolactin levels (Sourgens et al., 1982). The clinical relevance of these studies is unclear. Therapeutic trials have not been conducted in patients. Based largely on pharmacologic studies, Commission E recognized these indications for bugle weed in 1990: "mild hyperthyroid conditions with neuroautonomic dysfunction, also breast tension and tenderness (mastodynia)." In rare cases, thyroid enlargement can occur with long-term use. Sudden withdrawal should be avoided, because it may lead to increased prolactin secretion. Dose recommendations cover an extremely broad range from 0.2 to 2 g/day of the crude drug or equivalent.

The dried aerial parts of **silverweed** (*Potentilla anserina*, family Rosaceae) contain at least 2% tannins and have been approved for use in the supportive treatment of nonspecific diarrhea and for the local treatment of oropharyngeal inflammations. In 1985, Commission E additionally recognized the use of silverweed for "mild dysmenorrheic complaints." The recommended daily dose is 4–6 g of the crude drug. Stomach irritation has been reported as a possible side effect. The gynecologic indication for silverweed is based on pharmacologic studies showing that the herb increases the tonus of the isolated uterus in various animal species.

The aerial parts of **shepherd's purse** (*Capsella bursa-pastoris*, family Brassicaceae) are used in folk medicine for preventing or arresting hemorrhage. Commission E, in its 1986 monograph, recommends daily oral doses equivalent to 10–15 g of the crude drug for mild gynecologic bleeding. The active hemostatic principle in shepherd's purse is believed to be a peptide whose structure is still unknown.

The aerial parts of **yarrow** (*Achillea millefolium*, family Asteraceae) are used in folk medicine for the topical treatment of wounds and for gynecologic disorders. The Commission E monograph of February, 1990, approves its use in sitz baths for the treatment of pelvic autonomic dysfunction (painful spastic conditions of psychoautonomic origin involving the minor pelvis in women) and in oral dosage forms for dyspeptic complaints. The herb is reputed to have antispasmodic activity.

Rhapontic rhubarb root (*Rheum rhaponticum*, family Polygonaceae), besides containing small quantities of laxative principles (anthraquinone glycosides), also contains 4–11% stilbene derivatives, including the characteristic compound rhapontin, which reportedly has weak estrogenic effects. Given the risks posed by stilbene derivatives, the therapeutic use of this herb can no longer be recommended. Only one product containing the herb is still marketed in Germany.

Hops, the strobiles of *Humulus lupulus*, family Cannabidaceae) was found to have some estrogenic activity in earlier studies on small rodents (Koch and Heim, 1953). The authors believed that this accounted for the old observation that menstrual periods tended to arrive early in female hop pickers. Other investigators could not reproduce the results of Koch and Heim, however, and today it is generally agreed that hop does not have estrogenic effects (Fenselau et al., 1973). The psychotropic actions of hops are discussed in Sect. 2.4.2.

7.4
Therapeutic Significance

Gynecologic herbs cannot replace sex hormones, anti-infectious agents, or antispasmodic drugs that are medically indicated. So far, therapeutic efficacy has not been established for any herbal gynecologic remedies in a way that would satisfy current standards. In the treatment of premenstrual and menopausal syndromes, however, preparations made from chasteberries and black cohosh offer an alternative to higher-risk hormone therapies for a number of patients, especially when one considers that the subjective complaints of the syndromes in particular show a placebo response rate of approximately 50 %. Given the considerable practical importance of these preparations, reliable evidence of safety and efficacy is overdue.

7.5
Drug Products

The *Rote Liste 1995* includes a total of 19 single-herb products for gynecologic indications. Eight are preparations made from chasteberry, eight from black cohosh, and one each from silverweed, bugle weed, and rhapontic rhubarb. The chasteberry preparations are offered mainly for premenstrual complaints, the black cohosh preparations for menopausal discomforts, and the remaining three for dysmenorrheic complaints (silverweed), mastodynia and mild hyperthyroidism (bugle weed), and follicular hormone therapy (rhanpontic rhubarb). Three of these products are among the 100 most commonly prescribed herbal medications in Germany (see Appendix).

References

Bates GW (1981) On the nature of the hot flash. Clinical Obstetrics and Gynaecology 24: 231–241.
Daiber W (1983) Klimakterische Beschwerden: ohne Hormone zum Erfolg. Ärztl Praxis XXXV: 65.
Düker EM, Kopanski L, Jarry H, Wuttke W (1991) Effects of extracts from Cimicifuga racemosa on gonadotropin release in menopausal women and ovariectomized rats. Planta Med 57: 420–424.
Fenselau C, Talalay P (1973) Is estrogenic activity in hops? Fd Cosmet Toxicol 11: 597–603.
Frömbling-Borges A (1987) Intrathyreoidale Wirkung von Lycopus europaeus, Pflanzensäuren, Tyrosinen, Thyroninen und Lithiumchlorid. Darstellung einer Schilddrüsensekretionsblockade. Inauguraldissertation, Westfälische Wilhelms-Universität Münster.
Gumbinger HG, Winterhoff H, Sourgens H, Kemper FH, Wylde R (1981) Formation of compounds with antigonadotropic activity from inactive phenolic precursors. Contraception 23: 661–666.
Halbreich U, Assad M, Ben-David M, Bornstein R (1976) Serum prolactin in women with premenstrual syndrome. Lancet: 654–656.
Jarry H, Harnischfeger G, Düker, E (1985) Studies on the endocrine effects of the contents of Cimicifuga racemosa: 2. In vitro binding of compounds to estrogen receptors. Planta Med 51: 316–319.

Jarry H, Harnischfeger G (1985) Studies on the endocrine effects of the contents of Cimicifuga racemosa: 1. Influence on the serum concentration of pituitary hormones in ovariectomized rats. Planta Med 51: 46–49.

Jarry H, Gorkow Ch, Wuttke W (1995) Treatment of menopausal symptoms with extracts of Cimicifuga racemosa: In vivo and in vitro evidence for estrogenic activity. In: Loew D, Rietbrock N (eds) Phytopharmaka in Forschung und klinischer Anwendung. Steinkopff Verlag, Darmstadt, pp 99–112.

Jarry H, Leonhardt S, Wuttke W, Behr B, Gorkow C (1991) Agnus castus als dopaminerges Wirkprinzip in Mastodynon N. Z Phytother 12: 77–82.

Jarry H, Leonhardt S, Gorkow C, Wuttke W (1994) In vitro prolactin but not LH and FSH release is inhibited by compounds in extracts of Agnus castus: direct evidence for a dopaminergic principle by the dopamine receptor assay. EYP Clin Endocrinol 102: 448–454.

Lehmann-Willenbrock E, Riedel HH (1988) Klinische und endokrinologische Untersuchungen zur Therapie ovarieller Ausfallserscheinungen nach Hysterektomie unter Belassung der Adnexe. Zent Gynäkol 110: 611–618.

Merz PG, Schrödter A, Rietbrock S, Gorkow Ch, Loew D (1995) Prolaktinsekretion und Verträglichkeit unter der Behandlung mit einem Agnus-castus-Spezialextrakt (B1095E1). Erste Ergebnisse zum Einfluß auf die Prolaktinsekretion. In: Loew D, Rietbrock N (eds) Phytopharmaka in Forschung und klinischer Anwendung. Steinkopff Verlag, Darmstadt, pp 93–97.

Reuter HD, Böhnert KJ, Schmidt U (1995) Die Therapie des prämenstruellen Syndroms mit Vitex agnus castus. Kontrollierte Doppelblindstudie gegen Pyridoxin. Z Phytother Abstractband, p 7.

Schneider HPG, Bohnet HG (1981) Die hyperprolaktinämische Ovarialinsuffizienz. Gynäkologe 14: 104–118.

Schwabe U, Rabe T (1995) Gynäkologika. In: Schwabe U, Paffrath D (eds) Arzneiverordnungs-Report '95. Gustav Fischer Verlag, Stuttgart Jena, pp 228–235.

Sourgens H, Winterhoff H, Gumbinger HG, Kemper FH (1982) Antihormonal effects of plant extracts. THS- and prolactin-suppressing properties of Lithospermum officinale and other plants. Planta Med 45: 78–86.

Stoll W (1987) Phytotherapeutikum beeinflußt atrophisches Vaginalepithel: Doppelblindversuch Cimicifuga vs. Östrogenpräparat. Therapeutikum 1: 23–32.

Vorberg G (1984) Therapie klimakterischer Beschwerden. ZFA 60: 626–629.

Warnecke G (1985) Beeinflussung klimakterischer Beschwerden durch ein Phytotherapeutikum. Erfolgreiche Therapie mit Cimicifuga-Monoextrakt. Med Welt 36: 871–874.

Winterhoff H, Sourgens H, Kemper FH (1983) Pharmacodynamic effects of Lithospermum officinale on the thyroid gland of rats; comparison with the effects of iodide. Horm Metabol Res 15: 503–507.

Winterhoff H (1993) Arzneipflanzen mit endokriner Wirksamkeit. Z Phytother 14: 83–94.

Wuttke W, Gorkow Ch, Jarry J (1995) Dopaminergic compounds in Vitex agnus castus. In: Loew D, Rietbrock N (eds) Phytopharmaka in Forschung und klinischer Anwendung. Steinkopff Verlag, Darmstadt, pp 81–91.

8 Skin and Connective Tissues

This chapter deals first with plant drugs that are commonly used for dermatologic indications (local inflammations, eczema, neurodermatitis, acne, wound healing problems). A separate section deals with herbal remedies that are used externally or in some cases internally for the treatment of trauma and its sequelae (bruises, contusions, hematomas, fracture edema) and rheumatic complaints. The chapter concludes with a look at the potential uses of externally applied herbal preparations in the treatment of pain. Given the medical and economic importance of analgesic remedies, it is important to give due attention to possible phytotherapeutic alternatives.

8.1
Dosage Forms and Preparations

Every medication consists of the active drug and one or more excipients or diluting agents to give the drug a suitable form (see Sect. 1.4). With remedies for external use, the action of the medication depends much more on the vehicle than in the case of orally administered drugs. First, the vehicle may produce a marked effect of its own (cooling, drying, moisturizing, occluding) that contributes more to the overall effect of the medication than the drug substance itself. Second, the percutaneous absorption of the drug substance depends critically on the nature of the vehicle (Fig. 8.1).

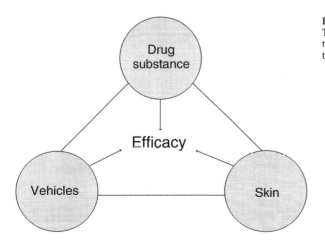

Fig. 8.1.
The efficacy of medications for topical use does not depend on the drug substance alone.

For example, petroleum jelly produces a strong occlusive effect that promotes absorption by increasing the degree of hydration of the epidermis. Other vehicles such as powders or detergents that draw moisture from the stratum corneum tend to retard penetration. Ethanol is a penetration enhancer, explaining why, for example, tincture of arnica has a much greater allergenicity than arnica cream.

As noted above, the vehicle can greatly affect the moisture content of the stratum corneum. Because of these intrinsic physicochemical actions, dermatologic agents should be administered in a base that is appropriate for the patient's skin type and for the particular stage of a skin disease. The basic rule is that formulations with a high water content, which have a cooling and drying action, are indicated for oily skin and acute inflammatory conditions, whereas fatty occlusive bases should be used for treating chronic or subcutaneous skin disorders (Fig. 8.2).

An important aspect in the treatment of inflammatory skin diseases is to protect the skin from external injury or irritation. This applies particularly to the various eczematous diseases, all of which, regardless of etiology, cause progressive damage to the stratum corneum. As the protective function of the epidermis is lost, the skin becomes increasingly susceptible to irritation. Demulcents and protectants serve to protect the skin, especially of the hands, from chemical agents and soap solutions. Plant oils, usually mixed with petroleum jelly or lanolin to form a fatty cream, are suitable for this purpose. Protection from organic solvents is afforded by botanically derived film-forming agents such as tragacanth and alginates.

It is beyond our scope to discuss the types of protective skin ointments that are recommended for different types of eczema or for individuals engaged in specific occupations. One example is palliative ointment, an ointment base with a creamy consistency and an excellent cooling action, an effective protectant and demulcent, and an excellent base for dermatologic formulations, especially those containing zinc oxide paste. Reportedly, its cooling action results from a change in the original w/o emulsion of the ointment to an o/w emulsion when the ointment is rubbed onto the skin. The pallia-

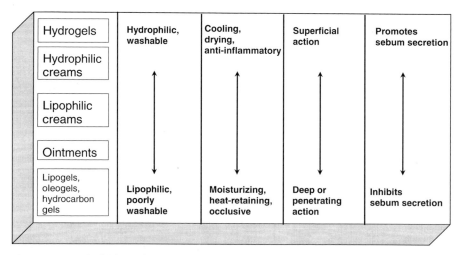

Fig. 8.2. Types of vehicles and excipients used in topical medications (after Beck, 1991).

Table 8.1. Galenic dosage forms for externally applied herbal remedies (modified from Stüttgen and Schaefer, 1974).

Dosage form	Brief characteristics
Moist compresses (moisture must be able to evaporate)	Fresh or distilled water containing plant extract; compress may be soaked in an infusion or decoction, or herb may be applied directly.
Tinctures	Herbal extract in an ethanol and water mixture (e.g., 30/70 to 70/30).
Hydrogels	Smearable, transparent preparation with a high water content and virtually free of fat and fatty substances.
Hydrophilic creams	Nontransparent preparations, smearable at room temperature, composed of fats or fatty bases and water and usually stabilized by the addition of emulsifiers. Type: oil in water emulsion. Cooling cream (vanishing cream) exerts a rapid cooling action.
Lipophilic creams	Creams of the water in oil type, so-called cold creams, exert a slow cooling action, are less drying.
Ointments	Smearable preparations, practically water free and often difficult to distinguish from lipogels.
Lipogels	Water-free gels with fatty or fatlike bases (hydrocarbons, waxes).
Pastes	Smearable preparations with a high content of suspended powder. Lipophilic pastes based on fat-containing ointments are distinguished from hydrophilic pastes based on hydrophilic cream bases or inorganic hydrogels.
Poultices	Usually hydrophilic pastes to which powdered herb or herbal extracts are added.
Lotion (applied with a brush)	Solid phase (powder) in an aqueous phase ("shaken mixture") or oily phase in an aqueous phase ("milk"). Useful for subacute inflammations with little exudation, also for extensive pruritus.

tive ointment described in the German Pharmacopeia 10 consists of yellow wax (7.0), cetyl palmitate (8.0), peanut oil (60.0), and purified water (35.0). Nowadays the semisynthetic compound cetyl palmitate is used instead of spermaceti, but the latter could also be replaced by the herbal product jojoba wax. Liquid jojoba wax is a clear, pale yellow, oily liquid that is expressed from the ripe seeds of the jojoba shrub *Simmondsia chinensis,* family Buxaceae; its properties are very similar to those of spermaceti.

The galenic dosage forms for external herbal applications (Table 8.1) are basically the same as those used in synthetic drug products for topical use. This chapter also deals with several plant drugs that are administered orally (medicinal yeast, pineapple [bromelain], devil's claw and European aspen preparations). These botanicals have been rated somewhat negatively in terms of their content of active ingredients, their absorption, or their efficacy.

8.2
Inflammations and Injuries of the Skin

Several dermatologic products contain active ingredients of plant origin that today can be isolated as pure compounds or produced synthetically in a modified form. These include compounds such as β-carotene, chrysarobin, anthralin, methoxsalen, and salicylates, which by definition are outside the bounds of phytotherapy (Chap. 1).

Of the approximately 300 medicinal herbs and herbal products that have been officially evaluated by Commission E, 47 are for dermatologic indications. The Commission has given a positive rating to 25 of these herbs, but only about half of the 25 play a significant role in therapeutic practice. The principal herbs and herbal preparations that are used topically for dermatologic indications are reviewed in Table 8.2.

Seven herbs with traditional applications in dermatology were given a negative rating because of serious risks and side effects. These are hound's tongue (contains hepatotoxic pyrrolizidine alkaloids), walnut hulls (contain the potentially carcinogenic juglone), pulsatilla (can cause very severe skin irritation), bilberry and oleander leaves (toxic in high doses), and common periwinkle leaves (hematologic changes). These herbs and their preparations should no longer be used. Commission E has published neutral monographs on 15 other traditional herbs, stating that their efficacy is unproven due to a lack of scientific evidence. Additionally, there are herbs that have received a positive rating from the Commission but have gained little practical therapeutic importance. Recent survey works may be consulted for further information on dermatologic plant drugs, particularly herbs that are not covered in this chapter (Hormann and Korting, 1994; Mennet-von Eiff and Meier, 1995; Willuhn, 1995).

Table 8.2. Important herbs and herbal preparations for external use, shown with year of publication of the Commission E monograph and the indications stated therein.

Monograph, source plant	Year*	Dermatologic indications
Chamomile (*Matricariae* flos)	1984	Skin and mucosal inflammations and bacterial skin diseases; diseases involving the anal and genital region (baths and douches)
Witch hazel leaves and bark (*Hamamelidis* folium et cortex)	1985	Mild skin injuries, local inflammations of the skin and mucous membranes; hemorrhoids, varicose veins
Podophyllin (*Podophyllum pelatum*)	–	For removal of pointed condylomata
Calendula flowers (*Calendulae* flos)	1986	Wounds, including poorly healing wounds; crural ulcers
Bittersweet (*Dulcamarae stipides*)	1990	Supportive treatment of chronic eczema
Purple coneflower (*Echinacea purpureae* herba)	1989	Poorly healing superficial wounds
St. John's wort oil (*Oleum hyperici*)	1984	Primary and secondary treatment of sharp and blunt injuries, myalgias, and 1st degree burns
Arnica flowers (*Arnicae* flos)	1984	Used externally for trauma-related conditions such as hematomas, sprains, bruises, contusions, fracture edema, and for rheumatic conditions of the muscles and joints
Comfrey, leaves, root (*Symphyti* herba/folium/radix)	1990	Bruises, strains, sprains.

* Monographs published in the *Bundesanzeiger*.

8.2.1
Chamomile Flowers

Used medicinally since ancient times, chamomile flowers were mentioned in the works of Hippocrates, Dioscorides, Galen, and Asclepius. Their use continued into the Middle Ages, and they are still considered to have therapeutic value today (Schilcher, 1987). A number of studies on the pharmacology of chamomile flowers, particularly their anti-inflammatory and antispasmodic properties, have been published in recent decades (Ammon and Kaul, 1992). By contrast, very few controlled therapeutic studies have been published on their clinical efficacy. The virtually un-questioned effectiveness of chamomile for a number of dermatologic indications is still based largely on empirical evidence, i.e., the experience of patients and physicians.

8.2.1.1
Crude Drug, Constituents, and Preparations

The genus *Matricaria* (family Asteraceae) includes several species of annual herba-ceous plants, most of which have numerous scientific synonyms. German chamomile (*Matricaria recutita* L., Fig. 8.3) is preferred in central Europe and the United States, while Roman chamomile derived from *Chamaemelum nobile,* which has larger flow-er heads, is increasingly used in other countries. Originally native to the Near East and eastern Europe, German chamomile now occurs throughout Europe, Australia, and North America. German chamomile is distinguished from the other chamo-miles, and especially from the unpalatable and allergenic dog chamomile *(Anthemis*

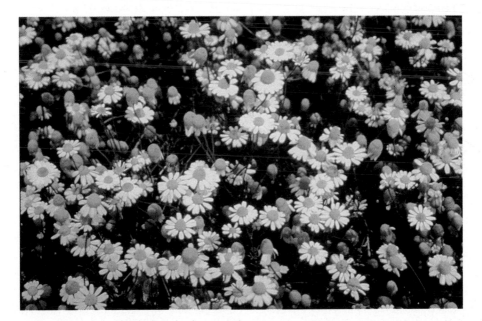

Fig. 8.3. German chamomile *(Matricaria recutita).*

cotula), by the conical receptacle on which the florets are arranged – it is hollow, not solid like that of the other chamomiles.

The active constituents of chamomile can be divided into two groups of compounds, one lipophilic and the other hydrophilic. The lipophilic group mainly includes the components of the volatile oil, whose content in the crude drug (dried flower heads) is 0.3–1.5%. The volatile oil, in turn, consists mainly (about 15%) of the dark blue chamazulene; the plant itself contains very little of this oil, most of which forms from its colorless precursor matricin during steam distillation. Another important component of chamomile oil is α-bisabolol, which is accompanied by its more oxygen-rich derivatives bisabololoxide A, B, and C. Different cultivated varieties of chamomile are characterized by different concentrations of the bisabolol derivatives (Mennet-von Eiff and Meier, 1995).

The most important hydrophilic constituents are flavonoids and mucilages. The total flavonoid content of the crude drug ranges from 1% to 3%. Experimental pharmacologic studies in isolated intestine indicate that the flavonoids, particularly apigenin, are chiefly responsible for the antispasmodic effects of chamomile preparations.

Today, chamomile flowers are obtained almost exclusively by cultivation of selected varieties. About 5000 tons are produced annually throughout the world, with an estimated 3000 tons being exported to Germany. The principal supplier is Argentina; Spain is one of several European countries that also grows chamomile. The German Pharmacopeia specifies that the crude drug must contain at least 0.4% volatile oil. It is used either in the form of aqueous preparations (chamomile tea: 1–2 teaspoons dried chamomile flowers in 200 mL boiling water, steeped for 10 min) or in the form of alcoholic extracts. The latter have a significantly higher content of the lipophilic constituents that have proven particularly active in pharmacologic models (Schilcher, 1987; Hänsel et al., 1992 a).

8.2.1.2
Pharmacology and Toxicology

Chamomile preparations are used mainly for their anti-inflammatory, antispasmodic, and carminative properties. Also, in vitro studies have demonstrated bacteriostatic and fungistatic actions that presumably contribute to the dermatologic uses of chamomile.

Anti-inflammatory effects have been demonstrated both for whole alcoholic extracts and for constituents isolated from them. The compounds have been tested in a number of standard pharmacologic models of inflammation (UV erythema, carrageenan-induced rat's paw edema, cotton-pellet granuloma, adjuvant arthritis in rats) using both topical and oral administration. Chamazulene, α-bisabolol, and flavones such as apigenin were the single components that were found to have the strongest anti-inflammatory properties, but most studies found that the whole extracts were more active than their individual components. The chamomile preparations and their isolated constituents acted mainly on the inflammatory mediators of the arachidonic acid cascade. They had an inhibitory effect on 5-lipoxygenase and cyclooxygenase.

Besides anti-inflammatory effects, alcoholic extracts of chamomile and isolated flavonoids have also exhibited antispasmodic properties in models such as the guinea pig intestine. When tested on spasms of isolated guinea pig ileum induced by barium chloride, 10 mg apigenin showed an antispasmodic potency roughly equivalent to that of 1 mg papaverine.

Chamomile preparations have also shown antibacterial and fungicidal activity, mainly against gram-positive organisms and *Candida albicans,* in microbial plate tests. Chamomile oil was active at concentrations of 25 mg/mL or higher, and bisabolol at concentrations of 1 mg/mL or higher. This could account for the positive therapeutic effects obtained with chamomile preparations applied topically to infected wounds, for example.

More information on the pharmacologic actions of chamomile and its preparations can be found in Schilcher (1987), Ammon and Kaul (1992), and Hänsel et al. (1992 a).

Experiments with chamomile oil in rabbits showed that the acute oral LD_{50} and acute dermal LD_{50} were greater than 5 g/kg, and the constituent α-bisabolol showed equally good tolerance (Jakovlev et al., 1983). There was no evidence of phototoxic effects, skin irritation, or allergenicity. Favorable findings such as these have prompted FDA approval of chamomile as a food additive in the United States. It therefore appears on the Generally Recognized as Safe (GRAS) list.

8.2.1.3
Therapeutic Efficacy
Chamomile preparations are used internally for inflammatory disorders and colicky gastrointestinal complaints (see Sect. 5.3), and they are administered by inhalation for inflammatory diseases and irritations of the respiratory tract (see Sect. 4.2). Chamomile preparations are also used to treat bacterial and nonbacterial inflammations of the skin, poorly healing wounds, abscesses, fistulae, and inflammations of the oral cavity and gums. Other indications are radiation-induced dermatitis and dermatologic conditions in children.

To date, specific evaluations of efficacy in the form of documented case reports, observational studies, and several controlled clinical trials have been based largely on one chamomile product, which has been marketed in Germany under the brand name Kamillosan since 1921. The case reports and studies have consistently shown positive results in the treatment of acute weeping skin disorders, decubitus ulcers, and dermatitis due to various causes (Schilcher, 1987).

Kamillosan has also been the subject of several controlled therapeutic studies (Albring et al., 1983; Aertgeerts et al., 1985; Nissen et al., 1988; Maiche et al., 1991; Korting et al., 1993). Though all these studies did not have a double-blind design with statistical analysis, most documented the therapeutic efficacy of a cream preparation of the standardized product in healthy subjects (cellophane tape stripping test) and in patients with contact dermatitis, various forms of eczema, and postirradiation dermatitis (survey in Hörmann and Korting, 1994).

8.2.1.4
Indications, Dosages, Side Effects, and Risks
The Commission E monograph of 1984 states that chamomile is indicated for "inflammations of the skin and mucous membranes and bacterial diseases involving the skin, oral cavity, or gums; also inflammatory diseases and irritations of the re-

spiratory tract (administered by inhalation) and diseases of the anogenital region (administered by bathing or douching)."

In a supplement to its 1990 monograph, the Commission gives these dosage recommendations: use a 3–10 % infusion for douches; as a bath additive, use 50 g of crude drug per 10 L of water; semisolid preparations should have a 3–10 % content of the crude drug.

No contraindications, side effects, or drug-drug interactions have been associated with chamomile. As for the risk of allergic reactions, Hausen et al. (1984) reviewed 50 scientific publications and concluded that contamination by dog chamomile (which contains the allergenic compound anthecotulide) could account for many cases of so-called chamomile allergy reported in the literature. Several true cases of sensitization by German chamomile have been documented, but the overall risk of allergy appears to be very low, especially with preparations made from specific varieties (e. g., Degumille) (Schilcher, 1987; Hörmann and Korting, 1994).

8.2.2
Witch Hazel and Other Tannin-Containing Herbs

Witch hazel (*Hamamelis virginiana*, Fig. 8.4) is a deciduous shrub or small tree that usually grows to 2–3 m and rarely may reach 7 m. Originally native to eastern North America, witch hazel was introduced to England in 1736 and since then has become a popular winter-flowering shrub in parks and gardens of central Europe. The leaves, bark, and twigs are processed to make the crude drug. The bark is particularly rich in tannins (hamamelitannin, gallotannins), containing up to 12 %.

Tannins have strong astringent properties. Applied topically to broken skin or mucous membranes, they induce a protein precipitation that tightens up superficial cell layers and shrinks colloidal structures, causing capillary vasoconstriction (hemostyptic action). The decrease in vascular permeability is tantamount to a local anti-inflammatory effect. The tightening (astringent) action on the tissues deprives bacteria of a favorable growth medium, producing an indirect antibacterial effect. Tannins also have a mild topical anesthetic action that soothes pain and itching. A number of other tannin-containing herbs besides witch hazel are used in the treatment of diarrhea and other ailments that respond to astringent medications (see Sect. 5.5.1 and Table 5.4). The usual preparations for external use (Table 8.1) have a yellow or brown color due to the presence of the tannins. The higher the tannin content, the darker the coloration. This may be why most witch hazel products are based on a distilled extract (hamamelis water) made by soaking the crude drug in water for about 24 h, then distilling the maceration and adding ethanol to the distillate. Unfortunately, these distillates contain almost no active tannins (Hänsel et al., 1993 a). Their astringency is generally attributed to the added ethanol.

Surprisingly, however, preparations made from hamamelis water were found to shorten bleeding time and induce vasoconstriction when tested in rabbits.

In two randomized double-blind studies, a hamamelis distillate cream significantly inhibited the development of erythema induced on the skin of the back by UV irradiation and cellophane tape stripping in two groups of 24 healthy subjects (Korting et al., 1993).

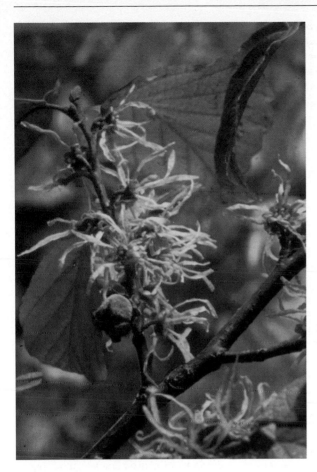

Fig. 8.4.
Inflorescence of witch hazel
(Hamamelis virginiana).

The same preparation was found to reduce inflammation and cutaneous hyper-emia in 22 healthy subjects and 5 patients with atopic neurodermatitis (Sorkin, 1980). Another randomized double-blind study compared hamamelis ointment with a glucocorticoid ointment in 22 patients with neurodermatitis. After three weeks' treatment, both ointments produced a significant (at least 50 %) improvement in cutaneous symptoms.

A common indication for hamamelis extracts and other preparations made from tannin-containing herbs is stage I or stage II hemorrhoidal disease. The efficacy of a combination product with a high content (10 %) of hamamelis bark extract (an ointment with the brand name Eulatin) was tested in two controlled clinical trials in 75 patients and 90 patients with stage I hemorrhoidal disease. A three-week course of therapy led to dramatic improvement in typical symptoms (bleeding, soreness, itching, burning) in 70–90 % of the patients. The potency of the hamamelis ointment was comparable to that of a corticoid ointment also tested in the double-blind studies (Knoch, 1991; Knoch et al., 1992).

The 1985 Commission E monograph with its 1990 supplement states the following indications for preparations made from hamamelis leaves, bark, and twigs: "mild skin injuries, local inflammations of the skin and mucous membranes, hemorrhoids, and complaints due to varicose veins." The recommended dosage is equivalent to 0.1–1.0 g of the crude drug applied topically to the skin and mucous membranes several times daily. No contraindications, side effects, or drug-drug interactions are known.

8.2.3
Evening Primrose Oil, Hypericum Oil, Podophyllin, Medicinal Yeast

Evening primrose (*Oenothera biennis*, family Onagraceae) is a biennial herb that grows to about 1 m. The plant is infertile for the first year, producing only a rosette of leaves close to the ground. During its second year, the plant bears seeds containing up to 25% of a fatty oil that is extracted with hexane for medicinal purposes. This extract contains 60–80% linoleic acid plus 8–14% γ-linolenic acid, an omega-6 fatty acid that is formed in the human body by the desaturation of linoleic acid. Reportedly, patients with neurodermatitis are deficient in the enzyme responsible for this conversion (Δ-6-desaturase), accounting for the therapeutic efficacy of evening primrose oil for that indication (Grimm, 1995).

Morse et al. (1989) performed a meta-analysis of four controlled parallel studies and five cross-over studies at various centers in which doctors and patients rated the efficacy of evening primrose oil in atopic eczema by scoring the degree of inflammation, dryness, scaliness, pruritus, and overall skin involvement. In the parallel studies, both the patient and doctor ratings showed a highly significant improvement in symptom scores relative to the placebo. Also, a positive correlation was noted between an improvement in clinical symptoms and a rise in the plasma levels of dihomo-γ-linolenic acid and arachidonic acid.

In Germany, capsules containing 0.5 g of evening primrose oil (corresponding to 40 mg γ-linolenic acid) have been approved for the treatment and symptomatic relief of atopic eczema. The adult dosage is 2–3 g of evening primrose oil daily. Occasional side effects are nausea, digestive upset, and headache (Hänsel et al., 1993b).

Hypericum oil is prepared by crushing the flowers of St. John's wort (*Hypericum perforatum*), placing them in olive oil (25:100 ratio), and steeping the herb in a warm place or letting it stand in sunlight for about 6 weeks until the oil acquires a reddish color. The exact composition of this "red oil" is unknown, but its ruddy color is caused not by the original hypericins but by naphthodianthrone compounds in the olive oil.

Hypericum oil is a traditional remedy for burns, and in former times, every village blacksmith kept a supply on hand for emergencies. The 1984 Commission E monograph on St. John's wort states that hypericum oil is used externally for the "secondary treatment of sharp and blunt injuries, myalgias, and first-degree burns." Today, however, the treatment of burns with a fatty oil is considered obsolete.

The antidepressant effects of alcoholic extracts of St. John's wort are discussed in Sect. 2.2.

Podophyllin, or podophyllum resin, is obtained from the rhizome and roots of the American mandrake *Podophyllum pelatum* (family Berberidaceae), a perennial plant native to the woodlands of eastern North America. The jointed and branched rhizome with attached roots is up to 1 m long and contains at least 4% resin with podophyllotoxin as the main constituent. Podophyllotoxin has a purgative action and is highly embryotoxic but nonteratogenic in experimental animals. The Commission E monograph of 1986 states that podophyllum resin is used externally for the removal of condylomata acuminata (venereal warts). It is applied locally once or twice a week in the form of a 5–25% alcoholic solution or equivalent ointment. The treated skin area should not exceed 25 cm², and adjacent skin areas should be carefully covered. There is evidence that preparations with a substantially lower concentration may be equally effective (Edwards et al., 1988).

Medicinal yeast consists of the fresh or dried cells of *Saccharomyces cerevisiae*, family Saccharomycetaceae. The Commission E monograph of 1988 states that medicinal yeast is approved as an adjunct in the treatment of chronic forms of acne and furunculosis when taken in an average daily dose of 6 g. Side effects consisting of migraine-like headache or flatulence may occur in susceptible individuals.

The use of live dried yeast as an antidiarrheal is discussed in Sect. 5.5.3.

8.2.4
Calendula Flowers, Echinacea, Dulcamara, Lemon Balm

Calendula flowers (*Calendula officinalis*, family Asteraceae are used in the form of an infusion, tincture, fluidextract, cold infused oil (calendula oil), or ointment to promote the granulation and facilitate healing of skin inflammations, wounds, burns, or eczema. Experiments in various wound models have demonstrated significant wound-healing properties, especially for a hydroalcoholic extract of the herb. The active principle that promotes wound healing has not been identified. One hypothesis is that this action is based on synergistic effects of the volatile oil and the relatively high concentrations of xanthophylls that are present in the herb.

The Commission E monograph of 1986 states that calendula flower preparations are used internally for inflammatory conditions of the oral and pharyngeal mucosa and externally for crural ulcers and for wounds with a poor healing tendency. The recommended dosage for internal use is 1–2 g of the dried herb. An ointment utilizing 2–5 g of the dried herb in 100 g of a suitable base is applied externally. No contraindications, side effects, or drug-drug interactions are known.

Isaac (1992) may be consulted for a comprehensive review of the pharmacy, pharmacology, and therapeutic use of calendula flower preparations.

Echinacea (coneflower) is an herbaceous plant of the family Asteraceae originally native to North America, where American Indians used the herb for a wide variety of conditions ranging from snakebite to infected wounds. A German settler, Dr. H. C. F. Meyer, used this indian herb in 1871 to produce the first commercial echinacea product. By the early 1900's, the herb was known in Europe as well. The original species (*Echinacea angustifolia* and *E. pallida*) were not grown in Europe, but the common purple coneflower *(E. purpurea)* was cultivated instead and used in various pharmaceutical products. According to the Commission E monograph of 1996, semi-solid preparations containing at least 15 % of the juice expressed from the aerial parts of the common purple coneflower are applied locally for the treatment of superficial, poorly healing wounds. Both the external use of echinacea and its internal use as an immune stimulant (Sect. 9.2) are contraindicated by progressive systemic diseases such as tuberculosis, leukoses, collagen disorders, and multiple sclerosis. Also, Commission E recommends the duration of use be limited to a maximum of eight weeks.

Dulcamara (bittersweet stem) is derived from the stems of the common nightshade (*Solanum dulcamara,* family Solanaceae) gathered in the spring and late fall after the plant has shed its leaves. Extracts of the herb contain steroidal saponins, which showed cortisone-like actions in experimental animals (Frohne, 1992). A multicenter clinical trial showed marked symptom relief in patients with chronic eczema and pruritic skin conditions (Hölzer, 1992). The 1990 Commission E monograph states that dulcamara is indicated for the "supportive treatment of chronic eczema." The recommended oral dose is 1–3 g of the dried herb daily. The monograph does not give specific dosage recommendations for the topical use of dulcamara in ointment form, and it mentions no known side effects or drug-drug interactions.

Lemon balm leaves (*Melissa officinalis,* family Lamiaceae) exhibited powerful virostatic properties in a study of tissue cultures treated with aqueous extracts from 178 medicinal plants (May and Willuhn, 1978). The active principle was thought to consist of tannins unique to the Lamiaceae. Based on these investigations, a cream was prepared from a balm leaf extract and tested in patients with herpes simplex (Vogt et al., 1991). The 1984 Commission E monograph on balm leaves and its 1990 supplement do not name herpes simplex as an indication, however.

8.3
Post-traumatic and Postoperative Conditions

Mild injuries sustained as a result of blunt trauma (bruises, contusions, strains, sprains) are associated with neurovascular injuries, hematomas, and edema leading in turn to painful limitations of motion. Physical therapy consists of immobilizing and elevating the injured part and may include the use of cold packs. Analgesics and anti-inflammatory agents may also be administered for swelling and inflammation. Two medicinal herbs – arnica and comfrey – have a long tradition in European folk medicine for external use in the treatment of injuries. Crude bromelain (from pineapple fruitstalk) and other herbal enzyme preparations are taken internally and are used mainly for the treatment of postoperative swelling.

8.3.1
Arnica

Arnica flowers are obtained from *Arnica montana* of the family Asteraceae (Fig. 8.5), an herbaceous perennial growing to 30–60 cm that is native to mountainous regions of Europe. Its large, orange flowers bloom from June to August. According to the

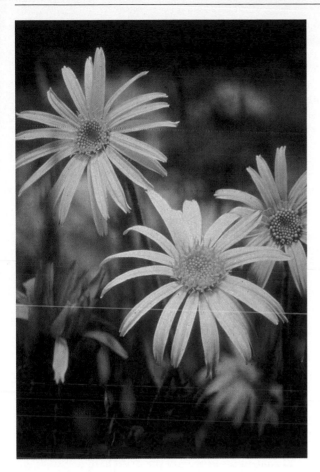

Fig. 8.5.
Arnica *(Arnica montana).*

1996 German Pharmacopeia, the flowers of *A. chamissonis* (subsp. *foliosa*) can be used in place of *A. montana* which is protected and cannot be cultivated. The crude drug contains 0.2–0.3% volatile oil. The constituents of arnica include helenalin and other sesquiterpene lactones that may be the active principles. The herb also contains about 0.4–0.6% flavones. Arnica has traditionally been used in the form of tinctures, particularly for external application. Several arnica-based ointments are currently marketed in Germany (see Sect. 8.5).

Experimental studies on the effects of arnica preparations have demonstrated antimicrobial, anti-inflammatory, respiratory-stimulant, positive inotropic, and tonus-increasing (uterus) actions. The therapeutically important anti-inflammatory effects of arnica preparations are attributed to helenalin, whose actions include a marked antiedemic effect that has been confirmed in experimental models (carrageenan-induced paw edema and adjuvant arthritis in rats). The external use of arnica preparations can cause contact dermatitis in individuals sensitized by sesquiterpenes of the helenalin type. The allergenic potential of arnica products depends both on the helenalin concentration and on the vehicle. The pharmacology and toxicology of arnica preparations have been reviewed by Hänsel et al. (1992b) and by Hörmann and Korting (1995). Today, arnica preparations are regarded somewhat critically in terms of their risk-to-benefit ratio (Hörmann and Korting, 1994).

The 1984 Commission E monograph states that arnica flower preparations are indicated for external use in the treatment of post-traumatic and postoperative conditions such as hematomas, sprains, bruises, contusions, fracture-related edema, and rheumatic ailments of the muscles and joints. Other indications are oropharyngeal inflammations, furunculosis, insect bites and stings, and superficial phlebitis. Allergy to arnica contraindicates its use. Edematous dermatoses and eczema may occur as side effects with long-term usage. Tinctures for compresses should be used in a 3:1 to 10:1 dilution, and ointments should contain a maximum of 20–25% tincture or 15% arnica oil.

Note: Internal use of the drug is not advised. The effects of arnica on the respiratory center, heart, and uterus have not been sufficiently tested to justify the risks associated with oral use. A fatal case of poisoning has been reported following the ingestion of 70 g arnica tincture.

8.3.2
Comfrey

Comfrey (*Symphytum officinale,* family Boraginaceae) is an indigenous European herbaceous plant growing to 50–100 cm with rough, hairy leaves and large purple-red flowers. The leaves and roots have a high mucilage content and also contain allantoin (up to 1.5% in the root). The mucilages have local demulcent properties, while allantoin promotes wound healing and accelerates the regeneration of cells. The 1990 Commission E monograph states that the aerial parts and roots are indicated for the treatment of bruises, strains, and sprains. Ointments or other preparations for external use only should contain up to 20% of the dried herb or equivalent amounts of extract. Comfrey contains unsaturated pyrrolizidine alkaloids, which have shown hepatotoxic, carcinogenic, and mutagenic properties in rats. Internal consumption of the herb has also been shown to induce veno-occlusive disease in humans. Thus, the monograph cautions against the external use of more than 1 mg of pyrrolizidine alkaloids daily or similar use of the herb for more than 4–6 weeks per year. If the pyrrolizidine alkaloid content of a product is not standardized or stated, it is best not to use comfrey or any other pyrrolizidine alkaloid-containing herbs (Michler and Arnold, 1996).

8.3.3
Bromelain

Crude bromelain is a mixture of proteolytic enzymes derived from the pineapple plant (*Ananas comosus,* family Bromeliaceae) and especially from the fruiting stems. Although it is widely believed that high-molecular-weight proteins must be broken down before they can be absorbed from the gastrointestinal tract, there is evidence that a certain percentage of orally administered bromelain enters the lymph and bloodstream unchanged in rats, dogs, and human beings (Seifert, 1983; Steffen and Menzel, 1983). The absorption rate in rats is approximately 50%. No data are yet available on the absolute bioavailability of bromelain in humans.

Orally administered bromelain has displayed anti-inflammatory and antiexudative actions in experimental models (rat's paw edema). Studies in rabbits and humans have shown a prolongation of prothrombin time and bleeding time (Hänsel et al., 1992 c). In 1993, Commission E reviewed a total of nine controlled clinical studies performed in patients with post-traumatic and postoperative edema. Of the five studies that could be statistically evaluated, three yielded a positive result and two a negative result. The Commission concluded that therapeutic efficacy had been satisfactorily established for "acute postoperative and post-traumatic swelling, especially of the nose and paranasal sinuses." The recommended daily dose is 80–320 mg bromelain taken in 2 or 3 divided doses. The duration of use generally should not exceed 8–10 days.

Hypersensitivity to bromelain is noted as a contraindication; side effects consist of gastric upset, diarrhea, and occasional allergic reactions. Bromelain may potentiate the effects of anticoagulants and platelet aggregation inhibitors.

8.4
Inflammatory and Degenerative Joint Diseases

8.4.1
Devil's Claw

Devil's claw (Harpagophytum procumbens) is a native South African plant of the family Pedaliaceae. The peripheral tubers of the plant grow up to 3 cm thick and 20 cm long and form the raw material for the crude drug. The tubers are chopped and dried in the sun for about three days. Natives used the herb as a bitter tonic (bitterness value 6000, see Sect. 5.1.2), antipyretic, and analgesic. Several iridoid glycosides occur in devil's claw, most notably the key active principle harpagoside, whose content in the crude drug is 0.5–1.6%.

Eight studies have been published to date on the pharmacologic actions of devil's claw. Both the herb and its constituent harpagoside exhibit anti-inflammatory and antiexudative activity. Most tests have been done in standard inflammation models in rats, and most have demonstrated anti-inflammatory effects, though some results are contradictory.

A total of 12 clinical reports have been published on efficacy in patients with rheumatoid and degenerative joint diseases, but only one study had a double-blind, placebo-controlled design. Eighty-nine patients with rheumatoid complaints received 2 g of the powdered herb daily for 2 months. The key criteria were sensitivity to pain (scored on a 0–10 scale) and the fingertip-floor distance (measured in cm). Both parameters showed significant improvement relative to the placebo when evaluated at 30 and 60 days.

The pharmacology and clinical aspects of devil's claw therapy are reviewed by Hänsel et al. (1993 d) and by Wenzel and Wegener (1995).

The Commission E monograph states that devil's claw is indicated for anorexia, dyspepsia (bitter!), and for the supportive treatment of degenerative musculoskeletal disorders. Gastric and duodenal ulcers are noted as contraindications. A daily dose of 1.5 g of the crude drug is recommended for anorexia and 4.5 g for joint ailments.

8.4.2
Aspen, Ash, Willow

The leaves and bark of the European aspen (*Populus tremula*, family Salicaceae), like ash and willow bark, contain salicylates. Extracts from European aspen leaves and bark exhibit anti-inflammatory effects in numerous experimental models. The only published clinical studies deal with a combination product (brand name Phytodolor) that contains extracts from goldenrod and ash bark as additional active ingredients. The manufacturer claims that 30 studies on this product have been carried out on a total of 1151 patients with rheumatoid and degenerative joint diseases. But due to methodologic deficiencies and uncertainty as to the contributions made by specific active components, Commission E discounted the therapeutic efficacy of European aspen bark in its 1992 monograph. Commission E has not evaluated the combination product in a separate monograph, and a critical meta-analysis of the therapeutic studies has not been published.

The analgesic and anti-inflammatory effects of willow bark are discussed in Sect. 4.2.1.4.

8.5
Transdermal Pain Relief

The practice of rubbing essential oils and rubefacients into the skin to relieve pain is deeply rooted in folk medicine. Conifer oils, camphor, wintergreen oil, and rubbing alcohol are commonly used for this purpose (see Sect. 8.6). Given the lack of controlled therapeutic studies on these preparations, it was assumed that all these agents had a similar mechanism of action, i.e., soothed pain by the counterirritation of organ-associated skin areas (Head's zones) via the corresponding spinal neurons.

In recent years, however, a number of controlled double-blind studies have been performed in healthy subjects and in patients to investigate the mechanisms of action and efficacy of peppermint oil and eucalyptus oil. These studies indicate that the external treatment of pain with essential oils is a more complex phenomenon than was originally assumed. A double-blind cross-over study using an experimental pain model in 15 healthy subjects has shown that the analgesic action of peppermint oil is apparently based on central inhibitory effects mediated by cold-sensitive A-Δ-nerve fibers (Bromm et al., 1995). Another placebo-controlled double-blind study investigated the effects of peppermint and eucalyptus oil preparations on neurophysiologic, psychologic, and experimental algesimetric parameters in 32 healthy subjects. Four different test preparations were used. The agents were applied to a large skin area on the forehead and temples using a small dose-metering sponge. It was found that peppermint oil in ethanol had a significant effect on sensitivity to pain (experi-

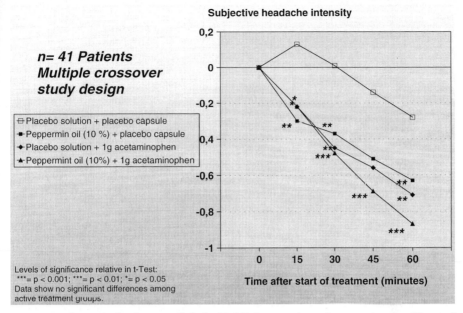

Subjective headache intensity

n= 41 Patients
Multiple crossover
study design

⊟ Placebo solution + placebo capsule
■ Peppermin oil (10 %) + placebo capsule
◆ Placebo solution + 1g acetaminophen
▲ Peppermint oil (10%) + 1g acetaminophen

Levels of significance relative in t-Test:
***= p < 0.001; ***= p < 0.01; *= p < 0.05
Data show no significant differences among
active treatment groups.

Time after start of treatment (minutes)

Fig. 8.6. Randomized, placebo-controlled, double-blind, crossover study comparing the efficacy of 10 % peppermint oil in ethanol solution, 1 g acetaminophen, and a placebo in 41 patients with tension headache. External treatment with the peppermint oil preparation proved as effective as acetaminophen (Göbel et al., 1995).

mentally induced by ischemia and heat), whereas eucalyptus oil did not (Göbel et al., 1994, 1995).

A placebo-controlled double-blind study was performed in 41 patients suffering from chronic tension headaches (most common form of headache, with a lifetime prevalence of about 30 % of the population). The headache episodes were treated according to a randomly assigned sequence using a double-blind format. Each episode was treated by giving the patient two capsules of an oral medication (1 g acetaminophen or placebo) and by the cutaneous application of 10 % peppermint oil in ethanol solution or small amounts of a placebo solution labeled as peppermint oil. The solution was applied to a large skin area on the forehead and temples; the application was then repeated at 15 min and again at 30 min. Compared with the placebo, the 10 % peppermint oil preparation produced a significant reduction in clinical headache intensity after just 15 min. Acetaminophen also proved effective relative to the placebo but did not differ significantly from treatment with 10 % peppermint oil (Fig. 8.6). This led the authors to conclude that peppermint oil is an acceptable and cost-effective alternative to oral analgesics in the treatment of tension headache (Göbel et al., 1995 c).

8.6
Formulations

Recurrent Herpes Simplex
Virtually all agents with a protein-coagulating and astringent action can improve the symptoms of a herpes lesion. Thus, claims such as "eau de cologne works wonders for fever blisters" (Medical Tribune of 24 Jan 1992) are entirely plausible. Eau de cologne consists of 90 % alcohol.

Rx   Eau de cologne   30.0 mL
      Directions: Dab externally onto affected area.

Alternative:

Rx   Ethanol 90 %   30.0
      Citronella oil   1 drop
      Directions: Dab externally onto affected area.

Noninfectious Dermatitis
Applied to acutely inflamed areas and small wounds, astringents tighten and dry the superficial cell layers, forming a protective barrier against bacterial invasion and soothing inflammatory symptoms. Herbal astringents contain tannins as their active principle (see Table 5.4).

Sample formula for acute eczema:

Rx   Tannic acid   1.0 (to 3.0)
      Purified water to   100.0
      Directions: Use externally; dilute with water and apply as a compress.

The following formula can be used in sitz baths for hemorrhoidal diseases and for anogenital fissures and erosions:

Rx   Tannic acid   5.0
      Glycerol to   100.0
      Directions: Use externally; dilute 1:10 with water.

Protective and Cooling Ointment
Jojoba wax, a plant product, can be used in place of spermaceti, which is no longer available. The wax is a clear, pale yellow, oily fluid expressed from ripe seeds of the jojoba shrub *(Simmondsia chinensis)*. A modified protective and cooling ointment to replace the older soothing ointment described in the German Pharmacopeia 10 can be formulated as follows:

Rx   Yellow wax   3.5
      Jojoba wax (liquid)   4.0
      Peanut oil   30.0
      Purified water to   50.0
      Mix and use externally.

Pain and Spasms
Rubbing alcohol, known in Germany as *Franzbranntwein*, was formerly a byproduct of cognac production and is now made by mixing diluted alcohol with essential oils

or aromatic tinctures. It has multiple uses in the treatment of muscle pain and spasms. An old pharmaceutical formula is given below:

Rx	Aromatic tincture	0.4
	Ethyl Nitrite Spirit	0.5
	Rhatany tincture	6 drops
	Ethanol (90 vol.%)	100.0
	Distilled water to	200.0

The rhatany tincture gives the product a cognac color. Modern products that are marketed under the name *Franzbranntwein* may be green or colorless. They usually contain juniper-berry oil, spruce-needle oil, dwarf-pine oil, menthol, camphor, and thymol. Both the essential oils and the alcohol have a rubefacient (hyperemia-inducing) action: alcohol in concentrations higher than 50 % causes mild skin irritation and acts as an antiseptic. Rubbing alcohol is rubbed into the skin to induce local hyperemia for muscle and joint pain, muscle soreness, strains, or bruises; it is also used in sports medicine and for connective-tissue massage. German rubbing alcohol is sold in various strengths (38–45 % v/v) and may be pure or blended with camphor or spruce-needle oil. In the United States, rubbing alcohol consists of denatured 70 % ethanol or 70 % isopropanol.

8.7
Drug Products

Herbal remedies used for the dermatologic indications in this chapter are subdivided in the *Rote Liste* into three different groups of indications: "Analgesics and Antirheumatics," "Anti-inflammatory Agents," and "Dermatologic Agents." Because the indications overlap, some chamomile preparations in the *Rote Liste* are placed under the heading of "Gastrointestinal Remedies."

References

Aertgeerts P, Albring M, Klaschka F, Nasemann T, Patzelt-Wenczler R, Rauhut K, Weigl B (1985) Vergleichende Prüfung von Kamillosan® Creme gegenüber steroidalen (0,25 % Hydrocortison, 0.75 % Fluocortinbutylester) und nichtsteroidalen (5 % Bufexamac) Externa in der Erhaltungstherapie von Ekzemerkrankungen. Z Hautkr 60: 270–277.
Albring M, Albrecht H, Alcorn G, Lücker PW (1983) The measuring of the anti-inflammatory effect of a compound of the skin of volunteers. Meth Find Exp Clin Pharmacol 5: 75–77.
Ammon HPT, Kaul R (1992) Pharmakologie der Kamille und ihrer Inhaltsstoffe. Dtsch Apoth Z 132 (Suppl 27): 3–26.
Beck P (1991) Identifizierung und Charakterisierung von Salben- und Gelgrundlagen, Pharm Z Wiss 136: 187–195.
Bromm B, Scharein E, Darsow U, Ring J (1995) Effects of menthol and cold on histamine-induced itch and skin reactions in man. Neurosci Lett 187:157–160.
Edwards A, Atma-Ram A, Thin RN (1988) Podophyllotoxin 0.5 % vs. podophyllin 20 % to treat penile warts. Genetnourin Med 64: 263–265.
Frohne D (1992) Solanum dulcamara L. – Der Bittersüße Nachtschatten. Portrait einer Arzneipflanze. Z Phytother 14: 337–342.
Göbel H, Schmidt G, Soyka D (1994) Effect of peppermint and eucalyptus oil preparations on neurophysiological and experimental algesimetric headache parameters. Cephalalgia 14: 228–234.
Göbel H, Schmidt G (1995a) Effekt von Pfefferminz- und Eukalyptusölpräparationen in experimentellen Kopfschmerzmodellen. Z Phytother 16: 23–33.

Göbel H, Schmidt G, Dworschak M, Stolze H, Heuss D (eds) (1995b) Essential plant oils and headache mechanisms. Phytomedicine 2: 93–102.

Göbel H, Stolze H, Dworschak M, Heinze A (1995c) Oelum menthae piperitae: Wirkmechanismen und klinische Effektivität bei Kopfschmerz vom Spannungstyp. In: Loew D, Rietbrock N (eds) Phytopharmaka in Forschung und klinischer Anwendung. Steinkopff Verlag, Darmstadt, pp 177–184.

Grimm P (1995) Neurodermitis: Was bewirkt Gamma-Linolensäure? Apoth J 17: 33–36.

Hänsel R, Keller K, Rimpler H, Schneider G (eds) (1992) Hagers Handbuch der pharmazeutischen Praxis. 5th ed., Vol. 4, Drogen A–D.Springer Verlag, Berlin Heidelberg New York, pp 817–831 (a); 342–357 (b); 272–280 (c).

Hänsel R, Keller K, Rimpler H, Schneider G (eds) (1993) Hagers Handbuch der pharmazeutischen Praxis. 5th ed., Vol. 5, Drogen E–O.Springer Verlag, Berlin Heidelberg New York, pp 367–384 (a); 929–936 (b); 476–479 (c); 384–390 (d).

Hausen HM, Busker E, Carle R (1984) Über das Sensibilisierungsvermögen von Compositenarten. VII. Experimentelle Untersuchungen mit Auszügen und Inhaltsstoffen von Chamomilla recutita L. Rauschert und Anthemis cotula L. Planta Med 50: 229–234.

Hölzer I (1992) Dulcamara-Extrakt bei Neurodermitis und chronischem Ekzem. Ergebnisse einer klinischen Prüfung. Jatros Dermatologie 6: 32–36.

Hörmann HP, Korting HC (1995) Allergic acute contact dermatitis due to arnica tincture self-medication. Phytomedicine 4: 315–317.

Hörmann HP, Korting HC (1994) Evidence for the efficacy and safety of topical herbal drugs in dermatology: Part 1: Anti-inflammatory agents. Phytomedicine 1: 161–171.

Isaac O (1992) Die Ringelblume. Botanik, Chemie, Pharmakologie, Toxikologie, Pharmazie und therapeutische Verwendung. Wissenschaftliche Verlagsgesellschaft mbH, Stuttgart.

Jakovlev V, Isaac O, Flaskamp E (1983) Pharmakologische Untersuchungen von Kamillen-lnhaltsstoffen. VI. Untersuchungen zur antiphlogistischen Wirkung von Chamazulen und Matricin. Planta Med 49: 67–73.

Knoch HG (1991) Hämorrhoiden 1. Grades: Wirksamkeit einer Salbe auf pflanzlicher Basis. Münch Med Wschr 31/32: 481–484.

Knoch HG, Klug W, Hübner WD (1992) Salbenbehandlung von Hämorrhoiden ersten Grades. Wirksamkeitsvergleich eines Präparates auf pflanzlicher Grundlage mit zwei nur synthetische Wirkstoffe enthaltenen Salben. Fortschr Med 110: 135–138.

Korting HC, Schäfer-Korting M, Hart H, Laux P, Schmid M (1993) Anti-inflammatory activity of hamamelis distillate applied topically to the skin. Influence of vehicle and dose. Eur J Clin Pharmacol 44: 315–318.

Laux P, Oschmann R (1993) Die Zaubernuß – Hamamelis virginiana L. Z Phytother 14: 155–166.

Maiche AG, Gröhn P Mäki-Hokkonen H (1991) Effect of chamomile cream and almond ointment on acute radiation skin reaction. Acta Oncol 30: 395–396.

May S, Willuhn G (1978) Antivirale Wirkung wässriger Pflanzenextrakte in Gewebekulturen. Arzneim Forsch/Drug Res 28: 1–7.

Mennet-von Eiff M, Meier B (1995) Phytotherapie in der Dermatologie. Ninth Swiss Conference on Phytothreapy. Z Phytother 17: 201–210.

Michler B, Arnold CG (1996) Pyrrolizidinalkaloide in Beinwellwurzeln. Dtsch Apoth Z 136: 2447–2452.

Morse PF, Horrobin DF, Manku MS, Stewart JCM, Allen R, Littlewood S, Wright S, Burton J, Gould DJ, Holt PJ, Jansen CT, Mattilas L, Meigel W, Dettke TH, Wexler D, Guenther L, Bordoni A, Patrizi A (1989) Meta-analysis of placebo-controlled studies of the efficacy of Epogam in the treatment of atopic eczema. Relationship between plasma essential fatty acid changes and clinical response. Br J Dermatol 121: 75–90.

Nissen HP, Blitz H, Kreysel HW (1988) Profilometrie, eine Methode zur Beurteilung der therapeutischen Wirksamkeit von Kamillosan®-Salbe. Z Hautkr 63: 184–190.

Schilcher H (1987) Die Kamille. Handbuch für Ärzte, Apotheker und andere Naturwissenschaftler. Wissenschaftliche Verlagsgesellschaft mbH, Stuttgart.

Seifert J (1983) Resorption von Makromolekülen aus dem Magen-Darm-Trakt. In: Caspary WF (ed) Handbuch der Inneren Medizin, Vol. 111, Part 3, Dünndarm, pp 394–418.

Sorkin B (1980) Hametum-Salbe, eine kortikoidfreie antiinflammatorische Salbe. Phys Med Rehab 21: 53–57.

Steffen C, Menzel J (1983) Enzymabbau von Immunkomplexen. Z Rheumatol 42: 249–255.

Stüttgen G, Schaefer H (1974) Funktionelle Dermatologie, Springer, Berlin Heidelberg New York, pp 397–398.

Vogt HJ, Tausch 1, Wöbling RH, Kaiser PM (1991) Melissenextrakt bei Herpes simplex. Allgemeinarzt 14: 832–841.

Wenzel P, Wegener T (1995) Teufelskralle. Ein pflanzliches Antirheumatikum. Dtsch Apoth Z 135 (13): 1131–1144.

Willuhn G (1995) Phythopharmaka in der Dermatologie. Z Phytother 16: 325–342.

9 Agents that Increase Resistance to Diseases

Herbal remedies fit very naturally into the natural and holistic system of medicine. As a result, all physicians and laypersons do not appreciate the kind of compartmentalized, organ-based approach to herbal healing that is followed in this book. Indeed, there are two classes of herbal remedies that do not fit into an anatomically oriented scheme: adaptogens and immune stimulants. Adaptogens are agents that are reputed to increase the body's resistance to physical, chemical, and biological stressors. Immune stimulants are agents that activate the body's nonspecific defense mechanisms against infectious organisms, particularly viral and bacterial pathogens.

9.1
Adaptogens

The life of every human being is marked by periods of increased physical and psychological demands. Recurring stresses of this kind generally are not harmful and are even beneficial to health, provided they are within manageable limits. But the degree of tolerance for these stresses varies greatly from one individual to the next. Also, every individual is subject to a life cycle in which overall stress tolerance is maximal from about 20 to 30 years of age. It is estimated that, by age 70, stress tolerance is diminished by approximately one-half (Hofecker, 1987). Critical peak stresses that are handled easily by a healthy young person may become disruptive in one who is debilitated due to age or illness. Irritable stomach, gastric ulcer, and irritable colon are but a few of the secondary disorders that may arise as a result of these critical stresses.

Adaptation syndromes are observed not only in the everyday practice of medicine but also have been investigated in various animal models. Selye (1946) showed in his classic study that previous exposure to a stressor can increase resistance not just to that particular stressor but to other noxious agents as well. In rats, for example, it was found that prior exposure to various stressors such as heat, cold, exertion, or trauma prevented the inflammation of the cecum that was normally induced by the intravenous injection of histamine. Prior exposure to psychological stressors also made rats more resistant to challenges such as papain injection, which normally causes a fatal degree of myocardial necrosis (Bajusz and Selye, 1960).

Hormonal influences are considered to play a major role in the pathophysiology of adaptation diseases. For example, rats are normally immune to infection by Mycobacterium tuberculosis but become susceptible when treated with immunosuppressive doses of cortisone (20 mg/day). When somatotropic hormone (6 mg/day) was administered concurrently with the cortisone doses, the animals retained their immunity to *M. tuberculosis* infection (Schole et al., 1978). This led the authors to conclude that hormones like cortisone whose secretion is augmented by stressful stimuli can act synergistically with other hormones to maintain homeostasis when the levels of the stress-related hormones bear a specific relation to the concentrations of the other hormones.

A number of substances of microbiologic (Farrow et al., 1978; Kaemmerer and Kietzmann, 1983) or plant origin (Brekhman and Dradymov, 1969; Ciplea and Richter, 1988) have shown adaptogenic effects in experimental animals. Most of these effects were measured in live, healthy animals, and the differences relative to controls were significant only in animals that were exposed to various stresses. The antistress effect was nonspecific for the nature of the stress, i.e., the effect did not depend on whether the stress was an infection, a toxin, radiation, trauma, or was physical or psychological in nature. The underlying mechanism of this effect has not been elucidated in animals or in man. Following Selyes' line of reasoning, we may assume that such substances help the body cope with stressful situations by expanding the adaptation phase while delaying or preventing the exhaustion phase.

9.1.1
Ginseng

Ginseng root and its preparations have had an established place in the traditional healing arts of eastern Asia for more than 2000 years. Furthermore, ginseng has generated what may be the most extensive body of scientific literature ever published on a medicinal herb. Two survey works on ginseng cited and abstracted no fewer than 482 (Ploss, 1988) and 151 (Sonnenborn and Proppert, 1990) books and papers on the use of the herb.

9.1.1.1
Plant, Crude Drug, and Constituents

The species *Panax ginseng* is the source of Asian ginseng root (Fig. 9.1). Ginseng is native to Korea and China, growing at altitudes of about 1000 m, but today it is extremely rare in the wild. As demand for the plant increased (by consumers that included the Chinese imperial court), the first ginseng plantations were established some 800 years ago (Hyo-Won et al., 1987). Today the plant is cultivated in Korea, China, and eastern Siberia. *Panax ginseng* is a perennial herb (family Araliaceae) with fleshy, pale yellow, often multibranched roots that have an aromatic odor and a bittersweet taste. The plant takes about six years to mature, the stem reaching a height of 60–80 cm. Ginseng powders and extracts are made from the dried roots, which contain 2–3% glycosidal saponins known as ginsenosides. At least 18 ginsenosides have been chemically identified and given special designations (R followed by a subscript small letter and often a numeral as well, e.g., R_c, $R_{g\text{-}1}$). American ginseng *(Panax quinquefolius)* is cultivated in the United States. The entire crop is exported to China where it is very popular. Roots of the different species are distinguished by their different saponin patterns. Ginseng also contains about 0.05% volatile sub-

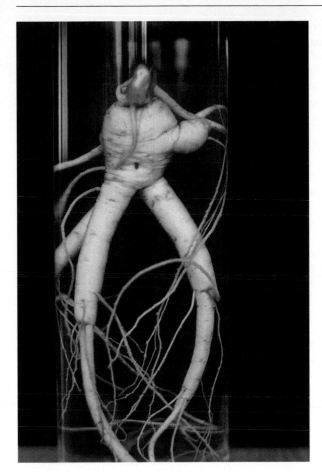

Fig. 9.1.
Ginseng root (from a plant approximately 6 years old).

stances that are soluble in ether (volatile oil) (Obermeier, 1980; Youn, 1987; Sonnenborn and Proppert, 1990). In the following sections, the discussion is limited to studies of Asian ginseng.

9.1.1.2
Pharmacology and Toxicology

Volumes have been written on the effects of ginseng extracts and ginseng saponins (ginsenosides). Among the effects demonstrated by animal experimentation are: CNS-stimulating effects; protective effects against various harmful agents such as ionizing radiation, infections, and toxins (lead salts, alloxan); protection from exhausting physical and psychological stresses; effects on carbohydrate and lipid metabolism and on RNA and protein biosynthesis; and immune-stimulating effects. It is difficult to draw any inferences from these studies regarding the efficacy of ginseng in humans. Neither the mode of administration (usually intraperitoneal) nor the dosage are comparable to ordinary ginseng usage in man. Ginseng extracts act on the human intestinal flora by promoting the growth of bifid bacteria while selectively inhibiting certain clostridial strains (Ahn et al., 1990). The anabolic (growth-promoting) effects observed in animal tests may also result from indirect effects of ginseng on the intestinal flora.

Acute toxicity studies were performed in mice and rats, and studies on acute to chronic toxicity (20–180 days) were conducted in rats, chickens, and dwarf pigs. Ginseng was tested for teratogenicity in pregnant rats and rabbits and for mutagenicity (carcinogenicity) in the Ames test. None of these studies showed any evidence of an increased toxicological risk (Ploss, 1988).

9.1.1.3
Clinical Studies in Humans

The results of a total of 37 clinical studies were published between 1968 and 1990, 22 during the period 1980–1985. Fifteen of the studies were controlled, and eight were double-blind. The studies covered a total of 2562 cases, including 973 healthy subjects (19 studies), 238 of whom were athletes, 943 geriatric patients (7 studies), 527 patients with various metabolic disorders (5 studies), and a total of 159 post-menopausal women (2 studies). The usual duration of treatment was 60–120 days. Powdered root preparations were administered in doses of 400–1200 mg/day and extract preparations in doses of 200–600 mg/day.

When the results of these studies were evaluated, it was found that subjects in 13 of the studies (1572 cases) showed improvements in mood while on treatment with the ginseng preparation. Seventeen studies (846 cases) also demonstrated improvements in physical performance. Improved intellectual performance was reported in 11 studies, and improvements in various metabolic parameters were noted in another 10 studies. All the studies emphasized the absence or near absence of side effects relating to ginseng therapy. There was only one reported instance of tachycardia. The results were statistically evaluated in only about half the studies. On the whole, it is unlikely that the design and conduct of these studies would conform to current scientific standards (study surveys in Ploss, 1988; Sonnenborn and Proppert, 1990).

9.1.1.4
Indications, Dosages, Risks, and Contraindications

The 1991 Commission E monograph on ginseng root states that the herb is used "as a tonic to counteract weakness and fatigue, as a restorative for declining stamina and impaired concentration, and as an aid to convalescence." The recommended daily dosage is 1–2 g of the crude drug. A dosage of 200–600 mg/day is recommended for extracts, based on the results of clinical studies. The Commission recommends limiting the duration of treatment to 3 months, as the possibility of hormone-like or hormone-inducing effects cannot be ruled out. Reports of possible addiction problems, blood pressure elevation, nervousness, sleeplessness, and increased libido (Palmer et al., 1978; Siegl, 1979, 1980) have now been thoroughly discredited. All such reports originated in English-speaking countries where ginseng preparations are sold as food products and are not subject to quality or dosage controls (Ploss, 1988; Sonnenborn, 1990). Some of the methodologies employed were also questionable.

9.1.2
Eleutherococcus Root

This herb, known also as Siberian ginseng but preferably referred to as eleuthero, consists of the dried root of *Eleutherococcus senticosus,* a shrub of the family Araliaceae that grows to 2–3 m; it is native to Siberia and northern China. The slender shrub is distinguished by its very thin, woody spines about 5 mm in length. The dried root of eleutherococcus has a sharp, aromatic, slightly sweet taste. Lignan glycosides of the liriodendrin and coumarin types, including isofraxidin, have been identified as key constituents. Unlike true ginseng, however, eleuthero is not a species of *Panax* and contains only small concentrations of saponins (Bladt et al., 1990).

Eleuthero root was tested and developed in the former Soviet Union during the 1960's as a substitute for ginseng. Pharmacologic studies there demonstrated an effect comparable to or even surpassing that of ginseng root (Brekhman and Dardymov, 1969). As a result, eleutherococcus root has been listed in the Russian Pharmacopeia as a tonic since the 1960's. It has also found use as an herbal tonic in Western countries since about 1975.

Animal studies on eleuthero extract were comparable in their design and results to the animal tests of ginseng extract. The studies confirmed the protein-anabolic action of both the extract (Kaemmerer and Fink 1980; Zorikov et al., 1974) and of the isolated constituent liriodendrin (Ro et al., 1977). Healthy subjects placed on a 4-week regimen of 10 mL/t.i.d. of an extract with the brand name Eleu-Kokk showed a highly significant increase in immunocompetent cells – principally T-lymphocytes of the helper/inductor type in addition to cytotoxic and natural killer cells (Bohn et al., 1987). This effect was demonstrated by flow cytometry. The implications of this finding for the clinical use of eleuthero extracts remains unclear (Lovett et al., 1984; Pichler et al., 1985).

Koch and Eidler (1988) may be consulted for a comprehensive survey and summary of the earlier literature.

The Commission E monograph on *Eleutherococcus senticosus* recommends its use "as a tonic to counteract weakness and fatigue, as a restorative for declining stamina and impaired concentration, and as an aid to convalescence." The recommended daily dose is 2–3 g of the crude drug or an equivalent dose of an extract-based preparation. As with ginseng, the Commission recommends that use be limited to 3 months. Hypertension is noted as a contraindication. There are no known side effects or drug-drug interactions.

9.2
Immune Stimulants

Immune stimulants are agents that increase the activity of the immune system. Unlike vaccines, however, immune stimulants have no antigenic relationship to specific pathogens. Consequently, their action is nonspecific and is believed to result from the stimulation of cell-mediated immune factors (macrophages, granulocytes, leukocytes) and of mediators that are released by the cellular immune system (Fig. 9.2). When immune stimulants are used, therefore, there is always a risk of physiologic

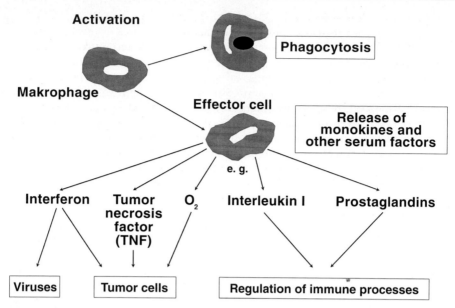

Fig. 9.2. Nonspecific stimulation of cell-mediated host defenses.

suppression of the immune response, leading to an exacerbation of chronic inflammatory processes. There is a danger that the desired stimulation of host immune defenses could activate previously quiescent autoimmune processes (Haustein, 1995).

The term immune stimulation is often used in phytotherapy in place of the traditional designation "stimulation and modulation (adaptation) therapy." Nonspecific stimulation therapy consists of inciting a focal or general reaction (inflammation, fever), stimulating the immune system, and/or modulating the autonomic nervous system in order to enhance the performance of natural regulatory processes.

In practice, species of two botanical genera stand out among the immune-stimulant herbs: coneflower *(Echinacea spp.)* and mistletoe *(Viscum album)*. Other herbs have assumed a degree of importance – boneset *(Eupatorium perfoliatum)*, wild indigo *(Baptisia tinctoria)*, and arbor vitae *(Thuja occidentalis)* – but only in combination products that also contain echinacea. Preparations made from birthwort *(Aristolochia clematitis)* and Venus flytrap *(Dionaea muscipula)*, once used in Germany as immune stimulants, are now banned due to their carcinogenic risks.

9.2.1
Coneflower (Echinacea)

Based on a total of four monographs published by Commission E in 1989 and 1992, two types of coneflower preparation can be recommended and prescribed today: alcoholic extracts made from the root of the narrow-leaf coneflower *(Echinacea pallida)* and juices expressed from the fresh aerial parts of the purple coneflower *(Echi-*

nacea purpurea). It is noteworthy that until about 1990, the root of *Echinacea pallida* appears to have been regularly confused with that of the species *Echinacea angustifolia* (Bauer and Wagner, 1988). Both species were formerly recognized as sources of the official drug in the United States.

9.2.1.1
Plant, Crude Drug, and Constituents

The genus *Echinacea* encompasses nine species in several varieties. The first species to be used medicinally was the narrow-leaf purple coneflower *(Echinacea angustifolia)* which may have been confused with the pale purple coneflower *(Echinacea pallida)*. These plants are native to eastern North America, where they grow to 40–60 cm and were used by the original inhabitants as a traditional wound-healing remedy and cure-all. European settlers introduced the plant to Europe in the early 1900's. Attempts to cultivate these two species were unsuccessful, so the common purple coneflower *(E. purpurea)* was grown instead and used for pharmaceutical products (Fig. 9.3).

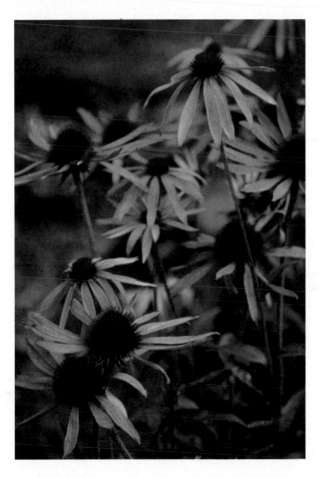

Fig. 9.3.
Common purple coneflower
(Echinacea purpurea).

Echinacea pallida root contains characteristic constituents such as echinacein, echinolone, and echinacoside in addition to water-soluble polysaccharides, some of which have exhibited immune-stimulating effects.

The juice of *Echinacea purpurea* is expressed from the fresh flowering plants. One hundred parts of juice contain water-soluble extractive from 40 parts of the fresh plant. The chemical composition of the expressed juices is not precisely known, but it may be assumed that its contents include the water-soluble polysaccharide fraction (Proksch, 1982; Stimpel et al., 1984).

A comprehensive review of the constituents and pharmacology of the echinacea herbs can be found in Bauer and Wagner (1990).

9.2.1.2
Pharmacology and Toxicology

A total of about 70 publications have dealt with the pharmacologic effects of echinacea preparations (survey in Bauer and Wagner, 1990). Most of the studies dealt with the stimulant effects of echinacea on immunocompetent cells in animals and humans. For example, in vitro studies were conducted on the phagocytic activity of human granulocytes incubated with yeast particles, and in vivo studies dealt with the phagocytosis of carbon particles by hepatic and splenic macrophages. Various echinacea preparations, either alone or combined with other herbal extracts (boneset, wild indigo, thuja), were found to stimulate phagocytic activity, as were a number of isolated fractions and pure compounds derived from echinacea herbs. It was also shown that certain echinacea polysaccharides stimulated the release of interleukin 1, tumor necrosis factor, and interferon (Bauer and Wagner, 1990; Wagner and Jurcic, 1991).

Toxicologic studies have not been performed on echinacea extracts, only on isolated polysaccharide fractions. The oral use of echinacea is considered to be without significant toxicologic risk.

9.2.1.3
Studies on Therapeutic Efficacy

Melchart et al. (1994) published a meta-analysis of 26 controlled clinical trials (18 randomized, 11 double-blind) on the immune-stimulant effects of echinacea. Six of these studies used a total of three single-herb extracts, and 20 used a total of four combination products. In all four combination products, echinacea extract (*E. angustifolia* or *pallida*) was the main quantitative ingredient and the most likely key active principle. Both single-herb and combination products used in a total of 26 studies are evaluated below.

The studies were evaluated by scoring each of 16 criteria and totaling the final scores. Only eight studies achieved more than 50% of the maximum possible total score. The best study (70%) used a combination product (brand name Resistan) that is not commonly prescribed by German physicians. No studies have been published on several products that are among the most commonly prescribed herbal medications in Germany.

Most of the studies reviewed by Melchart et al. tested the therapeutic efficacy of echinacea in patients with upper respiratory infections. The most highly rated study (Dorn, 1989) had a typical design. In a double-blind protocol, 100 patients with

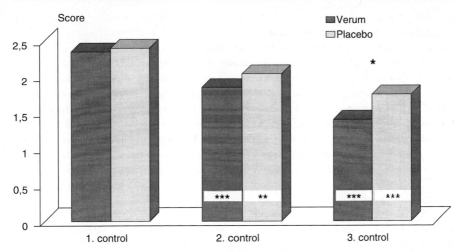

Fig. 9.4. Change in average severity of a typical flulike infection from admission (1st examination) to days 2–4 of treatment (2nd examination) and days 6–8 of treatment (3rd examination). Dark columns: echinacea preparation; light columns: placebo. Each column represents the mean values for 50 patients in a randomized double-blind study. * = p < 0.05; ** = p < 0.01; *** = p < 0.001 (Dorn, 1989).

acute flulike infections took 30 mL of the echinacea preparation or a placebo on the first and second days of treatment; then the dosage was reduced to 15 mL/day on days 3 through 6. The patients were examined on admission (term 1), at 2–4 days into the regimen (term 2), and at 6–8 days (term 3). Seven cold symptoms (lethargy, limb pain, headache, rhinitis, cough, sore throat, and pharyngeal redness) were rated for severity using a semiquantitative scoring system (Fig. 9.4). As one might expect, the scores declined rapidly during the roughly 8-day observation period in both the echinacea- and placebo-treated groups. The difference in the scores relative to the third and final examination was statistically significant for all seven symptoms in the echinacea group but for only three of the symptoms in the placebo group (p < 0.01–0.001). The results suggest that taking a suitable echinacea preparation when symptoms first appear can, in favorable cases, shorten the duration of a common cold by about 1/4 to 1/3 (i.e., from about 10 days to 7 days).

The same product (Resistan) was tested for possible prophylactic benefit as an herbal immune stimulant. In a placebo-controlled double-blind study, 646 students at the University of Cologne were placed a prophylactic course of treatment for at least 8 weeks during the 1989–1990 winter semester to test the possible effect of the product on the frequency of colds. A total of 609 subjects (303 echinacea and 306 placebo) completed the study. A total of 363 of the subjects had had more than three flulike infections during the previous 12-month period (the infection-prone subgroup). Comparison with the placebo indicated 15% fewer primary infections and 27% fewer recurrent infections overall in the subjects who took the echinacea product. The infection-prone subjects experienced a 20% reduction in total number of colds relative to the placebo. In contrast to the study population as a whole, the reduction achieved in the infection-prone subjects was statistically significant (p < 0.05).

9.2.1.4
Indications, Dosages, and Risks

Commission E revised its monographs on echinacea preparations in 1992, giving a positive rating only to alcoholic root extracts of the narrow-leaf coneflower *(E. pallida)* and pressed juice from the aerial parts of the common purple coneflower *(E. purpurea)*. Root extracts are indicated "for the supportive treatment of flulike infections" and echinacea juices for the "supportive treatment of recurrent infections of the upper respiratory tract and lower urinary tract." It is recommended that neither preparation be used for more than eight weeks. The recommended dose of root extract (1:5 tincture with 50% ethanol) is equivalent to 900 mg of crude drug daily. A dose of 6–9 mg/day is recommended for echinacea juice. Because echinacea may act at the oropharyngeal level (immune stimulation of tonsillar lymphoid tissues), it is possibly best administered in the form of a liquid preparation or buccal tablet. Due to the potential for stimulating autoimmune processes, echinacea is contraindicated by systemic diseases such as tuberculosis, leukoses, multiple sclerosis, collagen disorders, and other autoimmune diseases.

9.2.2
European Mistletoe

Rudolf Steiner introduced the use of mistletoe extracts for the treatment of cancer in 1916. Steiner is best known as the founder of anthroposophy, which is not a science but a philosophy. This historical background would seem to imply that treatment with mistletoe preparations has no place in a rational, scientifically oriented system of phytotherapy. However, efforts have been made to test the effects and efficacy of mistletoe preparations by means of orthodox pharmacologic studies and clinical trials. The following discussions are based purely on evidence furnished by modern testing and evaluation procedures.

9.2.2.1
Plant, Constituents, and Actions

European mistletoe *(Viscum album,* Fig. 9.5) is a semiparasitic evergreen shrub of the family Loranthaceae that extracts water and mineral salts from the host plant but is autotrophic for CO_2. Three subspecies are distinguished by differences in host specificity: broadleaf mistletoe, which grows on all European broadleaf trees except beech, preferring apple trees and poplars; fir mistletoe, which grows on silver fir; and pine mistletoe, which grows on pines, larches, and occasionally on firs.

Immunopharmacologic studies indicate that the lectins in mistletoe are the most important active principles; their effects include the stimulation of T-lymphocytes. The compound designated lectin 1 was found to induce macrophage cytotoxicity in experimental animals. It also stimulated the phagocytosis of various immune cells (Hajto et al., 1989, 1990a). In vitro testing of the same lectin stimulated monocyte cultures to release immune mediators such as tumor necrosis factor and interleukin (Hajto et al., 1990b). However, the content of lectins and immune-stimulating viscotoxins varies markedly among different mistletoe preparations (Wagner and Jordan, 1986). Some importance is also ascribed to the acid polysaccharides in mistletoe,

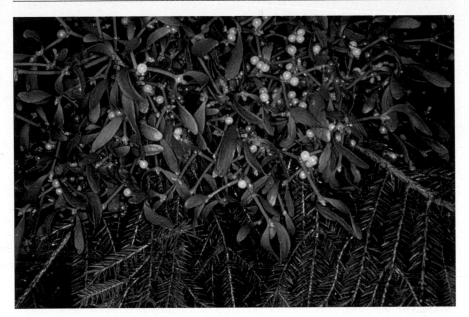

Fig. 9.5. European mistletoe *(Viscum album)*.

which stimulated complement-system activation and showed other activating effects in vitro (Wagner and Jordan, 1986; Beuth et al., 1992; Gabius et al., 1994).

The mistletoe preparations marketed in Germany are based on the fresh leaves, branches, and berries of European mistletoe. Different products use different processing methods, and some show a definite anthroposophic influence. Some products (o. g., Plenosol, Helixor) are produced by a relatively simple method that essentially yields an aqueous whole-plant extract. With other products (e.g., Iscador), the anthroposophic origins are unmistakable. One- to two-year-old shoots of the mistletoe shrub, complete with stems, leaves, buds, flowers, and berries, are processed in a fresh condition within 24 h after gathering. First, a kind of juice is prepared by grinding the plant parts, adding distilled water, and crushing the mixture between rollers to produce an aqueous extract in which 1 part extract weight corresponds to 1 part mistletoe weight. This extract is subjected to anaerobic lactic acid fermentation for 4–6 weeks. It is then diluted 1:5, and summer viscum juice is mixed with winter viscum juice to yield a 10% Iscador stock solution that is further diluted to make injectable solutions of varying strength. The ampules may be sterilized by heat or by filtration, depending on the legal requirements in the country of manufacture.

9.2.2.2
Clinical Efficacy Studies
Almost 50 clinical studies have been conducted on mistletoe preparations during the last 30 years. All involved parenteral administration, usually by subcutaneous injection. Given the heterogeneity of the preparation methods, only the results for spe-

Table 9.1. Meta-analysis of 11 controlled studies on mistletoe preparations in the treatment of cancer (after Kleijnen and Knipschild, 1994)

First author	Type of cancer	Product name	Statistical result	Total score
Dold, 1991	Bronchial carcinoma	Iscador	0	8.5
Douwes, 1986	Colorectal carcinoma	Helixor	Trend	6.0
Salzer, 1991	Bronchial carcinoma	Iscador	Trend	5.5
Douwes, 1988	Colorectal carcinoma	Helixor	Significant	5.0
Salzer, 1978, 1980	Bronchial carcinoma	Iscador	Significant	5.0
Salzer, 1979, 1983, 1988	Gastric carcinoma	Iscador	Trend	4.5
Fellmer, 1966, 1968	Cervical carcinoma	Iscador	Trend	4.0
Gutsch, 1988	Breast carcinoma	Helixor	Significant	4.0
Heiny, 1991	Breast carcinoma	Eurixor	Significant	3.5
Salzer, 1987a	Breast carcinoma	Iscador	Trend	3.0
Majewski, 1963	Genital carcinoma in women	Iscador	Trend	1.0

cific products can be meaningfully summarized. Surveys can be found in Kiene (1989) and Hauser (1993).

The 11 controlled clinical studies on mistletoe preparations were reviewed in a recent, comprehensive meta-analysis (Kleijnen and Knipschild, 1994). The authors used a scoring system based on 10 quality criteria to evaluate the study outcomes. The results of this meta-analysis, including types of tumor, products used, and statistical results, are summarized in Table 9.1. The authors rated the overall scientific quality of the studies as weak. None of the studies employed a double-blind design. One study was considered to be adequately randomized. The most highly rated study (Dold et al., 1991) was a multicenter study, commissioned by the German Federal Insurance Institute for Employees, in which the effect of Iscador was compared with a multivitamin preparation used as a placebo. The study involved 408 patients with a histologically confirmed diagnosis of advanced, non-small-cell bronchial carcinoma. The patients treated with Iscador had an average survival of 9.1 months, compared with 7.6 months for patients treated with the placebo. At 2 years, 11.5% of the Iscador patients and 10.1% of the placebo patients were still alive. The differences in average and 2-year survival were not statistically significant. The quality of life scores also showed no statistical differences, although the Iscador patients reported an improvement of general well-being significantly more often than the placebo patients. Nevertheless, the authors of this study did not believe that the outcome was sufficient to warrant a general recommendation for this therapy in patients with non-small-cell bronchial carcinoma.

9.2.2.3
Indications, Dosages, and Risks

Commission E published its monograph on European mistletoe in 1984. Although most of the controlled clinical studies (Table 9.1) were completed after that date, they did not yield any fundamental new discoveries. The 1984 monograph states that *Viscum album* is useful "for the segmental therapy of degenerative inflammatory joint diseases, based on the use of intracutaneous injections to induce local inflammation and elicit cutivisceral reflexes; also useful as a nonspecific stimulation therapy for the palliative treatment of malignant tumors." These applications are based entirely on the intra- or subcutaneous administration of the drug. The dosages should conform to manufacturer's recommendations. Iscador injectable ampules are supplied in up to 10 different concentrations, which are increased in increments during one treatment cycle, starting with the lowest concentration. They are also recommended for sequential regimens involving treatment with several subspecies (broadleaf, fir, and pine mistletoe); this reflects the anthroposophical origin of this therapy, which is only marginally related to orthodox scientific medicine.

Because the preparation is administered parenterally, it is contraindicated by protein hypersensitivity. Chronic, progressive infections such as tuberculosis also contraindicate the therapy due to the potential for immune effects. The monograph notes several possible side effects: chills, high fever, headache, chest pain, orthostatic hypotension, and allergic reactions.

9.2.3
Medicinal Yeasts

Yeast was used medicinally by the ancient Egyptians and later by the Greeks and Romans. Yeast has always been a popular folk remedy in beer-producing countries, where it has been used as a mild laxative, an antidiarrheal for enteral infections and poisonings, and as a preventive remedy for boils, acne, and eczema.

Dried brewer's yeast (medicinal yeast) is described in the German Pharmacopeia as a bottom-fermented yeast consisting of cells that can no longer replicate but which still retain most of their enzymatic activities. Because they are derived from fungal cultures (Saccharomyces cerevisiae), brewer's yeast preparations can be classified as phytomedicines. Crude bottom-fermented brewer's yeast has a high content of hop constituents, and the bitter principles must be removed from the yeast before it is processed further for medicinal purposes. By dry weight, brewer's yeast contains 50–60 % nitrogen compounds (proteins, nucleic acids, free amino acids, and biogenic amines), 15–37 % carbohydrates, and 4–7 % fats and lipids, chiefly phospholipids.

The therapeutic use of brewer's yeast is based largely on folk medicine and empirical healing. Several pharmacologic studies showed an increased phagocytic index for peritoneal macrophages in mice (Schmidt, 1977) and a decreased severity of experimental infections in mice and rhesus monkeys (Sinai et al., 1974). Dietary yeast supplementation promoted the more rapid clearing of edema in children with kwashiorkor (severe malnutrition), an effect presumably due to the content of B vitamins in the yeast (Gervais, 1973).

The 1988 Commission E monograph on medicinal yeast states that it is used for "anorexia and as an adjunct in chronic forms of acne and furunculosis." The average recommended dose is 6 g/day. As for side effects, the monograph notes that medicinal yeast can occasionally cause migraine attacks in susceptible patients and that the ingestion of fermentable yeast can cause flatulence.

9.3
Therapeutic Significance

Herbal agents that can enhance host defenses nonspecifically fill an important therapeutic niche, especially in outpatient settings where treatment options are extremely limited. This is particularly true of coneflower and mistletoe preparations. With a total of about 4 million prescriptions annually, coneflower preparations are still among the most widely prescribed phytomedicines in Germany (Haustein, 1995). They are prescribed for patients, including many children, who suffer from frequent recurring infections, particularly of the upper respiratory tract. The goal in such patients is to increase long-term resistance to infection mainly through nonpharmacologic means (e. g., Kneipp applications, exercise, the elimination of harmful agents). Often this approach is unsuccessful. Because there are very few pharmacotherapeutic options for these patients and it appears that echinacea preparations have very little risk potential, a trial with these preparations is justified. Available data, especially from clinical studies, suggest that echinacea products do have some efficacy in stimulating host defenses. Since immune responses are by nature episodic, there seems to be no rationale for the continuous use of these products. That is why the monographs recommend limiting the duration of use to eight weeks.

In the case of mistletoe preparations, data currently available cannot establish therapeutic efficacy in a provable, scientific sense. Nevertheless, the selective use of mistletoe preparations is justified in an anthroposophic sense for the palliative treatment of malignant tumors, inasmuch as orthodox medicine cannot offer suitable therapeutic alternatives.

Unlike herbal immune stimulants, herbal adaptogens (ginseng and eleuthero) generally are not covered by health insurance plans in Germany. But ginseng preparations still have an important role in physician-assisted self-medication. Eastern empirical medicine, the universal scope of ginseng use, and the relatively comprehensive scientific data base on the actions and efficacy of ginseng all suggest that the temporary use of ginseng products can be beneficial during convalescence and in other states of physical weakness, especially in older patients. The preparation should be taken in a sufficiently high dosage (1–2 g of crude drug or 300–600 mg of extract daily) for a period of no more than several weeks.

Preparations made from eleuthero have a less traditional and scientific foundation than ginseng. Although this botanical belongs to the same family as ginseng, its constituents are markedly different, indicating the generally low specificity of adaptogenic effects.

9.4
Botanical Antioxidants (Grapeseed, Green Tea, Pinebark)

Other botanicals that assist the human body in resisting various pathologic conditions are those acting as antioxidants. Polyphenolic oligomers of the bioflavonoid type, variously known as procyanidins, proanthocyanidins, leucoanthocyanins, pycnogenols, nonhydrolyzable tannins, or condensed tannins, occur widely in the plant kingdom. Common commercial sources include the seeds of grapes *(Vitis vinifera)*, the green leaves of tea *(Camellia sinensis)*, and the bark of the maritime pine *(Pinus pinaster)*. Some of these sources are extremely rich in procyanidins; green tea leaves contain up to 30 % by weight. The exact composition of the contained polyphenols varies from species to species; however, in most cases the mixtures are sufficiently similar to assume that their physiologic and therapeutic effects are also similar.

9.4.1
Pharmacology and Toxicology

Procyanidins are potent antioxidants, free-radical scavengers, and inhibitors of lipid peroxidation. They are also active inhibitors of collagenase, elastase, hyaluronidase, and β-glucuronidase, all of which are involved in the degradation of the main structural components of the extravascular matrix. By this mechanism procyanidins help maintain normal capillary permeability. Antimutagenic activity in *Saccharomyces cerevisiae* strain S288C has also been demonstrated for these compounds. These combined activities, all related directly or indirectly to the antioxidative properties of procyanidins, account for much of their purported therapeutic utility, including protection against pathologies such as cancer and atherosclerosis, normally associated with the aging process.

Tests in experimental animals have shown that procyanidins are well tolerated and devoid of toxic effects. The calculated LD_{50} in rats and mice exceeds 4000 mg/ kg. The compounds are also devoid of mutagenic and teratogenic effects.

9.4.2
Clinical Studies

Clinical trials with procyanidins include a double-blind study on 50 patients with symptoms of chronic venous insufficiency. Following administration of 150 mg/day for 1 month, measurements of subjective and objective criteria showed a more rapid and lasting effect than in patients treated with 450 mg/day of the bioflavonoid diosmin. Another double-blind placebo controlled study on 92 patients with the same symptoms showed that administration of 300 mg/day of procyanidin for 28 days was effective in 75 % of the patients in comparison to 41 % for the placebo group. Various clinical studies on ophthalmologic conditions, including resistance to glare, ocular stress, and retinal functionality, all showed favorable results following treatment with procyanidins (Bombardelli and Marazzoni, 1995).

9.4.3
Indications and Dosage

Available clinical evidence tends to support the effectiveness of procyanidins in treating venous insufficiency and conditions associated with alteration of blood rheology and capillary fragility. Claims of effectiveness for attention-deficit/hyperactivity disorder and arthritis are anecdotal in nature and require scientific verification. The exact degree of utility of procyanidins, and other antioxidants as well, in protecting against stress, cancer, various inflammatory conditions, and cardiovascular disease, remains to be determined.

Procyanidins are marketed in the form of tablets or capsules containing extracts ranging up to 97% of polyphenols. Dosage recommendations vary widely from 100 to 300 mg/day initially followed, in some cases, by a lower maintenance dose averaging 50 mg/day.

References

Ahn Y-J, Kim M-l, Yamamoto T, Fujisawa T, Mitsouka T (1990) Selective growth responses of human intestinal bacteria to Araliaceae extracts. Microbial Ecol Health Disease 3: 223–229.

Bajusz E, Selye H (1960) Über die durch Streß bedingte Nekroseresistenz des Herzens. Ein Beitrag zum Phänomen der "gekreuzten Resistenz". Naturwissenschaft 47: 520–521.

Bauer R, Wagner H (eds) (1990) Echinacea. Wissenschaftliche Verlagsgesellschaft mbH Stuttgart.

Beuth J, Ko HL, Gabius HJ, Burrichter H, Oette K, Pulverer G (1992) Behavior of lymphocyte subsets and expression of activation markers in response to immunotherapy with galactoside-specific lectin from mistletoe in breast cancer. Clin Invest 70: 658–661.

Bladt S, Wagner H, Woo WS (1990) Taiga-Wurzel. Dtsch Apoth Z 27:1499–1508.

Bohn B, Nebe C, Birr C (1987) Flow-cytometric studies with Eleutherococcus senticosus extract as an immunomodulatory agent. Arzneim Forsch (Drug Res) 37: 1193–1196.

Bombardelli E, Morazzoni P (1995) Vitis vinifera L. Fitoterapia 66: 291–317.

Brekhman II, Dardymov IV (1969) New substances of plant origin that increase nonspecific resistance. Ann Rev Pharmacol 9: 419–430.

Ciplea AG, Richter K-D (1988) The protective effect of Allium sativum and Crataegus on isoprenaline-induced tissue necrosis in rats. Arzneim Forsch/Drug Res 38: 1588–1592.

Dold U, Edler L, Mäurer HC, Müller-Wening D, Sakellariou B, Trendelenburg F, et al. (1991) Krebszusatztherapie beim fortgeschrittenen nicht-kleinzelligen Bronchialkarzinom. Georg Thieme Verlag, Stuttgart.

Dorn M (1989) Milderung grippaler Effekte durch ein pflanzliches Immunstimulans. Natur- und Ganzheitsmedizin 2: 314–319.

Farrow JM, Leslie GB, Schwarzenbach FH (1978) The in vivo protective effect of a complex yeast preparation (Bio-Strath) against bacterial infections in mice. Medita (Solothurn) 8: 37–42.

Gabius HJ, Gabius S, Joshi SS, Koch B, Schroeder M, Manzke WM, Westerhausen M (1994) From ill-defined extracts to the immunomodulatory lectin: Will there be a reason for oncological application of mistletoe? Planta Med 60: 2–7.

Gervais C (1973) Profitable effect of a lactic yeast in nutritionally deficient Biafran children. Bull Soc Pathol Exot 66: 445–447.

Hajto T, Hostanka K, Frei K, Rordorf C, Gabins H-J (1990a) Increased secretion of tumor necrosis factor α, interleukin 1, und interleukin 6 by Heiman mononuclear cells exposed to β-galactoside-specific lectin from clinically applied mistletoe extract. Canc Res 50: 3322.

Hajto T, Hostanka K, Gabius HI (1990b) Zytokine als Lectin-induzierte Mediatoren in der Misteltherapie. Therapeutikon 4: 136–145.

Hajto T, Hostanka K, Gabius HI (1989) Modulatory potency of the β-galactoside-specific lectin from mistletoe extract (Iscador) and the host defense system in vivo in rabbits and patients. Canc Res 49: 4803.

Hauser SP (1993) Mistel – Wunderkraut oder Medikament? Therapiewoche 43 (3): 76–81.

Haustein KO (1995) Immuntherapeutika. In: Schwabe U, Paffrath D (eds) Arzneiverordnungs-Report '95. Wissenschaftliche Verlagsgesellschaft mbH Stuttgart.

Hofecker, G (1987) Physiologie und Pathophysiologie des Alterns. Öster Apoth Z 41: 443–450.

Hyo-Won B, Il-Heok K, Sa-Sek, H, Byung-Hun H, Mun-Hae H, Ze-Hun K, Nak-Du K (1987) Roter Ginseng. Schriftenreihe des Staatlichen Ginseng-Monopolamtes der Republik Korea.

Kaemmerer K, Kietzmann M (1983) Untersuchungen über streßabschirmende Wirkungen von oral verabreichtem Zinkbacitracin bei Ratten. Zbl Vet Med A 30: 712–721.

Kaemmerer K, Fink J (1980) Untersuchungen von Eleutherococcus-Extrakt auf trophanabole Wirkungen bei Ratten. Der praktische Tierarzt 61: 748–753.

Kiene H (1989) Klinische Studien zur Misteltherapie karzinomatöser Erkrankungen. Eine Übersicht. Therapeutikon 3: 347–353.

Kleijnen J, Knipschild P (1994) Mistletoe treatment for cancer. Review of controlled trials in humans. Phytomedicine 1: 255–260.

Koch HP, Eidler S (1988) Eleutherococcus senticosus. Sibirischer Ginseng. Scientific report. Kooperation Phytopharmaka, Cologne.

Lovett EJ, Schnitzer B, Keren DF et al. (1984) Application of flow cytometry to diagnostic pathology. Lab Invest 50: 115–140.

Melchart D, Linde K, Worku F, Bauer R, Wagner H (1994) Immunomodulation with Echinacea – a systematic review of controlled clinical trials. Phytomedicine 1: 245–254.

Obermeier A (1980) Zur Analytik der Ginseng- und Eteutherococcusdroge. Dissertation Ludwig-Maximilians-Universität, Munich.

Palmer BV, Montgomery ACV, Monteiro JCMP (1978) Ginseng und mastalgia. Brit Med J 1: 284 (letter).

Pichler WJ, Emmendörfer A, Peter HH et al. (1985) Analyse von T-Zell-Subpopulationen. Pathophysiologisches Konzept und Bedeutung für die Klinik. Schweiz med Wschr 115: 534–550.

Ploss E (1988) Panax ginseng C. A. Meyer. Scientific report. Kooperation Phytopharmaka, Cologne.

Proksch A (1982) Über ein immunstimulierendes Wirkprinzip aus Echinacea purpurea. Dissertation, Ludwig-Maximilians-Universität, Munich.

Ro HS, Lee SY, Han BH (1977) Studies on the lignan glycoside of Acanthopanax cortex. J Pharm Korea 21: 81–86.

Schmidt Ch (1977) Unspezifische Steigerung der Phagozytoseaktivitäten von Peritoneal-Makrophagen nach oraler Gabe verschiedener Hefepräparationen. Dissertation, Freie Universität Berlin.

Schole J, Harisch G, Sallmann HP (1978) Belastung, Ernährung und Resistenz. Parey, Hamburg Berlin.

Selye R (1946) The general adaptation syndrome and the disease of adaptation. J Clin Endocrinol 6: 117–130.

Siegl RK (1979) Ginseng abuse syndrome – problems with the panacea. J Amer Med Assoc 241: 1614–1615.

Siegl RK (1980) Ginseng and high blood pressure. J Am Med Assoc 243: 32.

Sinai Y, Kaplan A, Hai Y et al. (1974) Enhancement of resistance to infectious disease by oral administration of brewer's yeast. Infection Immunol 9: 781–787.

Sonnenborn U, Proppert Y (1990) Ginseng (Panax ginseng C. A. Meyer). Z Phytotherapie 11: 35–49.

Stimpel M, Proksch A, Wagner H et al. (1984) Macrophage activation and induction of macrophage cytotoxicity by purified polysaccharide fractions from the plant Echinacea purpurea. Infect Immunity 46: 845–849.

Wagner H, Jordan E (1986) Structure and properties of polysaccharides from Viscum album (L.). Oncology (Suppl 1): 8–15.

Wagner H, Jurcic K (1991) Immunologische Untersuchungen von pflanzlichen Kombinationspräparaten. Arzneim Forsch (Drug Res) 41: 1072–1076.

Youn YS (1987) Analytisch vergleichende Untersuchungen von Ginsengwurzeln verschiedener Provenienzen. Dissertation, Freie Universität Berlin.

Zorikov PS, Lyapustina TA (1974) Change in a concentration of protein and nitrogen in the reproductive organs of hens under the effect of Eleutherococcus extract. Deposited DOC VINI, 732–774, 58–63, ref Chem Abstracts 86 (1977) 119732.

Appendix:
The 100 Most Commonly Prescribed Herbal Medications in Germany

The following tables reviewing the 100 most frequently prescribed herbal medications are based on the Public Health Insurance Drug Index as published in the *1996 Drug Prescription Report* (Schwabe and Paffrath, 1996). The nomenclature for herbs and herbal products follows the terminology used in the *Rote Liste 1995*. These 100 herbal products rank among the 1393 most commonly prescribed medications in Germany. They represent approximately 8% of the total German drug market, with gross pharmacy sales totaling 1.650 billion DM in 1995. Fifty-one of the 100 most commonly prescribed remedies are single-herb products (1.117 billion DM), and 49 are combination products (.533 billion DM). The latter include 22 two-herb products, 15 three-herb products, 3 four-herb products, 5 five-herb products, and 4 products containing from 6 to 13 herbs. The leading indications for herbal remedies listed in order of sales volume (Table A1) correspond to the eight chapter headings in this book. Ginkgo preparations are discussed primarily in Chap. 2 (Central Nervous System), and chamomile preparations for external use (pain, rheumatic conditions, bruises) and anti-inflammatory internal use are discussed in Chap. 8 (Skin and Connective Tissues). The 52 most commonly prescribed single-herb products can be reduced to 27 herbs and plant parts, which are listed in order of sales volume in Table A2.

Table A1.

Indications for the 100 most commonly prescribed herbal medications in Germany, listed in order of gross pharmacy sales in 1995.		
Indications	Products	Thousands of DM
Central nervous system disorders	19	621,686
Respiratory disorders	29	257,892
Urinary tract disorders	11	212,873
Cardiovascular disorders	10	208,370
Disorders of the stomach, bowel, liver, or biliary tract	10	147,647
Increasing resistance to diseases	6	91,350
Skin and connective-tissue disorders	11	79,574
Gynecologic indications	4	31,207

Table A 2.

> The 51 single-herb products that are among the 100 most commonly prescribed herbal medications in Germany. Products are listed by herb or active constituent in order of gross pharmacy sales in 1995 in thousands of DM. Any change since 1994 is shown in brackets.

1. Ginkgo biloba:	6 products	417,624	[−43,273]
2. St. John's wort:	5 products	97,519	[+38,771]
3. Horse chestnut:	4 products [+1]	87,664	[+5,036]
4. Sitosterol:	2 products [+1]	60,979	[+29,464]
5. Saccharomyces:	2 products	58,425	[−1.020]
6. Hawthorn:	2 products [−2]	51,232	[−13,717]
7. Saw palmetto:	2 products [+1]	42,600	[+12,354]
8. European mistletoe:	2 products [+1]	41,808	[+20,146]
9. Nettle root:	1 product	38,024	[+3,429]
10. Ivy leaf:	3 products [+1]	34,999	[+8,700]
11. Milk thistle:	1 product	30,078	[+588]
12. Echinacea:	2 products [−1]	24,371	[−9,451]
13. Bromelain:	2 products [+1]	22,435	[+11,852]
14. Chamomile:	2 products	16,077	[+1,062]
15. Chasteberry:	2 products [+1]	12,804	[+6,002]
16. Kava:	1 product [−1]	12,764	[−5,875]
17. Greater celandine:	1 product	12,675	[+723]
18. Cineole:	2 products	11,791	[+706]
19. Black cohosh:	1 product	11,181	[+1,641]
20. Comfrey root:	1 product [−1]	9,915	[−3,606]
21. Thyme:	2 products [+1]	6,763	[+2,675]
22. Colchicum:	1 product	4,514	[+119]
23. Valerian:	1 product	3,932	[+553]
24. Witch hazel:	1 product	3,898	[+726]
25. Alexandrian senna:	1 product	2,075	[−62]
26. Iceland moss:	1 product [+1]	1,352	[−]

Table A 3. Listing of the 100 most commonly prescribed herbal medications in Germany in 1995. **Abbreviations:** CT = coated tablet; DDD = prescribed in defined daily doses; E = extract; L = liquid; C = capsule; P = powder; J – juice; A rank = ranking by number of prescriptions among all herbal products; B rank = ranking by number of prescriptions among all drug products; O = ointment or cream; S = suppository; T = tablet; TDM = thousands of DM (gross pharmacy sales); TRx = thousands of prescriptions

Trade Name (preparation)	Active Constituants	A Rank	B Rank	TRx	DDD	TDM
Sinupret (CT, L)	Gentian root (P) Cowslip flowers (P) Sorrel (P) Elder flowers (P) Vervain (P)	1	10	4034	53806	52424
Gelomyrtol (C)	Cineol Limonen α-Pinen	2	17	3229	53807	48494
Tebonin (CT, L)	Ginkgo biloba (E)	3	29	2597	87121	155993
Perenterol (C)	Saccharomyces boulardi	4	34	2430	19373	54670
Prospan (T, L)	Ivy leaves (E)	5	67	1885	13976	24570
Rokan (T, L)	Ginkgo biloba leaves (E)	6	87	1625	55002	98999
Gingium (CT, L)	Ginkgo biloba leaves (E)	7	111	1415	46061	68866
Crataegutt (C, L)	Hawthorn leaves and flowers (E)	8	128	1303	59714	43295
Jarsin (CT)	St. John's wort (E)	9	138	1246	37219	48323

Trade Name (preparation)	Active Constituuants	A Rank	B Rank	TRx	DDD	TDM
Kytta Sedativum F (CT, L)	Valerian root (E) Hop strobiles (E) Passionflower tops (E)	10	150	1184	29837	29743
Ginkobil (L, CT)	Ginkgo biloba leaves (E)	11	159	1145	35127	54596
Esberitox N (T, L, S)	Arbor vitae tips (E) Purple coneflower root (E) Wild indigo root (E)	12	166	1098	13122	17947
Bronchium drops N (L)	Quebracho bark (E) White soaproot Thyme (E)	13	168	1084	17528	12235
Iberogast (L)	Wild candytuft (E) Angelica root (E) Chamomile flowers (E) Caraway (E) Milk thistle fruits (E) Lemon balm leaves (E) Peppermint leaves (E) Greater celandine (E) Licorice root (E)	14	175	1063	35288	16451
Sedariston concentrate (C)	Valerian root (E) St. John's wort (E)	15	209	900	26835	27398
Korodin (L)	Hawthorn berries (E) Camphor	16	222	870	57457	19880
Echinacin (CT, T)	Purple coneflower tops (E)	17	237	832	21693	19040
Transpulmin Balsam E (O)	Cineol Menthol Camphor	18	242	810	19318	12470
Bronchoforton N ointment	Eucalyptus oil Pine-needle oil Menthol	19	254	775	17933	11324
Venostasin retard/N/S (C, CT, T)	Horse chestnut seeds (E)	20	278	729	30242	51446
Sinuforton (C)	Anise oil Cowslip root (E) Thyme (E)	21	284	708	6451	9864
Aescusan 20 (CT)	Horse chestnut seeds (E)	22	305	683	21859	28910
Remifemin (T, L)	Black cohosh root (E)	23	321	656	16341	11181
Aspecton N (L)	Licorice root (E) Anise oil Eucalyptus oil Fennel oil Thyme oil	24	326	650	6525	8826
Harntee 400 (a urinary tract tea)	13 Ingredients	25	329	648	9043	9535
Iscador (L)	European mistletoe (E)	26	338	634	9386	31290
Hedelix (L)	Ivy leaves (E)	27	340	632	6618	7224
Kamillosan soln.	Chamomile flowers (E)	28	348	623	3957	11464
Bazoton uno (CT)	Nettle root (E)	29	361	606	32274	38024
Hyperforat (CT)	St. John's wort (E)	30	363	605	12782	11314
Azuprostat M	β-Sitosterol	31	381	581	37125	32665
Kaveri (CT, L)	Ginkgo biloba (E)	32	386	574	20386	31660
Soledum Balsam soln.	Cineol	33	393	562	8687	7095
Harzol (C)	Sitosterol/hypoxis	34	394	562	27711	28314
Luvased (CT)	Valerian root (E) Hop strobiles (E)	35	398	561	14383	7834
Eucabal Balsam/N (O)	Eucalyptus oil Pine-needle oil	36	424	530	8414	6569

Trade Name (preparation)	Active Constituants	A Rank	B Rank	TRx	DDD	TDM
Kytta Plasma F/Salbe F (O)	Comfrey root (E)	37	427	525	15123	9915
Bronchium Elixer N (L)	Quebracho bark (E) White soaproot (E) Thyme (E)	38	430	521	4927	5986
Sedariston drops	Valerian root (E) St. John's wort (E) Lemon balm leaves (E)	39	431	518	16497	14982
Tonsilgon N (CT, L)	Marsh mallow root (P) Chamomile flowers (P) Horsetail tops (P) Walnut leaves (P) Yarrow tops (P) Oak bark (P) Dandelion tops (P)	40	450	510	13370	6223
Echinacea ratiopharm	Coneflower root (E)	41	459	502	9588	5331
Babix inhalant N (L)	Eucalyptus oil Spruce-needle oil	42	481	482	29064	4503
Bronchipret liquid/drops	Thyme (E) Ivy leaves (E)	43	486	477	4516	3710
Phytodolor N (L)	Ash bark (E) Quaking aspen bark and leaves (E) Goldenrod tops (E)	44	513	451	23194	11462
Miroton N forte (CT, L)	False hellabore (E) Lily of the valley (E) Squill (E)	45	525	445	16243	22375
Prostagutt forte (C)	Saw palmetto berries (E) Nettle root (E)	46	532	442	29743	30918
Talso (C)	Saw palmetto berries (E)	47	538	438	34622	33313
Melrosum cough syrup N	Gumplant tops (E) Saxifrage root (E) Cowslip root (E) Rose blossoms (E) Thyme (E)	48	539	434	1381	3956
Transpulmin pediatric balsam S	Cineol Menthol Camphor	49	554	423	5643	4202
Esbericum (C)	St. John's wort (E)	50	558	420	15221	12188
Cystinol (L)	Birch leaves (E) Horsetail (E) Goldenrod tops (E) Uva ursi (E)	51	563	416	2315	5700
Kamillan plus (L)	Chamomile flowers (E) Yarrow tops (E)	52	587	399	3071	3640
Orthangin N (C, T)	Hawthorn leaves and flowers (E)	53	604	389	10762	7937
Bromelain-POS (T)	Bromelain	54	615	383	4427	13901
Neuroplant (C)	St. John's wort (E)	55	617	380	15640	12599
Psychotonin M/N (L)	St. John's wort (E)	56	631	371	17299	13095
Soledum cough syrup/ coughdrops	Cineol	57	639	368	1972	4325
Soledum capsules	Cineol	58	640	368	3245	4696
Legalon (C)	Milk thistle fruits (E)	59	697	334	13312	30078
Panchelidon (L)	Greater celandine (E)	60	709	328	7173	12675
Chol-Kugeleten Neu (CT)	Greater celandine (E) Aloe (E)	61	727	319	11015	13170

Trade Name (preparation)	Active Constituants	A Rank	B Rank	TRx	DDD	TDM
Cysto Fink (C)	Sweet sumac (E) Kava kava root (E) Hop strobiles (E) Uva ursi leaves (E) Pumpkinseed oil	62	739	311	10781	12461
Kamillenbad Robugen (L)	Chamomile flowers (E, oil)	63	783	293	5334	4613
Carminativum Hetterich N (L)	Chamomile flowers (E) Peppermint leaves (E) Caraway (E) Fennel (E) Bitter orange peel (E)	64	803	286	8852	3972
Thymipin N	Thyme (E) Camphor Eucalyptus oil	65	808	285	1476	3183
Pulmotin-N ointment	Anise oil Camphor Eucalyptus oil Thyme oil Conifer oil Thymol	66	846	274	1711	1520
Hametum ointment	Witch hazel (distilled)	67	859	270	6734	3898
Agnolyt (C)	Agnus castus berries (E)	68	868	267	14009	7818
Remifemin plus (CT)	Hypericum (E) Cimicifuga (E)	69	895	262	11896	7222
Tussamag cough syrup N	Thyme (E)	70	897	260	4671	2438
Baldrian Dispert (CT)	Valerian root (E)	71	911	254	3806	3932
Pinimenthol N (L)	Eucalyptus oil Pine-needle oil Menthol	72	932	249	4224	2951
Bronchoforton liquid/ drops	Ivy leaves (E)	73	941	246	2242	3205
Antares (T)	Kava kava rhizome (E)	74	962	240	11270	12764
Venopyronum N triplex (C)	Horse chestnut seeds (E) False hellebore (E) Lily of the valley (E) Squill (E)	75	970	237	20582	19233
Eucabal Balsam S	Eucalyptus oil Pine-needle oil	76	975	236	4162	3214
Santax S (C)	Saccharomyces boulardii	77	1002	228	3203	3755
Bronchoforton capsules	Eucalyptus oil Anise oil Peppermint oil	78	1003	228	2545	3348
Ivel (CT)	Valerian root (E) Hop strobiles (E)	79	1015	223	7680	6081
Transpulmin pediatric balsam N	Eucalyptus oil Pine-needle oil	80	1029	220	3150	2225
Kytta-Cor (T, L)	Hawthorn berries Hawthorn leaves/flowers	81	1050	215	6692	4668
Colchicum Dispert (CT)	Colchicine	82	1064	211	3996	4514
Prosta Fink N (C)	Saw palmetto berries (E) Pumpkin seeds (E)	83	1087	206	8779	9698
Agnucaston (CT)	Agnus castus berries (E)	84	1096	204	13389	4986
Miroton (CT, L)	False hellebore (E) Lily of the valley (E) Oleander leaves (E) Squill (E)	85	1140	195	6136	7843
Aristochol concentrate gran.	Greater celandine (E) Cape aloes (E)	86	1148	195	9994	5197

Trade Name (preparation)	Active Constituants	A Rank	B Rank	TRx	DDD	TDM
Helixor (FL)	European mistletoe (E)	87	1150	195	4460	10518
Hovenol (C)	Horse chestnut (E)	88	1155	194	2465	2783
Traumanase/forte (CT)	Bromelain	89	1218	182	636	8534
Reparil (FL, CT)	Aescin	90	1244	179	1985	4525
Cholagogum N drops	Greater celandine (E) Curcuma rhizome (E) Peppermint oil	91	1247	179	9426	5604
X-Prep	Alexandrian senna pods (E)	92	1253	178	178	2075
Cystium Wern (L)	Fennel oil Camphor tree oil	93	1264	175	4502	2958
Kamillobad (L)	Chamomile flowers (E) Chamomile oil	94	1286	169	4840	3108
Prostagutt mono (C)	Saw palmetto berries (E)	95	1294	166	13267	9287
Isla-Moos (CT)	Iceland moss (E)	96	1322	161	1193	1352
Ginkodilat (CT)	Ginkgo biloba leaves (E)	97	1327	160	4973	7510
Babix inhalant (L)	Eucalyptus oil Spruce-needle oil	98	1362	153	9637	1448
Liniplant inhalant (L)	Eucalyptus oil Cajuput oil	99	1383	149	5876	1536
Psychotonin sed. (C)	St John's wort (E) Valerian (E)	100	1393	148	6507	3809

Subject Index

Printing: Saladruck, Berlin
Binding: Buchbinderei Lüderitz & Bauer, Berlin